Talbot County Free L
Easton, Maryland 2

D0853574

# PBB: AN AMERICAN TRAGEDY

WITHDRAWN

Talbot County Free Library
Easton, Maryland 21601

# PBB:
## AN
## AMERICAN
## TRAGEDY

---

## EDWIN CHEN

Prentice-Hall, Inc.,
Englewood Cliffs, N.J.

55241

*PBB: An American Tragedy* by Edwin Chen
Copyright © 1979 by Edwin Chen

All rights reserved. No part of this book may be
reproduced in any form or by any means, except
for the inclusion of brief quotations in a review,
without permission in writing from the publisher.

Printed in the United States of America

Prentice-Hall International, Inc., London
Prentice-Hall of Australia, Pty. Ltd., Sydney
Prentice-Hall of Canada, Ltd., Toronto
Prentice-Hall of India Private Ltd., New Delhi
Prentice-Hall of Japan, Inc., Tokyo
Prentice-Hall of Southeast Asia Pte. Ltd., Singapore
Whitehall Books Limited, Wellington, New Zealand

10   9   8   7   6   5   4   3   2   1

**Library of Congress Cataloging in Publication Data**

Chen, Edwin
  PBB, an American tragedy.

  Bibliography: p.
  Includes index.
  1. Polybrominated biphenyls—Toxicology—
Michigan. 2. Food contamination—Michigan.
3. Feeds—Michigan—Contamination. 4. Veterinary
toxicology—Michigan.   I. Title.
RA1242.P69C43   1979   615.9'51   79-15982
ISBN 0-13-654608-0

Bro-Dart        10.95        10/25/79

# CONTENTS

*To Meredith*

# ACKNOWLEDGMENTS

This book was made possible by a four-month leave of absence from the Detroit *News*. My special thanks to Peter B. Clark, president and publisher; William E. Giles, editor and vice-president; Lionel Linder, managing editor; and Gary F. Schuster, Washington bureau chief. I also am grateful to many other colleagues at the *News* for their encouragement and helpful suggestions.

The genesis of this book came in 1977 when editors at the *Atlantic Monthly* urged me to write about the PBB incident; the result was an article published by that magazine in August of 1977. Peter McCabe, managing editor of *Harper's Magazine*, encouraged me to expand the piece into a book and then offered invaluable advice.

This book has numerous other contributors—concerned people both in and out of government who came forth generously with information, assistance and insights. I am deeply indebted to them. Rick and Sandy Halbert, for instance, were unfailingly gracious and patient throughout the long hours of interviews that spanned a period of more than two years. The contents of those conversations, and the Halberts' own book (*Bitter Harvest*, published by the William B. Eerdmans Publishing Company in Grand Rapids, Michigan), form the bases of chapters one and two.

Chapter 5 is based on portions of *Cancer and Chemicals* by Thomas H. Corbett, M.D., published by Nelson-Hall, Inc.; used by permission.

I also extend my gratitude to Alpha and Marlene Clark; to Steven J. Axelrod, my agent; to Oscar Collier, senior editor of the trade book division at Prentice-Hall, Inc.; and to Shirley Keir for her reliable help in preparing the manuscript.

Finally, I wish to thank all the members of the Chen and Ferguson families for their enthusiasm and unflagging support. Two such persons deserve a special tribute.

One is Nancy Tsai Chen, my mother. This book would be difficult to imagine were it not for the countless sacrifices she has made over the years. The other is Meredith Ferguson Chen, my wife. Her understanding, counsel and selfless contributions made it all possible.

# INTRODUCTION

Many top U.S. scientists and public health experts privately are predicting a sharp rise in Michigan's cancer rates fifteen to twenty years from now as perhaps the most alarming consequence of that state's PBB contamination, which began in mid-1973. But new evidence now suggests that Michigan's 9 million residents were not the only ones poisoned by PBB. Indeed millions of additional Americans may have been exposed to the toxic chemical fire retardant, for PBB has shown up now in the environment—including the food supply—of thirteen states besides Michigan. Yet, no concerted effort has been made to ascertain the true dimensions of the PBB contamination.

The Michigan incident began when several thousand pounds of PBB were inadvertently mixed into livestock feed, which then was sold to unsuspecting farmers all over the state. Many farm animals, primarily dairy cows, ate the contaminated feed and then died. But most did not; they ended up in Michigan's food channels. The accidental mix-up went un detected for nearly one year, and by then everyone in Michigan had been poisoned.

But the Michigan tragedy is more than merely a frightening episode of how a dangerous chemical seeps into the human food chain, poisoning 9 million people, causing widespread illnesses and social chaos. It also represents a shameful example of how the government not only failed to protect and help the people but, instead, inflicted further suffering. Even after the astonishing blunder became public, government, university and corporation officials steadfastly downplayed the significance of the accident. They consistently misread and ignored information that came pouring forth in the aftermath of the mix-up. These officials even ridiculed the farmers, accusing them of poor animal husbandry when their prize-winning registered herds sickened and died and, later, accusing them of being hypochondriacs and malingerers when they complained about their own ill health.

Instead of acting decisively to contain the contamination, the state pursued an undeviating course of suppression, obfuscation and outright deception in order to delay the emergence of the true proportions of the calamity—even as each nightmarish prediction by the "alarmists" became reality and as PBB spread throughout Michigan and beyond. Such stonewalling efforts prolonged, by years, human exposure to the chemical.

To make matters worse, there were no state or federal programs—such as federal disaster emergency funds—for the victims. The PBB accident did not involve an infectious disease or some "act of God" like a tornado, a drought or a flood. The affected farmers were simply left to their own resources, casting about for impossible solutions.

Incredibly, more than six years after the contamination began, the suffering continues. Accounts of such still-unfolding events, then, obviously would benefit from the passage of time. Yet, in endeavoring now to tell this tragic episode in American history, one must sacrifice the perspective time lends, for too many questions remain unanswered; and many more are simply unanswerable.

This book explains how Michigan became a vast test tube of 9 million human guinea pigs and examines the fascinating conduct of human affairs as this frantic struggle for survival unfolded. The cast of characters includes ill-informed politicians, overzealous attorneys, faceless corporations, aloof universities, bewildered veterinarians and country doctors, arrogant bureaucrats, world-famous scientists, a confused and frightened public and, finally, Congress and the Carter White House. Gerald Ford, a native of Grand Rapids, one of the hardest hit areas, did nothing to help the affected farmers—even after he became president.

However, Ford did sign the Toxic Substances Control Act less than one month before he was defeated in November 1976. The law is designed to constrict the flow of new and untested chemicals into the environment. Its passage represents a societal event because we finally had come to recognize the folly of imposing the rules of jurisprudence to chemicals in our environment—that is, presuming a chemical to be innocent of deleterious effects until proven guilty. So we have taken a modest step in the right direction. One can only hope that future generations will not condemn us for being so slow in acknowledging and caring about the integrity of the world that supports all life. There already are some sixty thousand chemicals in commerce today, with an estimated one thousand new ones coming into use annually. Of the chemicals now in use, about two thousand are suspected carcinogens; yet only a few hundred have been tested. The rest we know little, if anything, about in terms of their potential to damage living things.

"We've made a Faustian bargain with our chemical world," says Dr. Irving J. Selikoff, a leading environmental health scientist. "Now we have to learn enough so we can cut our losses."

The specter of poisoning by chemicals such as PBB, of course, is not a threat we alone in the United States face, as has been demonstrated so tragically over the last decade in Japan and, more recently, in the Italian town of Seveso, about thirteen miles north of Milan. There an explosion occurred in an unattended reactor at a chemical plant on July 10, 1976, releasing into the open air a vaporous plume containing an extremely toxic chemical called dioxin. Soon after the cloud had cleared, many of the children and adults in the area began to feel nauseated. Later they grew dizzy and developed headaches, diarrhea and marked skin irritation. Chickens, cats and other domestic animals began to sicken and, by the middle of the following week, many died. Little research had been available concerning dioxin, and public concern that the chemical could cause malformations in babies born to women exposed to it prompted many pregnant women to obtain abortions. Earlier this year, Italian officials reported a 41 percent rise in birth defects in the Seveso area—from 38 in 2,774 live births in 1977 to 53 in 2,749 live births in 1978.

Dioxin made its toxic debut around 1950 as an inevitable and useless by-product in the manufacture of herbicides such as 2,4,5-T, which itself has been implicated as a significant fetus-deforming chemical. Yet, it was used extensively in the United States to destroy unwanted vegetation around homes and on farms, to defoliate vegetation on power line, highway, pipeline and railroad rights-of-way, and to kill shrub and broad-leaved plant life on rangeland, pastureland and forestland. In all, millions of acres were sprayed each year—even after dioxin began turning up in human breast milk in Oregon and Texas. Finally, the U.S. Environmental Protection Agency in March 1979 banned 2,4,5-T after studies turned up a rate of miscarriage in the sprayed areas three times greater than the norm. The ban came nine years after Dr. Jesse L. Steinfeld, the U.S. surgeon general, announced a series of government actions aimed at limiting the use of 2,4,5-T.

Yet, even in cases where the government has taken swift and unilateral action to remove a toxic chemical, genuine concern may be expressed as to whether such action has come too late. A good example involves the chemical PCB, or polychlorinated biphenyl, which happens to be a close relative of PBB, or polybrominated biphenyl. PCB also is a fire retardant and because it comes in a liquid form it has been much more widely disseminated in the environment. PCB became widely recognized as an environmental hazard in 1968 when rice oil in Yusho, Japan, became contaminated by it and then went on to poison about a thousand persons. By 1976, five of the Yusho victims had died of liver cancer—representing a rate of five hundred such cases for every one hundred thousand persons, compared with the normal expected rate of thirty-one cases out of every one hundred thousand persons. PCB now is believed to be in the fat tissues of nearly every resident of the United States. Congress has banned its manufacture as of January 1, 1979, but the chemical is already so widespread that it is found in virtually every major body of water on this planet.

Often causes of strange outbreaks of widespread illnesses are never discovered. The recent cases of cancers in Rutherford, New Jersey, appear to be a case in point. A wide-ranging examination into the circumstances surrounding the highly improbable cluster of cancer cases in that city of twenty thousand so far has turned up nothing. Yet in a five-year period, there were six leukemia cases in young people between the ages of five and nineteen. The six cases represented six times the expected national average for that age group.

More susceptible to chemical poisoning than the general population are those who work in close contact with such substances. They are, says Dr. Selikoff, like "canaries in a coal mine" for the rest of the population because they are intensively exposed to many substances that are widespread in the general environment in less concentrated amounts. Thus the disease experience of workers often can help zero in on chemicals that contribute to cancer and other illnesses in the general population. One such substance is asbestos. By following, for decades, the medical and death records of asbestos workers, Dr. Selikoff proved that the substance is one of the most potent carcinogens known. Extraordinary numbers of workers exposed to asbestos even for a short time developed lethal cancers, often decades later. Dr. Selikoff's continuing studies led to more stringent regulation limiting exposure to asbestos, which enters the environment at a rate of 4 million tons each year. Today scientists believe nearly every urban resident has asbestos fibers in his or her lungs. Clearly, then, the need to study workers is well established. Yet merely counting the number of victims is hardly the satisfactory answer.

In the Tidewater area of Virginia, for instance, the Life Science Products Company in Hopewell for sixteen months in the 1970s made a chemical pesticide called Kepone without ever warning its employees that the chemical is quite toxic. A series of job-related illnesses finally raised workers' suspicions, and, in July 1975, the plant was shut down—but not before seventy workers had been identified as victims of Kepone poisoning, twenty-nine of whom required hospitalization. Their symptoms included tremors, liver damage and at least one case of sterility. Two children of the employees also were contaminated merely through contact with their fathers at home. Today vast tracts of the James River and the seafood-rich mouth of the Chesapeake Bay have been declared off limits to fishing.

More recently, the case of Love Canal in 1978 comes to mind as another grisly ecological monument to the irresponsibilities of the petrochemical industry, and highlights another related problem: that of disposal of toxic substances. In the 1940s and early 1950s, the Hooker Chemicals and Plastics Corporation in Niagara Falls, New York, buried its toxic wastes in the unused dry channel. The land in 1953 was sold to the Niagara Falls Board of Education for one dollar. Then the dump and the surrounding area became a school and a residential area. Persistent complaints about noxious odors eventually led to the discovery that toxic chemicals had begun leaching out of the soil and was contaminating homes in the area. More than two hundred compounds have been identified from the wastes in Love Canal, including dioxin. More than two hundred families had to abandon their homes. More than a dozen children in the area had been born with birth defects; and on one block alone, four mentally retarded children were born. Pregnant women miscarried at a rate 50 percent higher than normal. "The Love Canal situation is just the tip of the iceberg," says Dr. Clark W. Heath, a medical epidemiologist at the U.S. Center for Disease Control. "There are thousands of these dumps all over the country. Love Canal could be a front-runner of similar incidents to come." In Michigan, as an example, PBB wastes and contaminated feeds were buried haphazardly in landfills scattered around the state, and their existence was not even known by state officials until years later.

Michigan's PBB tragedy is important because it represents the prototype of a new large-scale public health menace we as a civilization face in the years and decades ahead: the silent, invisible chemical time bomb. Thus the lessons the Michigan incident has taught us must not be forgotten. When such a tragedy strikes, government leaders must fully and promptly inform the citizens of the potential health hazards. Only then can the public insist upon the appropriate protective measures. The PBB debacle clearly has demonstrated that no amount of affirmation or denial of health risks will suffice until independent research is done. Procrastination and wishful thinking must not replace good, sound science.

_____

*The health of the people is
really the foundation upon which
all their happiness and all their
powers as a state depend.*
                    *—Disraeli*

_____

# 1
# SEASONS
# OF DEATH

The cold wet touch of death made Rick Halbert shudder. But there was no time to waste. Thankful for the pocketknife's sharp blade, he hacked through the calf's abdomen and rib cage. Soon the front of the calf was severed, and it dropped to the ground, splattering the pool of blood on the straw bedding.

At once, Halbert turned to the other half of the calf, still lodged in the birth canal of the exhausted motionless cow. The only way to save the cow was to shove the remaining portion of the calf back into the cow's uterus, turn it around and then pull it out backward. He knelt behind the cow and gingerly pushed on the sharp stump of the calf's spine. It began sliding back toward the cow's uterus. But suddenly the 1,400-pound cow began straining once more, trying to expel what was left of her calf. The sharpness of the calf's severed spine worried Halbert; it easily could puncture the uterus and cause death. But the cow sensed there would be no progress, and she slackened her muscles. Slowly, Halbert turned the severed hindquarters around so its rear feet were nearly protruding from the cow, and its sharp severed spine pointing away from him. The moment of truth was at hand. Halbert stood up to take several deep breaths and flex his blood-drenched arms, numb with fatigue.

More than an hour had elapsed since the young dairy farmer walked into the maternity stall to find this cow in labor. Normally it took perhaps several hours from the start of labor until a calf emerged, its front hooves bracketing its nose. Although most calves on his farm are born without help, Halbert liked being on hand when cows showed signs of impending delivery. If labor took too long or if some other calving complication developed, simply rotating the calf or attaching obstetrical chains to its hooves and then pulling with

1

each contraction of the cow's uterus would suffice. For the truly difficult cases, Halbert would call Dr. Ted Jackson, his veterinarian. Halbert had been on his way home when told that the cow was experiencing calving troubles. He encountered the cow, already two weeks overdue, stretched out on her side in a large straw-bedded stall, nearly overcome with fatigue. Her contractions were weak and she was breathing rapidly, periodically uttering a loud moan. Halbert realized that if the cow strained much longer, the unrelenting nerve-pinching trauma could paralyze her. The problem seemed obvious: The calf was too large and its head was caught in the cow's birth canal. All Halbert could see were its forefeet and nose. The cow was making no progress, and so he decided to intervene. He attached the obstetrical chains to the calf's protruding front feet, hitched the chains to a sturdy post and slowly began applying tension. The cow responded with several strong contractions, and soon the calf's head emerged. But after a foot or so, the calf stopped moving and progress came to a halt once more. Halbert waited. It wasn't unusual to see a brief respite before the final delivery. But the seconds ticked away. The unborn calf's midsection was in its mother's cervix. Soon it would suffocate if it stayed in that position. The calf began gasping, unable to expand its lungs. It should have been delivered by Caesarean section, but it was too late. The calf stopped gasping. But instantly a new struggle began—to save its mother. Halbert ran for a knife, a bucket of water and some soap. He knew his only option was to dissect the dead calf and then remove the other half—and quickly. Calling Dr. Jackson would mean perhaps an hour's delay. So without hesitation, Halbert had performed the amputation. Now, as he washed his bloody hands and arms, Halbert was momentarily struck by the ghastly scene.

He attached the calf's hind feet to the obstetrical chain and slowly began to tighten the hand-operated winch, a powerful instrument with a drum around which the chain was coiled. Nothing happened. Again he tightened the winch, hitched to a post. This time the cow began sliding backward across the straw bedding; she was being pulled along with the remainder of her calf. Halbert stopped, and considered tying the cow's neck to another post to keep her in place. But once more, in desperation, he tightened the winch. Finally the calf's mangled rear quarters began to emerge from the birth canal. Soon it dropped unceremoniously to the straw bedding.

The November night had fallen by the time the handsome young farmer left the barn, unaware that in the upcoming months the musty smell of death increasingly would permeate his barns—and the barns of countless other farmers throughout Michigan. "The PBB story didn't start as a wave, sweeping death and destruction over Michigan farms," Halbert would recall later. "Rather, it slipped onto most farms almost unnoticed. Lying hidden, it would rise up when animals came under stress. It struck its victims in bizarre ways, unpredictable."

# 2
# IF SOMETHING ODD HAPPENS

"Lunch will be ready in about five minutes. Why don't you read the paper while you're waiting?" Sandy Halbert said to her husband, Rick, as he entered the house through the kitchen. But her smile dropped when she saw his face. "The cows still won't eat a thing. They just stand in their stalls at the milking stations, and they won't even look at the parlor feed," Halbert said, referring to the high protein supplement fed to cows while they are being milked twice a day. When lunch was ready Sandy found him absorbed, reading a veterinary textbook. "We've lost hundreds of pounds of milk in a few days, and I can't figure out why the cows won't eat. I just don't understand it," he said. "Trained in literature and art," Sandy recalls, "I realized with frustration that I could be of very little help to Rick during the crisis that was engulfing us."

Soon Halbert was headed back to the farm, five miles away, so preoccupied that he forgot to say good-bye to Stephanie, his daughter, who was standing under a maple tree in the brilliant September sunshine. He was intrigued by the sudden milk production decline, but realized that even the best of dairymen from time to time encounter inexplicable ups and downs in milk production.

Halbert, a farmer who kept up with the latest research and innovations in dairy agriculture, wondered if perhaps something was wrong with the special feed he had purchased recently. In the late 1960s and early 1970s, animal nutritionists began to learn that adding magnesium oxide to dairy feeds increased a cow's milk production as well as the butterfat content of the milk. The higher the butterfat content, the higher the price a farmer was paid for his milk. And so in early fall of 1972, Halbert had ordered dairy feed containing four pounds of magnesium oxide per ton of feed. By December, he

4

was so pleased with the results that in his next order Halbert doubled the amount of magnesium oxide per ton. The feed supplier began production of this custom feed in March 1973 and called it dairy feed #402, as other farmers also began buying the special formula feed. It was shortly after Halbert received and began using the thirty-five tons of dairy feed #402 in mid-1973 that his animals started suffering illnesses and drastic declines in milk output. Was there a connection?

Several years earlier, Halbert surprised many of his friends and colleagues, and disappointed his mother, when he resigned from a choice position as a Dow Chemical Company engineer to return to his family farm near Battle Creek. After receiving a master's degree in chemical engineering from Michigan State University, he had joined Dow as a chemist under "corporate special assignment." That meant Halbert was given the flexibility to move around within the giant corporation for up to two years while making up his mind which area interested him most. Thus many folks were surprised when the Halberts sold their subdivision home in Midland, Michigan, home of Dow Chemical's headquarters, and bought an old farmstead five miles north of the two hundred-acre dairy farm the Halbert family had owned for thirty years. "My dad decided to build a new farm and undergo a major expansion; I got involved in that even while living in Midland. Then I decided to come back and get my feet dirty again. So we just cut loose. Sandy followed me along. I guess I always viewed myself as being somewhat vulnerable working for a big corporation or an institution. When you live in the country, you sort of develop a free spirit which is somewhat shackled by being an organization person," the young farmer explained, his pale blue eyes twinkling. "His parents," Sandy recalled, "had been disappointed at what seemed to them an abandonment of his natural appetite for science. But he fit easily into the routine of managing the farm with his father, a life he had known from childhood." With some four hundred cows, the morning milking began as early as midnight and lasted up to six hours, requiring two men to handle the rhythmic chore. A third worker would show up around six A.M. to feed the cows as they finished milking. At seven, the rest of the men came to work, receiving their job assignments from Halbert in the barn office. The milking is repeated twelve hours later. On weekends, Halbert and his younger brother, Mark, would do the milking. The daylight hours often are spent tending to the assorted needs of the animals, such as hauling manure out of the barns to the fields, repairing machinery, fences and barns, and moving animals from one barn to another, depending on their age and productivity. When Halbert was a boy, his father and grandfather had had two farms, totaling almost three hundred acres of choppy, partially wooded land. But within two years after Halbert left Midland, the family farm had grown to two thousand acres, with more than four hundred cows, making the farm among the bigger dairy operations in the entire state. The only tip-off to Halbert's previous career training and interests was the monthly deluge of engineering and amateur radio magazines.

Arriving back at the farm after lunch that September day, Halbert went straight to the shiny giant metal milk tank. Production had dropped another four hundred pounds within the past twenty-four hours. Halbert, troubled, went to a filing cabinet in his barn office to check his herd's feed records. His father, Ted, walked in. Halbert told him the news. "I know," Ted told his twenty-eight-year-old son, "I checked it, too. Don't get excited. You know how daily production can vary. Things will probably turn around in a day or so."

"But it's been three days already," Halbert replied. "And I don't see the cows eating anything. There just doesn't seem to be any improvement. Maybe something will show up in the next day or so. But if nothing improves we'd better call Dr. Jackson." Then Halbert went to inspect the cows. He was struck by the silence as he entered the barn where the best-producing cows were kept. He walked quickly down the center alley. He stopped suddenly. A cow in front of him looked as if she had been crying. Tears were streaking down her cheeks. He checked her for infections, especially pinkeye. He resumed down the barn alley. He encountered another tear-streaked face. And then another. And another. Almost every one of the one hundred cows in the barn was afflicted, whatever the problem was. Then he noticed something else even more alarming. Not one of the cows was chewing her cud. Normally cows chew their cud even while sleeping. "As ruminates, cows have a fermentation stomach filled with microbes, which digests the cellulose found in plant leaves and stems," Halbert explained. "In order to prepare this roughage for their digestive system, cows regurgitate the coarse material and chew it over and over until it can pass on to the conventional stomach for further digestion." A barn full of cows not chewing their cud suggested one thing: Their digestive system was not functioning, Halbert thought as he dialed Dr. Jackson's number. Within an hour, the wiry energetic veterinarian was unloading his instruments at the Halbert farm.

"There's no reason for these cattle to have IBR [a flulike disease which can cause abortions in cattle]," said the stoop-shouldered animal doctor. "I vaccinated them all myself, and the vaccine came from several suppliers, so we can't blame it on a bad batch of vaccine. But I'll be hanged if I know what it is. These cattle don't act like any I've ever seen before. No cuds, no appetites, no fever. I don't know what they've got."

"Dr. Jackson was too dedicated a veterinarian, too tenacious a diagnostician to let the mysterious ailment go unexplained," Halbert recalls. He said to Halbert as they walked back to the milk parlor, "I think it might be a good idea to have the vets from the Michigan Department of Agriculture come around and take a look at your herd, Rick. There might be something in their experience that could help get this pinned down. What do you think?" Halbert nodded. "I think I'll give Farm Bureau Services a call," he said. Dr. Jackson, packing his equipment, replied, "Good idea." For years, the Halberts had purchased their livestock feed from Farm Bureau Services, a statewide cooperative organization set up by the Michigan Farm Bureau to meet the assorted needs of farmers, such as supplying fuel, equipment and feed. Still troubled that the cows refused to even touch their parlor feed, Halbert dialed the Farm Bureau Services number in Lansing, the state capital. "Could I speak to your staff nutritionist, please?"

Dr. James McKean came on the line.

"My name is Rick Halbert. My father and I have a dairy herd near Battle Creek, and we've been using Farm Bureau's number 402 complete ration pelleted feed in the parlor," Halbert began.

"I'm familiar with that feed, yes," Dr. McKean replied.

"Well," Halbert said, "since shortly after we took delivery of the last load of number 402 five days ago, the cattle have been refusing to eat the pellets or their other feed. Their production has dropped drastically for the last several days; we've lost four hundred more pounds of milk each day since then." Dr. McKean said the problem sounded like a lack of appetite. "Your corn is probably moldy." Earlier that year about

7

forty dairy herds in Wisconsin had experienced problems similar to those Halbert was describing and eventually molds were identified as the cause. McKean asked Halbert what other feeds and minerals he was using, then concluded, "Well, there can be a lot of problems associated with loss of appetite. Since we haven't had any other complaints about number 402, I suspect one of your other rations is at fault. If it'll make you feel any better, I'll send somebody over to take samples of the feed so we can analyze it. Can you get it ready by tomorrow morning?"

"Yes, we'll be waiting," Halbert replied. Before hanging up, Halbert asked one further question. "Because our soil here is low in magnesium, the forage we harvest is low in it, too. So we asked that the batches of feed made up for our herd have magnesium oxide added to make up for this natural deficiency. Could someone at the feed plant have made a mistake and added manganese oxide instead? The chemical symbols are similar, after all."

"Absolutely not," McKean replied.

Still not satisfied, Halbert called Paul Mullineaux, manager of Farm Bureau Services' main feed plant in Climax, a small town midway between Kalamazoo and Battle Creek just south of the busy U.S. Interstate 94, the main Detroit-to-Chicago highway. "Paul, I'd like to know what lubricant you're using on your pelleting machine," Halbert asked.

Mullineaux, surprised, answered, "They're approved for this use. Why do you ask?"

"Well," Halbert said, "we're having an appetite problem with our cattle, and the source of it may be the number 402 pellets you delivered a few days ago. In the 1940s and 1950s, there was a mysterious disease in cattle called X Disease. Somebody noticed some animals who showed signs of the disease licking the grease off a feeder truck. Tests on the cattle for chlorinated naphthalenes, which are found in machine lubricants, came out positive. But a second source of lubricant had also contaminated the feed itself—and that was from the pelleting machine. Since then the U.S. Department of Agriculture has controlled all lubricants used in feed equipment."

Mullineaux replied, "We follow those regulations, Rick. You can be sure nothing like that happened here."

Halbert continued. "How about the magnesium oxide? Where does it come from?"

8

"Michigan Chemical Corporation of St. Louis [Michigan]. I can assure you it's pure; it's the same stuff they use on antacid tablets for humans," Mullineaux said.

After several more questions, Halbert apologized for "grilling" the feed plant manager. As he returned the telephone to its cradle, Halbert was impressed by the straight answers Mullineaux had given, even though many questions remained unanswered. Most of that evening, Halbert was stretched out on the sofa, reading from his veterinary textbooks, impervious to the noise made by his young daughters, Stephanie, Kristen and Lisa. "The children went to bed unnoticed," Sandy would remember of that night.

Just before ten o'clock the next morning, Halbert looked up from his desk in the barn office to see two Michigan Department of Agriculture veterinarians turning into the farm from M-37 in a green car with a state seal on either side. As they were putting on their coveralls, Dr. Jackson also arrived. Halbert and his father took the animal doctors for a tour of the barns. "Couldn't miss those symptoms," Dr. Donald Grover exclaimed. "Just look at those eyes!" The cows' temperatures proved normal, however. Halbert next led them to the manger. "This is the current silage ration," he said, running his hands through the corn silage. "Everything seems normal here, not spoiled or moldy," Dr. Grover commented. The other state veterinarian, Dr. Frank Carter, nodded in agreement, as the two gathered some feed samples to take back to Lansing for testing. "It should be about a week before these samples can tell us anything," Dr. Grover said. "We'll have to let the cultures grow before we read them. Call us in about a week. We should have the results for you. This is probably a virus of some sort. It is still warm enough outside for flies to transmit disease from cow to cow."

As Dr. Grover was putting his last supplies into the car, Halbert said, "We're planning to have samples of the feed tested this week for nitrates and excess urea. I've also requested that a dairy nutritionist come down from Michigan State and go through our feeding program to see if something is wrong with the nutrition in the cow's diet.... I also notified Farm Bureau shortly after the whole thing began. I thought they should know in case something's wrong with the pelleted feed. If you happen to see someone else who has the same set of problems, let me know. I'd sure like to know what this is and how to

9

get over it." Dr. Grover, climbing into the state car, said, "We will—though you're the only ones who have come up with this so far."

After they left, Halbert resumed fretting. If laboratory testing showed a problem with the feed, it might mean dumping $250,000 worth of silage, more than enough to last through the winter.

The next day, Dr. Donald Hillman, a Michigan State University dairy nutritionist, stopped by. "He read through the nutrition statement supplied with the pelleted feed and said it sounded good to him. He wants us to stop using that top dressing of high-moisture corn," Halbert told his wife during lunch. "There's a crust of mold on it just from last week's rain. He took a sample of it to test, but I'd already decided to take it out to the field with the manure spreader; and we haven't fed any of that corn since it got wet anyway."

Dr. Hillman also took feed samples from the silo for testing, and advised Halbert to take all the cows off their regular feed immediately, and put them on dry hay instead. The next morning, Halbert relayed the changes in ration to his work crew. Soon a large farm truck returned to the barn with the first load of chopped hay. Halbert watched intently to see what would happen. "They went at the green hay as if they hadn't eaten in a lifetime!" he recalls. "The scene was repeated in all the barns, and the cows were voraciously hungry." Elated, Halbert shouted to the driver of the second truckload of hay as it arrived, "Tell Gordon to chop another round! They've eaten everything we've given them!" He felt better than he had in days. "We had begun to turn the corner at last!" Halbert thought.

The herd's milk production began to stabilize. "The improvement was welcome but it did not mean that the troublemaker was one of the three previous feeds. It wasn't easy at that time of the year to go out and chop forage, but it worked."

Several days later, the cows on the all-hay diet began increasing their milk production. Halbert and his father then decided to reintroduce the #402 feed as milk parlor feed to see what would happen.

On the first day, the cows ate the pellets routinely. The next day, however, they began to ignore the feed, and their milk output again plunged. "That's it," Halbert said to his father, and they agreed to stop using the #402 feed. By mid-October, the

10

cows' conditions again stabilized, but their milk production showed no improvement.

"Now we had the cows stabilized and we could initiate action which might shed some light on this mystery. The two fermented feeds were exonerated by feed trials on the farm," Halbert said. "This left the pellets." Meantime, the Department of Agriculture laboratory reports were starting to come back; they showed no identifiable infectious agents. A private laboratory in Kalamazoo indicated no excessive urea or nitrates in Halbert's feed. Dr. Hillman's tests at Michigan State on the high-moisture corn indicated that the organisms present in the moldy-looking pile were only yeast.

In early November, Halbert decided to feed twelve weaned calves nothing but the #402 pellets as an experiment. Within six weeks, the calves began to die. "But since we did not have a control group, the results could not be considered conclusive or scientific," he said. One day while the feeding experiment was still in progress, but before the feed's lethal effect had manifested itself, Halbert walked past the five tons of feed he was saving for the experiment. The feed had been so expensive that he bought thirty-five tons while he could get a good price. Now he walked up to the pile, scooped up a handful and walked out into the late-afternoon autumn sunlight. He rolled the feed reflectively between his palms. It's got to be here, he thought. He pinched several pellets, weighing perhaps two ounces, put them in his mouth, chewed them and then swallowed the feed. "Looking back," Halbert said later, "it seems so stupid to have done that. But I guess it was my intense curiosity as to why the animals wouldn't eat."

The twelve weaned calves in his feeding experiment did not just "up and die," Halbert said. "Essentially, they stopped eating. After a week of ceasing eating, they'd die, clearly of malnutrition. We took some of those calves to the [Michigan State University] diagnostic lab in East Lansing. The lab concluded the animals died of malnutrition! We realized the animals were suffering malnutrition, but not because there was no feed offered. What we wanted to know was why they wouldn't eat. Pathologies didn't really reveal anything. We were somewhat infuriated, dismayed and upset that, implicitly, they felt we weren't caring for the animals—or at least that was the way we were reacting to the lab reports."

As the November days grew shorter, Halbert thought the

11

worst of the crisis might be over. The cows were eating again; the unusual tearing had stopped; milk production was stable, although still far below the previous daily output of thirteen thousand pounds. But soon other symptoms appeared among the cows, such as abnormally rapid hoof growth and lameness.

"We weren't sure what was happening except it was clear that it was something unusual. And many things crossed my mind, including sabotage by an employee we had let go." The man had been hired at a busy time during the summer and, by the time Halbert got around to checking the man's references, Halbert discovered the new employee had a history of chronic alcoholism and a prison record for assault. But Halbert and his father decided to keep the man on, if he would promise not to operate machinery or show up for work drunk. Around midnight in late August, shortly after being paid, the man was found slumped over the steering wheel in the driveway. He was fired the next morning. The likeliest way to sabotage livestock would be to poison the two-hundred-gallon water tank in each barn. So Halbert and his brother, Mark, emptied each tank, scrubbing the interiors with cleansing solution. In the last tank, they found a goldfish. One of the employees had placed his children's goldfish in the water tank after it grew too big for the fish bowl. The brothers smiled; the tanks could not have been poisoned if a fish had thrived in the water. Halbert also wondered, he said, "if someone working for the feed company didn't like us. I suppose there was a certain paranoia involved. And as things went on, we got a little more desperate and the paranoia increased."

One night, Sandy woke up with a stab of pain, marking, she later recalled, "the beginning of a spreading kidney infection. Before that was taken care of, Lisa's cough had gotten worse instead of better, and what we thought was a common cold tracked home from kindergarten by her older sister turned out to be pneumonia and required ten days in the hospital. Things fell into a quiet routine finally, but it was December before all of us were healthy again."

One December morning, Halbert was cleaning the milk parlor when Karl, his second cousin, entered. "Have you seen those two rats in the milkhouse lately?" he asked Karl. "I just realized I haven't seen a mouse or rat in here for several days." Karl, a super handyman around the farm, had a special interest in the rats because it was he who usually repaired the wiring that rodents gnawed. "No, I haven't seen any rats for over a week. But it's not because of the poison; I've given up on that," Karl said. The sudden disappearance of rats intrigued Halbert.

That afternoon Halbert posed the same question to Mark. "No," his brother replied, "I haven't seen them. I haven't seen any of my cats either—not even the white one. I've put milk out for them the last two or three days and they haven't shown up to drink it."

"One day it just sort of hit us: Where did all the rodents go? There was no Pied Piper in evidence. Now this was before the calves we fed the pellets began to die. So I put ten pounds of this pellet feed under the kitchen of another building where rodents had been. There, too, they disappeared. It was a dramatic indication of something unusual in the feed," Halbert said. Rodents are an inevitable fact of farm life, man-made rat poisons notwithstanding. So what, then, could have caused their sudden disappearance? Halbert continued to wonder. Later in the week, he was walking through the big barn when he started at something that lay in his path. Two cats were stretched out near the pile of the pellets. One was the white cat Mark especially liked. Both were stiff. "It was unusual to see one dead cat, let alone two, which had apparently succumbed to the same nameless thing about the same time," Halbert said. On his way home that late November afternoon, Halbert found himself alone in the maternity stall trying desperately but unsuccessfully to save a calf that was being born. He finally had to dissect it in order to save its mother.

In December, Halbert decided to call the Michigan Department of Agriculture again for help, having seen so much death on his farm—the experimental calves, the cats, the rodents. "We asked them if they would run tests on the calves or on laboratory animals under their direction to verify our findings. They said that calves would not be practical but mice could be fed the feed in question. The feed trial began in mid-December."

In the meantime, Michigan State University's diagnostic laboratory agreed to conduct postmortems on some of the twelve calves in Halbert's own feeding experiment. A week or so after the autopsies began, an official university envelope arrived at the Halbert house. "Surely this would be the explanation we were awaiting, the answer that would put an end to the plague that had struck the cows," Sandy thought as her husband tore open the envelope. His eyes moved quickly down the page and by the time they reached the bottom of the letter, he exploded in anger. "Malnutrition?! You've got to be kidding. Malnutrition?! The poor calf wouldn't eat for two weeks before it died. What I wanted to know is why," Halbert shouted in exasperation. Soon similar reports arrived on the other calves. Several had ulcers, others inflamed kidneys. All showed severe loss of body fat. Yet no clear pattern emerged.

Halbert once more picked up the telephone to call Michigan State University, this time dialing sciences department. He explained his feed problem and even offered to supply the calves and the feed if the department would look into the matter. "But they said that, since we were the only people who had this problem and being a tax-supported institution, they could not help us," Halbert recalls.

Next he called Dr. N. J. Gatzmeyer at the Michigan Department of Agriculture's Geagley Laboratory in East Lansing to inquire how the mice were doing on the #402 feed. Dr. Gatzmeyer said they appeared normal. But when Halbert called back several days later, just before the end of 1973, the situation had drastically changed. "All of the mice in the experiment have died," Dr. Gatzmeyer told him. "They went from thirty grams to twenty of body weight in ten days. But they ate the feed heartily. Some of them died with feed in their mouths."

That evening, December 28, Halbert called Donald Armstrong, the executive vice-president of the Farm Bureau Services, Inc., the feed company. Halbert started at the beginning, ending with the dead mice in Dr. Gatzmeyer's experiment. Armstrong listened patiently and then gave a surprised whistle when Halbert finished. "I'm not qualified to say how adequate those pellets are as rodent feed," Armstrong said. "But it sounds like there may be something there that cattle don't like to eat. Can you send me those test results, Rick? I should have them for my records. We take such care in formulating, processing and handling at the feed plant that I can't believe those pellets could be causing any trouble. I'm going to ask Jim McKean, our staff vet, to repeat the mouse trials to see if he can find out what's going on. Maybe there was something about the way you stored or handled the feed that caused some spoilage. I'll get back to you in a few days or so."

The year 1973 ended with $80,000 in losses.

In January, many more calves were born dead. Moreover, many of the cows, after giving birth, had to be sold for meat, or culled, because their udders went dry and began looking like raisins—shrunken and without milk. That month alone, more than thirty cows were sent to the market. Normally, Halbert might cull perhaps a hundred cows all year. An attempt to improve milk production by milking three times a day proved fruitless.

On January 6, Farm Bureau Services officials scheduled a meeting with Halbert and his father. The Halberts meticulously assembled all the evidence they had available to support their case against the #402 feed, including even computerized milk production records from the three previous years to demonstrate that theirs was an outstanding dairy operation. For the meeting, Sandy even polished her husband's briefcase. As Halbert put on his tie, he could still feel the ache in his arms from having struggled to help deliver three more calves. When father and son arrived at the Farm Bureau office in Battle Creek, they were greeted by Armstrong and Tony Grusczynski, the gregarious manager of the co-op's store in Battle Creek. Ted Halbert began by recounting their experiences with the feed. Then his son described his own feeding experiments, the mice studies by Dr. Gatzmeyer and even the inexplicable disappearance of rats and mice from their farm. When they finished, Armstrong disclosed that his organization also had arranged for some experiments with the #402 feed to be done by the Agway Research Center just outside Syracuse, New York. The experiments, he said, would involve four groups of calves, each consisting of four animals. Additional feed analyses, Armstrong added, would be done by the Wisconsin Alumni Research Foundation, a laboratory known by its acronym WARF. "If anything turned up, Rick would be notified," he told the Halberts. "You can be sure that we'll get to the bottom of this." The Halberts would not learn until late March that Armstrong, alarmed by the scattered evidence of the toxicity of his co-op's #402 feed, had already launched a recall of the feed. They felt reassured, when the meeting ended, by Armstrong's willingness to unravel the mystery. And the morning's tension dissipated as the four adjourned for lunch in a nearby cafeteria, with Armstrong reminiscing about the days when he was manager of the Farm Bureau store in Battle Creek. But further experiments meant more waiting.

Not long after the meeting, Halbert learned that Dr. Gatzmeyer, at the request of Farm Bureau Services, had repeated his mice experiments using the #402 feed and the

15

results confirmed the feed's deadly effects. He called Dr. James McKean, the Farm Bureau Services' veterinarian. "I hear that the mice who were fed the number 402 pellets in your test died," Halbert said. "Don't you think that proves something's wrong with the feed?" Dr. McKean replied evenly, "This is cattle feed, not mouse food."

Halbert returned to the veterinary books, many of them borrowed from Dr. Jackson, his veterinarian. The two men often held long telephone discussions late into the night, exchanging information and speculation. The weird ailments that became widespread in Halbert's animals so puzzled Dr. Jackson that "he was putting in time on it 'after hours' despite Rick's insistence that he bill us for whatever time he was spending on the problem," Sandy recalled. Dr. Jackson in the summer of 1968 had undergone open heart surgery at age forty-six, and was advised to shift his practice from farm animals to household pet work, a less physically demanding job. "So he took on two young men," Mrs. Jackson said. "But it ended up they did the pet work and Ted continued doing farm animals. And when Halbert's cow problems began showing up, you couldn't get Ted to slow down." To try to take the pressure off her husband, Lois Jackson even went back to school and obtained a master's degree in library science and then took a full-time job. They had three children on the threshold of college. "But it didn't make any difference," she recalls. "He never let up. I'm sure he would have lived longer if he had paced himself. But you couldn't get him to stop." In May 1975, Dr. Jackson died of a heart attack at age fifty-three. However, he did live to see the discovery of PBB in Halbert's feed in May of 1974. And for the animal doctor, the last year of his life was his happiest. "He was so elated," Lois Jackson recalls, "That whole year, he was practically euphoric. That was the high point of his career. Even when Rick Halbert began getting all the credit, Ted was satisfied merely to have pursued the diagnosis to the end. When Ted's friends suggested that he claim some of the credit, he was too busy; he was off on his legislation kick, trying to help pass laws to prevent similar mix-ups."

One night after Christmas of 1973, Dr. Jackson called Halbert. "I just read a journal article by a Dr. Allan Pier of the National Animal Disease Laboratory in Ames, Iowa," Dr. Jackson told Halbert. "This article is about his work with mold toxins—mycotoxicosis—in feed. I thought I might give him a call, with your permission, of course, and see if he'd be interested in working on your feed problem. From this article it seems as if there's a chance that a mold toxin might be your problem."

"I'd wondered about that myself," Halbert replied. "But I didn't know where to look for someone really qualified to analyze the feed for mold." Molds were a prime suspect not only because many of the animal symptoms suggested moldy feed but also because corn harvested in Michigan in the fall of 1972, as in Wisconsin, had been contaminated with molds due to long delays in harvesting caused by nonstop rains. After Dr. Jackson persuaded Dr. Pier to analyze the #402 pellets, Halbert began calling Dr. Pier every few days, "trying to keep our project on the front burner."

"Ted not only made all the contacts with laboratories," recalls Lois Jackson, "but often he also had to call these people to placate them because they would get mad at Rick, who called them constantly. I guess Rick was a very impatient and brash young man. But I can't blame him." Dr. Pier in Ames first wanted to duplicate the mice experiments Dr. Gatzmeyer had done. Within two weeks, the mice all died. "They showed a certain 'refusal factor.' In many cases, the mice would rather starve than eat the feed," he told Halbert. Meantime, the surviving calves in Halbert's own feeding experiment had begun to have their calves. "We had quite a mess," Halbert recalls. "The poor animals would have overterm calves, and they would develop no mammary tissue, and their pelvic ligaments would not adjust to allow for normal calf presentation."

Near the end of January, Dr. Pier informed Halbert he would no longer work on the problem. But he did give Halbert the name of a colleague at the National Animal Disease Laboratory, a toxicologist named Dr. Al Furr who was willing to test the feed further. Dr. Furr asked Halbert to send him some of the pelleted feed. About a week later, Halbert and Dr. Furr were chatting rather aimlessly and were about to end the telephone conversation when Dr. Furr said, "By the way, we did discover something that may be significant, though we can't interpret the result."

"What is it?" Halbert asked.

"We've been running some tests on your feed with a gas liquid chromatograph. Are you familiar with that equipment?"

17

Halbert was. He had seen fellow chemists at Dow use the marvelous piece of machinery. In essence, the machine is capable of producing the "fingerprints" of each compound in an unknown substance. First the substance is heated and vaporized into a gas. The vapor then passes through a long coiled tube. As the vapor passes through the tube, molecules of different compounds separate from one another and emerge from the far end as distinct compounds. As they emerge, they are exposed to radiation that creates a tiny electric current. Different compounds absorb, or "accept," different amounts of electrons. The more they accept, the more the current is diminished. Each change in the current then is registered by the movement of a tracing needle on a revolving cylinder of graph paper. Chemists know that the lighter the molecules the earlier they show up on the printout, and they have learned to identify chemicals by the various peaks, or fingerprints, on the graph.

"Well," Dr. Furr told Halbert, "when we left the chromatograph on for eight hours, after all the known peaks for pesticides and polychlorinated biphenyls [PCBs] would have shown up, we began to get a series of peaks on the printout that looked like the Rocky Mountains. The pattern is something I haven't seen before, and I haven't any idea what it is. I can't say that these peaks are the mystery ingredient that caused your problem, but I thought you'd like to know we did find something."

Normally, a gas liquid chromatograph might be left on for a few minutes, maybe even one hour. But Dr. Furr said the machine in Ames had been accidentally left on for eight hours by a lab technician.

"Are you sure you've never seen this pattern before?" Halbert asked. Dr. Furr said no, adding, "On the other hand, many of the peaks are repeated in the cow tissue samples we got from Dr. Jackson. Whatever it is, the animal and the feed had something in common." Halbert was intrigued by the new lead, although he was not at all certain what it meant.

The cows continued to die. Halbert calculated that each animal sold to the slaughterhouse—due to inadequate milk production—represented an annual loss of $900, since he was in the business of selling milk, not beef. But there was no choice but to continue culling nonproductive cows. Total milk production now had stabilized at eight thousand pounds daily, down from thirteen thousand pounds a day before the feed problem

18

developed. Yet the cows continued developing illnesses. Many had hooves that curled upward and inward uncontrollably; some began losing hair, then their skin thickened and wrinkled. With each death, Dr. Jackson would do a postmortem. The signs always seemed the same: enlarged livers, inflamed kidneys, nearly a total absence of fat. One day, as he was cleaning up after another postmortem, Dr. Jackson snapped, "You'd think the diagnostic lab at Michigan State University would have found something. They've got the equipment there to do tests that I just can't run. I don't know why they didn't send out the state police to shut down that feed plant when those mice died. You'd think the state government doesn't know—or doesn't care—what's going on. Their own vets and labs have been involved in this from the start."

As the experiments continued, evidence mounted against the #402 feed. At the National Animal Disease Laboratory, where Dr. Furr was giving the feed to steers and pigs, two of the pigs died, one bleeding from the ears and the other from nearly every orifice in its body. When Dr. Furr had only one week's worth of #402 feed left for his experiments, Halbert offered to ship more to Iowa. "Well," Dr. Furr interrupted, "we've been discussing whether we ought to drive out to Michigan to pick up some more feed ourselves. Then we could take a look at your herd, so that we could compare the symptoms with those our animals are showing. Maybe that would suggest some tests that we haven't tried." Halbert could hardly believe what he heard. "Finally I think we've got some heavyweights interested," he told his wife when he got home. The Ames group was due to arrive on a Friday afternoon and Halbert waited for the group in his barn office until nine that night, finally giving up and returning home for supper, thinking perhaps he had gotten the days confused. The next morning, he sprang out of bed and drove back to the farm. Again, no one showed up. "I'm terribly sorry, Rick," Dr. Furr explained over the telephone early Monday morning. "Friday, after we got packed to come to Michigan we got word from our director in Washington that absolutely no more funds could be spent on the project and that we had to stop any further work on it. We had to cancel the trip and the project. Period." Pausing, Dr. Furr added, "I wonder if the Farm Bureau had anything to do with this."

"I hope not," Halbert said. He then called Dr. Francis J. Mulhern, administrator of the Animal and Plant Health Inspection Service of the U.S. Department of Agriculture. Dr.

19

Mulhern, who was Dr. Furr's superior, listened patiently as Halbert once more poured out his story. Finally, Dr. Mulhern spoke. His voice was cool and formal. "This is all very interesting, Mr. Halbert. But why hasn't anyone else in Michigan complained of problems with the feed? Why haven't other veterinarians seen anything unusual?" Mulhern's decision was a polite but firm no. Years later, Mulhern explained his decision: "In such investigations we never know when the end point will be found and, in many cases, we never find the cause. So such expenses might have gone on indefinitely." Dr. Mulhern said when he further looked into the activities of the Ames laboratory he discovered complaints were being received that work at the center "was not being carried out because of personnel being diverted to this [Michigan] problem." Thus, he ordered the work stopped.

Several days after his futile plea with Mulhern, Halbert called Dr. Furr again in Ames. Perhaps Mulhern had changed his mind? The answer still was no. But Dr. Furr gave Halbert a list of laboratories around the country with the capability perhaps to solve the mysterious "Rocky Mountain peaks" that appeared in the National Animal Disease Laboratory gas liquid chromatograph. Among those on that list was the Wisconsin Alumni Research Foundation [WARF]. Halbert commissioned WARF to perform a gas liquid chromatograph reading of the #402 feed. Again, the mystery peaks appeared. Don Hughes, the scientist at WARF who performed the analysis on Halbert's feed, told him the compound contained a halogen—meaning either a fluorine, chlorine, iodine or bromine—and had a high molecular weight. Halbert now was sure the still unidentified substance had to be a man-made compound.

Several nights later, the entire Halbert family was leaving the house after dinner to get ice cream cones in town when Dr. Jackson called. "One of my rabbits died," he told Halbert. Dr. Jackson's rabbit experiment was his own idea. He picked up two rabbits from a friend who raised rabbits for meat, put them in his garage and started feeding them the #402 pellets. The three Halbert girls were getting restless waiting for their father, and Sandy had her hands full trying to placate them. Yet she remembers thinking, "How could we ever pay the veterinarian for his dedication? It seemed clear that he was putting in many more hours on our behalf than were showing up on the bills." On the way into town, Halbert no longer had any doubt that the mysterious ingredient in the #402 feed was lethal. Yet, solving the problem seemed to depend solely on his own efforts to identify the agent. "Rick was getting the strong impression that Farm Bureau Services was less than eager to proceed," Sandy recalls.

The experiments the co-op had promised back in January had been postponed several times at Agway Animal Research Center near Syracuse. They finally began in late February just before a second meeting Ted and Rick Halbert held with Don Armstrong, Dr. McKean and Farm Bureau Services' risk manager, Ken Jones. By then, however, the number of calves in the Agway experiments had been reduced from sixteen to four. The second meeting between co-op officials and the Halberts, again held in Battle Creek, was less cordial than the first. The Farm Bureau Services people seemed self-assured as they put on the table before them volumes of test data they had commissioned the Wisconsin Alumni Research Foundation to perform. But when the young Halbert saw what tests had been requested, he was deeply disappointed. Only the standard pesticide screenings had been done. "As you can see," Armstrong said expansively, "there is nothing here to indicate that the feed is anything but wholesome and pure."

Halbert replied pointedly, "Don't you think that the death of the mice in Dr. Gatzmeyer's experiments proves the opposite?" Armstrong and his cohorts held their ground. Their attitude confused both Halberts, who had assumed coming into the meeting that Farm Bureau Services had been genuinely interested in finding out what was wrong with their #402 feed; instead, the co-op seemed more interested in demonstrating its goodness. Again, as in the first meeting, Farm Bureau Services hid the fact that it had begun a massive recall of the #402 feed.

The Halberts' suspicions did not diminish when, a short time later, Ken Jones visited their farm with a tape recorder seeking more information. "I hope you don't mind my bringing this along to help me take notes," Jones said, "but getting it right the first time does save a lot of time." Reluctantly, Halbert assented. But the machine turned out to be malfunctioning in any case. As Jones prepared to leave, Halbert asked casually, "Heard anything about the animals in the Agway study yet?"

Jones stopped, looked at Halbert, and said, "Didn't you know? Three of them died."

Finally, there is proof—from Farm Bureau Services' own

experiment—that the number 402 pellets are harmful to the animals they are supposed to nourish, Halbert thought as he reached for the telephone after Jones departed.

"Rick Halbert here," he said when the familiar voice of Dr. James McKean came on the other end of the line. "Have you seen anything in those Agway calves yet?"

"No," Dr. McKean replied. "They're doing all right."

"No problem?" Halbert persisted.

"I'm sure there's no problem," the veterinarian said.

"I just got word that three of the four have died," Halbert said. Dr. McKean said nothing. Halbert added, "Ken Jones was just here. He told me about the calves."

"If he wanted to tell you, I guess that's okay. It's not my place to give out information," Dr. McKean said.

At about the same time, Halbert received some intriguing—and frightening—test results back from the WARF laboratory in Madison. He had sent it two samples of Farm Bureau Services feed he bought in November 1973 and in February 1974. "We had asked the co-op that no magnesium oxide be added to those feeds because it was suspect in our minds," Halbert said. He instructed WARF to check the #112 feed samples for the presence of the "Rocky Mountain peaks." To his astonishment, the peaks were still present. Could the lethal agent be in all the other Farm Bureau Services feeds as well? For the first time in twenty years, the Halberts contemplated switching feed suppliers. "Does this mean that the cattle have gotten another dose of the toxin?" Sandy asked. "If the peaks are the result of the presence of a toxin," her husband answered, "it means we've had that toxin in all the batches of feed since mid-September. I just wish I knew what these peaks are. We might be worrying about something completely harmless."

Again, Halbert dialed Dr. James McKean's number in Lansing. The Farm Bureau Services' staff veterinarian dismissed the possibility that the peaks in the #112 feed meant all the co-op's feeds might be contaminated. "We don't even know what the peaks mean," he said. "They might be something totally ordinary." Halbert could no longer contain his anger. He snapped, "You promised us an insurance settlement. Where is it? If we don't start seeing some progress on this problem soon, I'm going to call the FDA," referring to the U.S. Food and Drug Administration. Halbert had contemplated calling the regulatory agency earlier. "But whenever I asked people with whom I was working whether the FDA should be notified, the answer was a firm and uniform no. I was told they would only create trouble," Halbert said. One scientist told him, "Don't call them expecting help. The best they might do is hinder the progress you're making. They don't research the causes of problems; they just police them." And now Dr. McKean was echoing those warnings: "You can go ahead and call the FDA. But I think you'll be sorry."

Many years later, Halbert still would distinctly remember his agony that day as he sat in the barn office, watching the traffic go by on M-37, a busy two-lane state highway connecting Grand Rapids and Battle Creek, debating whether or not to call the U.S. Food and Drug Administration. "It seemed that institutions, in order to take action, needed something spelled out, in the form of a cookbook or a dictionary. If you can tell them what to do, they will do it, maybe; if you can't, they won't. There's really not that initiative one'd expect. It was difficult getting access to people, the professional scientists; they were all working on their own pet projects. Yet people kept saying to me, 'Nobody else in Michigan is having a problem.' The inference was that it must be related to something I was doing rather than something somebody was doing to me. There really seemed to be no daylight. It seemed that no matter who touched this project, it never was followed through. And the companies were no different from the government. Well, of course, there were nagging doubts that it was something we were doing," Halbert said. "During this time period, when you have animals that are not producing—and this was beginning to happen to farmers all over the state—you send them to the market; that's what you'd call culling cows. This happened all over the state during the time period when we were struggling with this. By mid-March Halbert's own cows began showing new symptoms. Many began dying before giving birth to calves. Losing both a cow *and* her calf became more frequent. "I was getting desperate. The people in Iowa said they couldn't work on it anymore. The phone bills were running into the thousands of dollars. So I called the Detroit FDA office and said we were having a problem. What I was really trying to do was get access to some laboratory facilities, you know, somebody that could do the work." What Halbert hoped for was access to a mass spectrometer, another exquisitely fancy piece of scientific gadgetry, which sorts out and then identifies the atoms in a

23

sample of material. A "mass spec," as chemists call the machine, might determine the composition of the "Rocky Mountain peaks."

Using a mass spectrometer has been likened to panning for gold. Panning for gold involves scooping up gravel from a stream bed, sloshing it around so that the running water washes away all the lighter sand and stones, leaving behind the heavier gold nuggets. Similarly, a mass spectrometer sorts out molecules according to their weights, or masses, by ionizing the molecules so they can be manipulated within electrical or magnetic fields. The ionized molecules are sorted according to mass by varying the intensity of the electrical or magnetic fields to which they are subjected. The amount of molecules in each mass category is then measured. The resulting information then is presented in the form of a graph with many peaks and valleys. The location of each peak on the horizontal axis indicates the mass, or weight, of the substance represented by the peaks. The height of the peak indicates the amount of the substance present. Nowadays, scientists can detect as little as one picogram (one trillionth of a gram) of a substance. The basic techniques of mass spectrometry, however, date back to the turn of the century when it was used to measure the masses of the basic elements, leading to the discovery of isotopes, which are forms of an element that differ only slightly in atomic weight. During World War II, mass spectrometry was used to isolate the radioactive isotopes of uranium for use in the first atomic bomb.

Calling the agency's Detroit office, Halbert spoke to John P. Dempster. "I sort of needed a mechanism to lead into a dialogue with the FDA," Halbert recalls. "I specifically didn't tell them about the mice and calves dying in the experiments at Agway and at the Michigan Department of Agriculture lab. I wanted them to get a fresh start." The next day, FDA inspector Clarence Bozarth, based in Kalamazoo, visited Halbert's farm and collected a truckload of feed samples to take back for analysis. Halbert had told Dempster that he thought his problem might be related to excessive lead in the #402 feed. As Bozarth drove off, Halbert was pleasantly surprised by his first contact with the Food and Drug Administration, particularly after so many scientists had counseled against calling in the agency and after getting the runaround from so many other institutions. But his optimism was short-lived.

"Basically I learned very little from the FDA, and I began to call the office in Detroit trying to find out how things were coming. As time passed, I offered them hints as to what they might look for, other than heavy metals. Their attitude was that they were not a research agency but a regulatory agency, and unless we knew what was wrong, there was little they could do for us," Halbert said.

One aspect of his contacts with the agency troubled Halbert. In his initial telephone conversation with Dempster, the FDA official promised a full investigation and then added casually, "We'll want your full cooperation, of course." Since then, Halbert felt slightly uneasy because he had not disclosed to the agency the history of feeding experiments others already had performed with the #402 feed. But Halbert said he hoped the agency would "break some new ground in the case." And so he kept feeding the FDA hints. One of them was a description of the "Rocky Mountain peaks" seen at both the National Animal Disease Laboratory and the Wisconsin Alumni Research Foundation. "The scientist who ran the tests," Halbert told Dempster, "said it should be looked into further, but they had no more funds for testing,"

"I'm sorry, Mr. Halbert, we're just not a research organization," Dempster answered.

By the end of March only two of Halbert's original twelve calves in the feeding experiment were still alive. Now the two survivors were beginning to lose their hair in huge patches; soon there was no hair left on their faces and necks, and the hairless patches were spreading quickly. Before long both calves were totally hairless. Then their skin began to develop a condition called hyperkeratosis, which makes it resemble elephant hide. The calves failed to respond to all treatment. Halbert's accumulating financial losses now soared well into six figures. But money was not all that occupied his thoughts. His wife, Sandy, had developed a bleeding ulcer and inexplicable chest pains. The strain on Dr. Jackson also was beginning to show. The doctor's shoulders seemed more stooped, and his features increasingly more grim. Both he and Halbert were increasingly troubled by Farm Bureau Services' seemingly cavalier attitude toward the feed problem. The two had sent sheafs of test results to the co-op's veterinarian, Dr. McKean, but they never heard from him. Later, when Halbert pressed him, Dr. McKean admitted he decided the data, which included vital information on each animal's health history, was useless and threw them away.

The end of March meant the arrival of Farmers' Week at Michigan State University, an annual event featuring meetings highlighting the latest developments in agriculture. Halbert, as usual, attended. As he neared the outskirts of East Lansing, he took a detour to see Dr. McKean at Farm Bureau Services' office on the north side of Lansing. "Well," he said to the veterinarian, "I don't understand why you're not hearing from other farmers about this feed. You said there was only one farmer, around Allegan, who complained about a palatability problem with it. Have you heard from anyone else?"

"No," Dr. McKean said.

"That seems inconceiveable to me," Halbert replied.

He then coaxed Dr. McKean to go through the distribution records of the co-op's feed plant in Climax. And he noticed that the name of the elevator in Yale showed up many times as a distribution center for the co-op's feeds. Yale is located clear across the state in the Thumb area near Port Huron.

"And you haven't heard anything from that area about the feed?" Halbert asked.

"No. Absolutely nothing," Dr. McKean replied. If the animal doctor had been annoyed with Halbert, he didn't show it. Yet Dr. McKean already had come to the conclusion that "feeding and management programs" were partly to blame for the Halbert herd's problems, as he told others, including his boss, Don Armstrong.

Halbert had one final question before he left for Michigan State University. "What about the magnesium oxide? What is your source for that? Our feed tested low in magnesium oxide each time it was run."

Dr. McKean told him, "We get it from Michigan Chemical Corporation in St. Louis, Michigan. It's the same grade of stuff they put in antacids for humans."

"Do you consider Michigan Chemical an unimpeachable source?"

"Absolutely," Dr. McKean replied. "They're the best source of mag oxide in this country."

The night Halbert returned home from the Farmers' Week seminars, he called a neighbor, Laverne Bivens, whose brother, Bill, was an agricultural agent near the Yale elevator. Halbert and Bill Bivens had met each other several years earlier, and when Halbert identified himself over the telephone and explained his problem, Bill Bivens' first reaction was one of surprise. "I thought you had become a scientist, not a farmer," Bivens said. "You always were running chemistry experiments and building radios in your spare time, as I recall."

Halbert laughed. But he got to the point of his call. "I'm wondering whether you've seen any problems up there or if you know of anyone in your area who has been using the number 402 feed."

Bivens cleared his throat. "I know you're not the kind of person to make all of this up to conceal a management problem, Rick. I wish I could be of more help, but I've only got one name I can give you. A farmer by the name of Bob Demaray was going to try the number 402 with his silage this year. Let me give you his phone number."

During lunch hour the next day, Halbert called Demaray. Careful not to ask leading questions, Halbert inquired how he liked the #402 feed.

"We've had some problems with persistent infections after calving," Demaray replied candidly. "The vet can't get them to respond to antibiotics. We've never seen anything like it."

But it turned out that Demaray had used very little of the suspect feed—about one or two pounds daily per cow; Halbert had given each cow twenty pounds a day. "That stuff is terribly expensive, so we just gave them a little of it. The elevator says that it isn't making any more, so we haven't had any since January," Demaray said.

"Do you know of anyone else in your area who has been using the number 402 feed?" Halbert asked.

"There is one neighbor, Art Laupichler. Let me look up his number. At first, we were having such good results from feeding the number 402 that we got him interested in it as well." Like most farmers, Demaray had taken his problems philosophically, as "just one of those things."

Art Laupichler's animals had many of the same health problems Halbert's animals had. "I sure do remember that stuff," Laupichler said. "Bob Demaray had good luck with it, so I decided to try some, too. The cows dropped right down in milk production; they just weren't doing well at all."

"What about calving?" Halbert asked.

"Some of the best cows were having problems with it. When I saw all of that happening, I called the local elevator here in Yale, and told them something was wrong," Laupichler answered.

"What did they say?" Halbert continued.

"The elevator people told me they'd come out and pick up the number 402 feed and repay me for the milk I'd lost. Well, they did pick up the feed, but I haven't been paid for the milk yet," Laupichler said.

Halbert was stunned. He thought, all along the people at Farm Bureau Services had been trying to portray our problems as an isolated case with no parallels. Now here was someone who had complained and had had his feed picked up and compensation offered—if not paid—for lost production. Halbert thanked Laupichler. His voice was trembling as he called Dr. McKean.

"What do you have in your records about an Art Laupichler and a Bob Demaray?" Halbert asked.

"I don't recognize either of those names," Dr. McKean answered.

Halbert said, "Laupichler claims to have fed number 402 with some of the same results we had: lost production, difficult calving. So he called the Yale elevator to complain, and they came right out to haul it away and promised to repay him for that lost milk. Demaray had similar problems."

Dr. McKean did not respond.

"I guess I shouldn't be surprised—after the cover-up about the Agway calf experiment—that I wouldn't get straight answers about other complaints about the feed. Don't you people realize that this is our business, our lifeblood, that you're willing to sacrifice rather than admit a mistake?" Halbert said with righteous indignation.

Again, Dr. McKean didn't respond. He hung up.

The arrival of April meant spring planting, one of farmers' busiest times of the year. "Some vague hints from Farm Bureau Services renewed the hope that an insurance settlement would be just around the corner; with that in mind, Rick had virtually dropped the idea of spending any more of his own time and money on research into the feed problem. The efforts to find a mass spectrometer had not been successful," Sandy Halbert recalls.

But before Halbert abandoned his efforts entirely, he learned the name of a government research center in College Station, Texas, that might be interested in his feed problem.

28

There, a toxicologist named Dr. Harry Smalley sounded genuinely interested as Halbert once more related his story. "These are strange symptoms—like nothing I've ever encountered," Dr. Smalley told Halbert. "Would you be able to send some of the feed down here? I'd like to set up an experiment using some pregnant ewes." For the first time, Halbert thought, here was someone who immediately was interested in the mysterious problem. "Why don't you call the USDA [Department of Agriculture] vet in Lansing," Dr. Smalley was saying, "and have him obtain a government bill of lading to ship five hundred pounds of the feed down here?"

Halbert was shoveling the #402 feed pellets into two cardboard drums when, a short time later, the federal government veterinarian called back to tell him that a supervisor in Ohio had denied the request for a government bill of lading. "I don't understand why, Mr. Halbert," the veterinarian said. "I've never had this happen before."

Halbert sighed wearily. He had lost track of the amount of money he already had spent. But he was sure the shipping costs to Texas would not significantly add to that sum. "Thanks for trying. I guess I'll contact a freight company and ship it myself," Halbert replied. That afternoon, the two drums of feed were on a truck enroute to Texas. The cost was $45; Halbert hoped to hear from Dr. Smalley by the end of June. Then his thoughts once more turned to the spring planting.

But death continued to plague the farm. One victim was Supercow, so named because she was the best animal the Halberts had ever bred. "As a two-year-old," Sandy Halbert recalls, "she had set a state record in butterfat production, and we had been hoping her progeny would carry on her outstanding traits." But two days after Supercow died, her week-old calf also died.

In early April, when Halbert called the Michigan Department of Agriculture for information about vaccinating calves, he spoke to Dr. George L. Whitehead, the department's deputy director and chief veterinarian. Just as the routine conversation was about to end, Dr. Whitehead lowered his voice. "Did you say you're from around Battle Creek?" he asked.

"Yes, our farm is a bit north of there," Halbert said.

"Have you contacted the FDA in Detroit recently?"

"Yes. We contacted them about a problem we had with some dairy feed we bought from Farm Bureau Services,"

Halbert answered, puzzled by Dr. Whitehead's apparent knowledge.

"A few weeks ago," the veterinarian explained, "while I was in a meeting with a legislative committee, I was called out to discuss something urgent with an FDA representative. He said that we at the Department of Agriculture should withhold your milk because there was lead in it."

Halbert was stunned. No wonder everyone advised him not to call the FDA. "Well, what did you do?" he asked Dr. Whitehead.

"We went into our records of your milk samples. We found that we had tested your milk for lead and other heavy metals last fall and that we had found nothing. So we notified the FDA in Detroit that your milk samples contained no lead. They said, 'Okay,' and took our word for it. The matter was dropped."

Halbert, still flabbergasted, thanked Dr. Whitehead and hung up. So, he thought, this was the bottom line of the investigation that had started with Clarence Bozarth's diligent sample-collecting; FDA wanted to shut off my milk just because of a conversation I had with them just to get them interested in the problem.

A few days later, Halbert learned from Louis Newman, a Michigan State University veterinarian, the name of a U.S. Department of Agriculture Laboratory in Beltsville, Maryland, just outside Washington. Dr. Newman told Halbert that a Dr. George Fries, an animal research scientist at the National Pesticide Degradation Laboratory, might have access to the facilities to further analyze the #402 feed. But when Halbert called, Dr. Fries was attending a conference in California. Halbert called again when Dr. Fries returned in mid-April. Dr. Fries listened sympathetically, and then jotted down the telephone numbers of five scientists who had worked with Halbert and whom Halbert suggested Dr. Fries could call for corroboration or further information.

Dr. Fries, a large affable man with a penchant for Stetson hats and leather boots, was cautious and spoke in guarded tones. Complaints of this sort were not uncommon to him. Indeed he had just gone through one unpleasant experience in which he learned that a Wisconsin farmer he was trying to help had not told him the entire truth involving a problem with pesticides.

30

"So then I did a little checking. I called all the names on the list Halbert gave me, except Dr. McKean of Farm Bureau Services; I wanted to avoid any involvement with the companies," Dr. Fries said.

Dr. Fries' discussions with Dr. Furr of Ames, Dr. Gatzmeyer in Lansing, Dr. Hillman at Michigan State University, who also was his classmate in graduate school, sufficiently aroused his curiosity.

Halbert on Wednesday, April 17, called back Dr. Fries, who agreed that Halbert should send him a sample of the #402 feed. That afternoon, Halbert put the feed in the mail, special delivery.

On Friday, Halbert called Dr. McKean at Farm Bureau Services to see what progress was being made in the research sponsored by the co-op. "We've found out that the halogen is a bromine," he told Halbert. That came as a surprise to Halbert; he had expected a chlorine because chlorine is used much more widely as an industrial chemical. A bromine, on the other hand, suggested a special-use material. "Can you give me the molecular weights of the peaks?" he asked.

"The material has two major peaks and five minor peaks," Dr. McKean said, reading the figures to Halbert. "That's all the information I have."

Halbert immediately called Dr. Fries in Maryland. As he repeated the molecular weights, Dr. Fries did the same.

"That sounds like something I've run into before," Dr. Fries said after a slight pause. "A fire retardant. Let me check my files."

Halbert could hear paper rustling at the other end of the line as well as his own heart beating. He barely was able to contain himself. Soon Dr. Fries returned to the line. "Okay. Let me read these molecular weights back to you to check," Dr. Fries said. "I got this material as a sample from a chemical company. They had advertised a new fire retardant in a trade magazine, *Chemical Week*," Dr. Fries continued. "The trade name of the stuff is Firemaster BP-6. Chemically, it's basically polybrominated biphenyl, PBB." Dr. Fries and Joel Bitman, a colleague in the adjacent laboratory, had done work previously with PCBs, and so they decided to test PBB as well, since both are so similar in structure.

"What companies manufacture PBB?" Halbert asked.

"I got this sample from Michigan Chemical Corporation in St. Louis, Michigan," Dr. Fries said.

Halbert's search was over.

"Our feed was supposed to have magnesium oxide added to it; and the feed company got their magnesium oxide from Michigan Chemical. We hadn't been able to account for the low test for magnesium in the feed. What apparently happened was that Michigan Chemical sent the wrong stuff to Farm Bureau, and the fire retardant was added to our feed in place of magnesium oxide."

Dr. Fries was more cautious, however. "Well," he said, "I don't have your feed sample yet. So I can't state positively that PBB is in it. But it certainly looks like it. I'll give you a call when I run a test on the feed itself and let you know."

Dr. Fries's go-slow approach didn't deter Halbert from immediately calling the corporate offices of Michigan Chemical in Chicago. He spoke to a man in the marketing department and when he finished his explanation, the man gasped audibly. Then Halbert called Dr. McKean, telling the Farm Bureau Services veterinarian, "I've found out what the contaminant in the feed is. Dr. Fries at Beltsville identified the material as being a fire retardant called Firemaster BP-6, manufactured by Michigan Chemical Company. I'll call you back next week, when the confirmation is complete."

On the next working day, Monday, Dr. Fries told Halbert, "I ran your sample this morning and compared it with the Firemaster chromatogram. There's no doubt about it; the peaks in your feed are the chemical fingerprints of polybrominated biphenyl." Dr. Fries then added, "I hope I haven't created a problem for you, but I felt that it was my duty to call the U. S. Department of Agriculture and tell them that there might be a contamination problem in Michigan."

Two days later, Dr. Fries ran the feed sample through a mass spectrometer for confirmation. "I wanted a hundred percent confirmation," he said. "I knew it would become a messy legal problem, and I didn't want there to be any question what the material was."

Halbert was elated. The search was over. But little did he know that the nightmare was really just beginning, and not only for him and his family but for millions of other Michigan citizens.

# 3
# BAGS OF TROUBLE

The surrender ceremonies aboard the Missouri in September of 1945 marked the official end of World War II. And for the first time since September of 1939, no war communiqué had been issued anywhere in the world. But peace also meant an abrupt end to the millions of wartime jobs. Few industries were hiring the hordes of returning servicemen. One exception, however, was the fast-growing chemical industry, fattened during the war by lucrative government contracts and spurred in peacetime by unquenchable consumer demands for new and dazzling synthetic products. And so through the late 1940s and continuing today, research chemists from coast to coast worked feverishly to keep their industry's wartime productivity—and profitability—thriving. There seemed no end to the products they invented, which, aided by another growing industry, advertising, and by increased consumer spending, would become the staples of American life. Each month, hundreds of new formulas, compounds and products emerged from laboratories to catch the public fancy.

There were countless new detergents that came in handy-squeeze bottles. There were nylon stockings, sheer, seamless and somehow more fashionable than the old-fashioned silk ones. Quick-drying paint made every newlywed couple do-it-yourself decorators. Plastics and pesticides revolutionized farming, made backyard picnics more pleasant and changed the automobile industry, the construction business and just about every other American industry. In just one decade, from 1953 to 1962, U.S. chemical sales rose from $18.8 billion to $32.8 billion. Chemicals were emerging so rapidly that there was little time or incentive to test whether they were safe for workers and consumers.

By 1971, the National Institute of Occupational Safety and Health had 8,000 entries on its "Toxic Substances List." By 1975, that list had grown to 16,500; several thousand of these substances were toxic chemicals in the workplace for which exposure standards were needed. But many chemicals had come and gone so quickly that they escaped regulation altogether. One such product was PBB, or polybrominated biphenyl, a synthetic fire retardant manufactured in the early and mid-1970s by a small chemical firm called the Michigan Chemical Corporation. The company, with some four hundred workers, was the largest employer and biggest taxpayer in the town of St. Louis, a community of four thousand in one of Michigan's most depressed areas. The town calls itself "The Middle of the Mitten," a handy reference to its location in Michigan, which resembles the back of a left-handed mitten.

Michigan Chemical, like its giant neighbor to the east, Dow Chemical, was drawn to Michigan by the state's vast deposits of underground salt. The beginnings of large-scale salt production in Michigan go back to the Civil War. Michigan long had been a thriving lumbering state, and soon the idea was advanced to use the scrapwood left over from lumber sawing as fuel to evaporate brine. Among the products derived from Michigan brines are bromine and magnesium, both of which had tremendous versatility in the magic world of chemistry.

Michigan Chemical was the direct outgrowth of the salt wells sunk by the numerous sawmills that were built on the scenic Pine River in Gratiot County when pine lumber was being produced. Soon the company began pumping brine from the earth of Michigan, now the nation's leading producer of salt. And so where hardy woodsmen once swung their axes and transient sawmills briefly had their heyday, new resources had been found to meet the public's ever-changing demands and needs; the transformations also turned Michigan into the home of some of the world's leading pharmaceutical companies, such as the Upjohn Company in Kalamazoo and Parke, Davis and Company in Detroit.

Once the various salts are extracted from deep-water brine, sodium chloride is removed from the brine by filtration. Some of the brine can further be processed to extract bromines for use in the manufacture of brominated products. Bromine is an element that possesses the exquisite capability of breaking a chemical chain reaction known as fire. After bromine is ex-

34

tracted, the brine is routed to the magnesia plant at Michigan Chemical's St. Louis facility, where the end result of still further processing is magnesium oxide. The remaining salt solutions are sold to cities and counties around Michigan for wetting down roads after snowfall. The magnesium oxide is sold to Michigan Farm Bureau Services, Inc., which blends the magnesium oxide into livestock feed as an additive nutrient. Research at a number of agriculture colleges, including Michigan State University, had shown that magnesium oxide sweetens sometimes acidic feed and help increase milk production as well as the butterfat content in that milk.

In 1970, Michigan Chemical began to develop polybrominated biphenyls for use as a flame retardant in thermoplastics products. The company decided to call the product Firemaster BP-6. But before it began full commercial marketing of the new product, Michigan Chemical in April 1970 commissioned Hill Top Research, Inc., a toxicology laboratory in Miamiville, Ohio, to assess the acute toxicity of Firemaster BP-6. On May 22, Carol L. Daniels, the laboratory's supervisor of toxicology, told Michigan Chemical that BP-6 was "nontoxic by ingestion or dermal application." The Ohio laboratory had experimented with rabbits and rats, giving them various amounts of the chemical orally as well as by inhalation and by dermal application.

"The results of the Hill Top study," said Paul Hoffman, later president of Michigan Chemical, "indicated that BP-6 was suitable for incorporation in such things as typewriters, calculator housings, radio and TV parts and hand-tool housings."

In 1971, the company began the fateful commercial production of Firemaster at its St. Louis plant, along the Pine River in central Michigan. The firm selected a site within the plant and said it set it aside solely for the production and storage of Firemaster BP-6. "This location is physically separate and distinct from other manufacturing operations conducted by the company in St. Louis," Hoffman said.

Apparently in spite of the reassurances of Hill Top Research, Inc., Michigan Chemical's own scientists, upon further examination of the Ohio test data, began having doubts about the laboratory's conclusions. And by the time the first commercial sales of BP-6 were made to various product manufacturers, Michigan Chemical cautioned its consumers on the handling of BP-6. In a letter titled, "Firemaster BP-6: Health and Safety," the company repeated Hill Top's finding that "the acute toxicity of BP-6 is relatively low," but added prophetically: "BP-6 should not be incorporated in any product that might be expected to come in contact with food or feed and reasonable care should be taken to protect plant workers from dust and fumes of BP-6." The two-paragraph, December 28, 1971, letter also warned, "If ingested or inhaled in small quantities over a period of time, we would expect BP-6 and similar materials to accumulate in fatty tissue and in the liver, which certainly is undesirable and possibly could be dangerous." Michigan Chemical's concern had not been overly cautious, for the test results furnished by Hill Top showed that some rats fed BP-6 at higher dose levels died, and autopsies revealed congested lungs and kidneys, and irritated intestines and depleted body-fat stores. Michigan Chemical said it received no health or safety complaints from its 130-odd industrial customers who used BP-6 in their products.

Scientists both in government and in industry became increasingly interested in fire retardant chemicals after the congressional passage in December 1967 of an amendment to the Flammable Fabrics Act of 1953. The amendment called for more studies on how to decrease flammability of all fabrics, particularly children's sleepwear. And two giant chemical corporations—Dow Chemical Company of Midland, Michigan, and the E.I. duPont de Nemours and Company of Wilmington, Delaware—immediately began testing a number of brominated products, particularly a class of chemicals called PBBs.

Dow eventually withdrew from the development of PBBs in the early 1970s after extensive studies on two particular PBBs—octabromobiphenyl and decabromodiphenyl oxide, including thirty-day dietary feeding studies that began in late 1970—to evaluate both substances. In January 1971, test results suggested that octabromobiphenyl might have more serious toxicological consequences than the decabromodiphenyl oxide. Further studies were pursued at Midland. In January 1972, a two-year rat-feeding study on both compounds began. Preliminary results became available in May 1972. Again, the octabromobiphenyl seemed the more worrisome of the two. And Dr. Perry J. Gehring, then Dow's assistant director of the toxicology laboratory, said of octabromobiphenyl, after reviewing the data, "This compound must be considered to have a high potential for producing chronic toxic effects. It is likely

36

that liver injury will occur in rats receiving even lower daily doses for two years." He added, "The continued development and use of this compound as a fire retardant appears very unwise." The corporation three months later terminated plans to produce a pilot production of a thousand pounds of octabromobiphenyl. Although the two-year experiment involving decabromodiphenyl oxide continued, it later was determined that this substance was much less effective than octabromobiphenyl as a fire retardant in fabrics and textiles. So decabromodiphenyl oxide also was shelved by Dow. On November 29, 1972, Dow reported its findings and conclusions at the Conference on Polymeric Materials for Unusual Service Conditions at the Ames Research Center of the National Aeronautics and Space Administration in Moffett Field, California. This paper was delivered a second time on May 23, 1973—the very month that shipments of Firemaster arrived at Michigan Farm Bureau Services' mixing plant in Climax—at the Polymer Conference Series, sponsored by the Polymer Institute of the University of Detroit. The two-year feeding study also was published in a paper entitled "Results of a Two-Year Dietary Feeding Study With Decabromodiphenyl Oxide (DBDPO) in Rats," in the November 1975 issue of the *Journal of Combustion Toxicology*.

DuPont, the other chemical company that tested and then shied away from PBBs, also published its findings. The duPont paper was presented on March 8, 1972, at the Society of Toxicology meeting in Williamsburg, Virginia. The study's conclusion: "Because of the toxicity picture presented here and the likelihood that it would accumulate in the environment, duPont has discontinued efforts to develop flame retardant synthetic fibers based on brominated biphenyl."

But Michigan Chemical paid little heed to such warnings issued by two of the world's leading chemical companies concerning the potential hazards of PBBs.

Shortly after it began marketing Firemaster BP-6, Michigan Chemical received a number of requests from customers asking for the flame retardant in a powdered form, which would make the substance more "dispersible" and adaptable for incorporation into a greater variety of consumer products. At the time, BP-6 emerged from the dusty production line as irregular amber-colored chunks, resembling peanut brittle. In response to those requests, Michigan Chemical through the first half of 1972 sent BP-6 to the Cincinnati Chemical Processing Company for pulverization. Almost all the powdered BP-6, code-named Firemaster FF-1, then was returned to St. Louis both in two-hundred-pound drums and in fifty-pound bags. The last shipment—consisting of 202 fifty-pound bags—arrived back at Michigan Chemical on July 19, 1972. A few of the fifty-pound bags had been shipped to Michigan Chemical's customers directly from Cincinnati Chemical's plant in Batavia, a suburb east of Cincinnati. The FF-1 was packaged in fifty-pound bags as well as in the larger drums because, due to its experimental nature, many Michigan Chemical customers only wanted small amounts at first. In fact, by February 1973, Michigan Chemical decided to change all shipping containers to the smaller fifty-pound bags.

The FF-1 in bags that were returned to Michigan Chemical were stacked on pallets at the company's St. Louis plant. On each of the plain brown bags, the name Firemaster FF-1 was stenciled in block letters.

PBB turned out to be a phenomenal success. Sales leaped from 185,000 pounds in 1971 to 2,221,000 pounds in 1972. By 1973, Michigan Chemical sold 3,889,000 pounds of PBB to its 130-odd customers all over the United States.

It was in 1973 that Michigan Chemical perceived "a substantial increase in the market" for magnesium oxide as a result of agricultural research suggesting that the substance markedly enhanced milk production in dairy herds. Before 1973, Michigan Chemical's sales of magnesium oxide to agricultural customers had been insignificant. The company wasted no time in stepping up its production of magnesium oxide, which it called Nutrimaster. The company ordered preprinted blue bags to package the magnesium oxide; but to avoid losing potential sales, Michigan Chemical on March 7, 1973, began selling Nutrimaster in plain fifty-pound brown bags, with the brand name stenciled on the bag, also in block letters, just like the bags of Firemaster. Once the preprinted, blue bags for Nutrimaster arrived, they were used up rather quickly and, by October, the plain brown bags again were used to bag magnesium oxide until a fresh supply of the blue bags arrived the following month.

"Company procedures at the time specified that these two products were to be stored in separate and distinct locations," said Paul Hoffman, who did not become head of Michigan Chemical until September 26, 1975, well after the accident had occurred and come to light. "Our records do not reflect, and no one associated with Michigan Chemical recalls, any shipments of Firemaster FF-1 to Farm Bureau."

Ironically, shortly before the PBB-magnesium oxide mix-up apparently occurred, the U.S. Food and Drug Administration had been planning a special visit to Michigan Chemical to obtain samples of Firemaster. "We wanted to learn more about this potential contaminant," said John R. Wessel, scientific coordinator of the agency's office of regulatory affairs. "But I don't know that an inspection [then] could have prevented this Michigan contamination." That assessment, however, is subject to speculation, for a number of FDA inspections—including before the shipping accident occurred—repeatedly uncovered shoddy practices and procedures at the chemical company plant. Although the Food and Drug Administration had no direct legal jurisdiction over Michigan Chemical's PBB manufacturing processes (because the chemical was not intended as a drug, food, feed or cosmetic ingredient), it did have the authority to inspect the company's procedures in the manufacture of feeds, such as magnesium oxide. So as early as November 7, 1969, inspectors for the FDA, exercising the agency's authority to inspect such firms at least once every two years, toured the Michigan Chemical plant. At the facility—an aging, rusting tangle of cheap buildings, molding vats and weedy fields on the edge of St. Louis, coiling along the scenic Pine River— the federal inspectors found numerous problems in Michigan Chemical's production and labeling of certain products. Deviations from good manufacturing practices included failure to use batch production records, failure to code medicated products, lack of written production and control procedures, and excessive dust residues in the manufacturing areas. Also tests revealed that certain medicated trace mineral animal salt products did not contain the amount of drug ingredient specified in the labeling. A follow-up inspection eleven months later, on October 6, 1970, showed the company still was producing a medicated salt product that fell below the label claims for the active ingredient. This time, FDA inspectors took a sample analysis and, based on test results, charged Michigan Chemical with misbranding a medicated animal salt product containing less than the declared amount of medication, and misbranding the label because it lacked adequate directions for use and adulteration.

Still another FDA inspection was held on May 24, 1973. This inspection covered the company's magnesium oxide and other mineral salt products. The FDA's only objection was excessive dust build-up in the production area. FDA's next inspection of Michigan Chemical took place on March 14, 1974, just one month before the shipment mix-up was discovered by Rick Halbert. The government inspectors reported finding the weighing scales covered with "heavy build-ups of residue, and open containers of trace elements in the premix area, allowing for potential cross-contamination." Still, no evidence was turned up to suggest a shipping accident had taken place at the plant, which touched off the worst man-made agricultural disaster in U.S. history.

FDA inspectors made a number of additional inspections soon after it learned of the PBB–magnesium-oxide mix-up, beginning on April 26, and again on April 29 and 30. Michigan Chemical, of course, knew about the mix-up a week earlier, when Halbert informed the company on April 19, right after he had spoken with Dr. Fries in Maryland. The inspectors found no explanation as to how the mix-up might have occurred. The magnesium oxide and the PBB, they reported, were being manufactured, bagged and stored in different buildings a quarter mile apart. Michigan Chemical's plant officials professed astonishment at the accident. The Food and Drug Administration conducted six more inspections through August of 1974, but learned very little substantive information to shed light on the mix-up.

To this day there still is no full explanation as to how ten to twenty bags of Firemaster FF-1 were shipped in lieu of Nutrimaster to the Farm Bureau Services feed plant in Climax, about 120 miles southwest of St. Louis. But the final, irrefutable evidence came in late April of 1974, right after PBB was identified, when an open bag of Firemaster was found at the Farm Bureau's co-op in Mendon, about 15 miles south of Climax in the southern region of Michigan. What probably happened was that part of the Firemaster FF-1 production, after it was pulverized and returned by Cincinnati Chemical, somehow became separated from the rest of the FF-1 inventory at the Michigan Chemical plant in St. Louis—ending up where

40

magnesium oxide was being stored. Later it became known that the final FF-1 shipment from Cincinnati, totaling 10,100 pounds of PBB, had been stored in at least two different places at Michigan Chemical before ending up in the proper location, the BP-6 warehouse.

At the Farm Bureau Services' towering feed plant in Climax, the autumn of 1973 was an unusually hectic time. Business was so brisk, in fact, that Paul Mullineaux, the manager, began keeping the plant in operation around the clock. The price of grain had risen sharply. A ton of soybeans, for instance, was up from $120 to $500. But farmers doing business with the co-op liked to purchase grains through advance booking, a purchasing method whereby they would commit themselves to buy an order of feed at predetermined prices, but to be picked up or delivered at various times according to individual needs. But beginning early that fall, partly because grain prices were still climbing, countless farmers began taking every pound of feed allocated to them at the lower preset prices.

One such farmer was Rick Halbert, who had read in scientific and dairy journals that magnesium oxide could increase milk production in dairy cows. So in October 1972, Halbert ordered dairy feed supplemented with four pounds of magnesium oxide per ton. The innovation not only was progressive but successful. Halbert was so pleased with the results that soon he doubled the magnesium oxide content per ton of dairy feed #402. By the time Halbert's order came in for eight pounds of magnesium oxide per ton of feed, several other farmers also had decided to try the change, including Peter Crum of Coopersville and Jerome Petroshus of Allegan. Soon they were followed by other farmers from throughout Michigan, thereby setting the stage for a statewide disaster.

Farm Bureau Services is one of many interrelated farmer-oriented corporations in Michigan. In essence, it is a farmer-owned cooperative. And it provides nutritional and veterinary advice and information and sells fertilizers, hardware supplies, chemicals, petroleum products, building material and, of course, feeds, such as corn, oats, rye and soybeans.

A dairy farmer has a variety of ways to provide his cattle with the necessary nutritional requirements such as fat, fiber, roughage, protein, minerals and vitamins. One is to buy commercially prepared feed; but that often gets too expensive. So most farmers raise much, if not most, of their own grain and roughage, purchasing only salt, minerals and vitamin supplements. There are many variations, stemming from individual factors such as personal experience and theory, available acreage, size of herd and the fluctuations in supply and demand, and prices.

Since the 1920s, the company has operated its own feed plant in Saginaw. Then in the late 1960s, the Saginaw facility was destroyed by a fire—but, luckily, at a time when a second facility was already under construction in Climax, a small community midway between Kalamazoo and Battle Creek just off Interstate 94. The new plant's location would make it easily accessible to other highways leading to the company's ninety-seven dealer outlets throughout Michigan. And so because of the Saginaw fire, the production capacity of the Climax plant, even while it was still under construction, was expanded in order to handle the company's entire feed output. Today Farm Bureau Services has some five thousand customers. The Climax plant is fully automated and computerized, and considered one of the most efficient feed-mixing facilities in the country. With the exception of minute quantities, which are weighed and mixed by hand, feed ingredients flow from storage bins via automated scales to a mixer and then to bulk storage bins all under electronic control. Nutritional formula is transferred to computer punch cards that activate the batching system, adding each ingredient in the proper sequence and amount. A standard three-ton batch of feed, such as dairy #402, takes as little as seven minutes to mix. At each stage of mixing, an electronic control panel shows the total weight in the mixer, corresponding to a cumulative weight figure on the nutritional formula. If the mixing errs by more than five to seven pounds, the system will automatically shut down. The flow of feed through the yellow-and-brown cereal-box-shaped plant is enormous. For the fiscal year 1973–1974, for instance, the plant produced more than 100 million pounds of feed. Bins holding up to 300 tons of high volume ingredients, such as soybean meal or corn may be emptied in a matter of two or three days.

Magnesium oxide, as with other feed ingredients that are hand-added, was stored on pallets in the feed plant's warehouse, which adjoins the mixing room. If the production schedule called for only a few batches of feed requiring magnesium oxide, Charles Szeluga, the plant's day-shift mixer operator, would simply carry a bag of Nutrimaster from the warehouse, place it by the hand scales and weigh out the specified amount for each batch. But if the production schedule called for many batches with magnesium oxide, Szeluga would have a number of bags of Nutrimaster brought in with a forklift truck. By May of 1973, according to Szeluga, he and other mixers had grown accustomed to using magnesium oxide under a variety of different names and bags. But whatever the name or container, there was a designated area in the open warehouse where the magnesium oxide was to be stored. So when a Michigan Chemical shipment of four thousand pounds of Nutrimaster (which, unknown to anyone at the time, also contained Firemaster, or PBB) arrived at the feed plant on May 2, 1973, it was routinely stocked where magnesium oxide customarily is kept. It was there that Szeluga and the plant's other mixers learned for the first time yet another name: Firemaster. Earlier, they had become familiar with the name Nutrimaster. On June 29, Szeluga was taking inventory when he saw two pallets near one another, each only partially stacked to capacity. He saw at least three fifty-pound bags bearing the unfamiliar name Firemaster on one of the pallets. So he called his boss, Mullineaux, the plant manager. According to Szeluga, Mullineaux told him that both Firemaster and Nutrimaster were magnesium oxide and to stock and inventory the two together, as one. Szeluga said he followed Mullineaux's orders. For the next several months, despite regular inventories, despite periodic use of the bags by different plant employees and despite Mullineaux's twice-a-day walks through the warehouse, the presence of PBB escaped detection—even though bags of Firemaster sat in plain view on a pallet in the middle of the aisle between the warehouse and the feed-mixing area. "I do not recall seeing any bags labeled Firemaster," said Mullineaux. Even if he had, he said, "I would not have known what it was." About a year after the fateful arrival of PBB at the feed plant— that is, when the mix-up had begun receiving considerable publicity—Szeluga heard a radio account of the accident. "At first," he said, "PBB didn't mean anything to me. I didn't put anything together until I heard the word Firemaster mentioned." Szeluga said he then reminded Mullineaux about their June 29, 1973, telephone conversation in which Szeluga had asked about Firemaster. Mullineaux told him to keep the matter "inside the company," Szeluga later testified in court, under

43

oath. But Mullineaux had a different story, also given in court, under oath: "When Szeluga told me a year later about the call, I was shocked." Mullineaux said he could not even remember that June 29 telephone call, much less the content of the conversation.

In any case, from June 29 on, so far as Szeluga and Farm Bureau Services' other feed mixers were concerned, Firemaster was magnesium oxide—to be used when livestock feeds called for magnesium oxide as an additive.

But not all eighty of the fifty-pound bags that arrived on May 2 at the feed plant were Firemaster; indeed the majority probably were not. The best guess, made by both Michigan Chemical and Farm Bureau Services, is that ten to twenty bags of Firemaster were involved in the actual feed mixup.

Not surprisingly, Michigan Chemical had evidence strongly suggesting that such a mix-up indeed had occurred well before June 29, when Charles Szeluga detected the presence of Firemaster in the Farm Bureau Services feed plant. But there, too, that evidence was ignored. Michigan Chemical records show that it had no Firemaster left from prior productions on July 19, 1972, when the final 202 bags of pulverized FF-1 were returned from Cincinnati Chemical. Over the next nine months or so, however, FF-1 sales were slower than expected, largely because sales of BP-6 had begun soaring. By late April 1973, a Michigan Chemical inventory showed forty-six bags of FF-1 still unsold, sitting in the company's St. Louis plant warehouse. William W. Thorne, Michigan Chemical's plant operations manager, then obtained permission from officials in the Chicago headquarters to recycle the pulverized fire retardant. That opportunity came on June 7 when Thorne saw that some of the bags containing FF-1 had been torn open, apparently by accident, which was not an uncommon event at Michigan Chemical. Forklifts were forever ripping bags open. Such torn bags usually would be stacked in a corner until enough accumulated to be recycled. The warehouse had no signs to keep such products straight. Thorne instructed Richard Jeffries, the assistant plant manager, to reprocess the remaining forty-six bags of FF-1 into the BP-6 production. But Jeffries could not locate all forty-six bags of FF-1. Nor could anyone else. Later Jeffries and other Michigan Chemical officials put the number of unaccounted bags at thirteen.

At Farm Bureau Services, Paul Mullineaux, in reconstructing all the uses of magnesium oxide in order to trace the shipments of feeds that had been contaminated by PBB, discovered that magnesium oxide also was to have been added in February 1974 to several other feeds, including #405, #407 and #410, as well as the #402 that Halbert had ordered. That meant many, many more cattle herds—all over Michigan—had been poisoned by the chemical. "I don't blame our employees for the accident," said Donald Armstrong, Farm Bureau Services' executive vice-president. "We assumed that we got what we ordered, especially when the products looked so much alike." So, of course, did the co-op's thousands of customers throughout the state.

"But what we got," said Roy Tacoma, a Falmouth, Michigan, dairyman, "were bags of trouble."

# 4

# NEEDLESS SUFFERING

"May began with a lifting of our spirits," Sandy Halbert recalls. "Now that the contaminant was no longer a phantom but an identifiable chemical compound, Rick began to relax for the first time in months." The people at Farm Bureau Services were equally relieved. "Something approaching euphoria seemed to reign at Farm Bureau Services now that the origin of the plague had been shifted to the Michigan Chemical Corporation," Halbert recalls. But whatever sense of relief the Halberts felt quickly dissipated.

Twice during the first week in May 1974, officials of the Michigan Department of Agriculture and the U.S. Food and Drug Administration showed up at the Halbert farm to collect milk samples to test for PBB. Then on May 10, the Halbert telephone rang. "Mrs. Halbert, is Rick there? This is Ken Van Patten. It's really very important that I speak with Rick before the milk hauler comes today." Van Patten, the state Agriculture Department dairy division chief, did not want simply to leave a message when Sandy told him Rick was out plowing. "No," Van Patten said ominously, "I'm afraid I have to tell him myself. The news isn't good, and I know he'll have some questions."

Sandy wrote down Van Patten's number in Lansing, then piled the three girls into the car and drove to a distant field where her husband was plowing. She waved him down, climbed up onto the large tractor and gave him the message. Without a word, he shut off the engine and followed her back to the car. They drove home in silence.

When they got home, Sandy stayed outside in the warm afternoon sun with the children as her husband went in to call Van Patten. "I'm sorry," the bureaucrat said when Halbert identified himself. "I'm going to have to ask that you not ship your milk today," Van Patten continued. "We've found a

46

substantial amount of PBB in your milk: forty parts per million."

When Halbert emerged from the house a few minutes later, Sandy knew the substance of the telephone conversation by his grim expression. "We've been shut off," he said. "I've got to drive to the barn to stop Pete Schrantz from picking up the milk."

"What are we supposed to do now?" Mark Halbert asked his older brother. "Did Van Patten say what we're supposed to do with the milk?"

"There was no word on that," Rick Halbert answered. "They're primarily interested in cutting off the sources of the contaminant. I guess that we'll have to drain the milk into the holding area waste tank, and haul it out with the manure tank."

When Peter Schrantz arrived, he was stunned when Halbert told him the news. "They called you this morning?" he asked Halbert. "I've never seen anything like this—it's so sudden. I've lost two big stops this morning, and I've only gone to six farms!" The quarantines had begun. Halbert no longer was alone in his anguish. "My dad," Halbert recalled years later, "said hundreds of farms could be involved in this. But I told him, 'That doesn't seem possible. Maybe thirty farms; certainly not hundreds.' Dad doesn't usually overemphasize things. Well, it turns out even he was way low."

After Schrantz departed, Halbert returned to the milk-house, where the two bulk storage tanks were. He knelt on the cool concrete floor, checked to make sure the floor drains beneath the tanks were open, and then opened the tank drain. He stood up slowly, watching eight thousand quarts of the white liquid disappear.

In the coming days, Halbert and his crew continued to milk the cows, fully knowing their milk would have to be dumped. The identification of PBB in the feed, instead of ending the problem, brought even more havoc to the farm. "I haven't slept more than a few hours a night since the quarantine began," Halbert said to Sandy one night, after trying unsuccessfully for hours to go to sleep. "There's no end to this thing. My mother is getting so depressed doing our bookkeeping that Dad says he finds her in tears when he comes home to eat. Money is just running through the account like water through a sieve."

"Has the Department of Agriculture said anything definite?" Sandy asked. "I called them yesterday," he answered. "They have a bill introduced in the legislature that would condemn the quarantined cattle. They would, in effect, buy the tainted cows, and pay the farmer for them when they were hauled away. The cattle would go to a site where they would be humanely destroyed and buried. And the farmers would have the money to settle mounting overdue bills and begin cleaning the farm up. Then the Department of Agriculture would go to court against Farm Bureau Services and Michigan Chemical to recover the money it would cost to run the program and the animal burial site."

The legislation didn't have a chance. "We were accused of wanting to bail out Farm Bureau Services and Michigan Chemical Company," said B. Dale Ball, director of the state Agriculture Department, "when in fact we wanted to prevent farmers from going bankrupt and suffering financial loss and mental anguish when the state, through quarantine, had prevented the sale of their livestock and products to protect the general public. Senator [Alvin] DeGrow, for one, said people asked him if this legislation I had drafted was an effort to bail out Farm Bureau. I said, 'No. It's an effort to keep farmers from going down the tube until it can be decided in court.'" Ball's early effort to help the affected farmers also got no support from Governor William G. Milliken, who wanted the companies responsible to pay for the damages. It was obvious Ball's proposal would get nowhere. Next the Agriculture Commission, the department's policy-making body, authorized Ball to draft a bill providing low-interest loans to the affected farmers. "I went to a hearing in the House with that bill in my suitcase, a hearing on the first bill. The farmers who at that time had contaminated cattle and were under quarantine said, 'We don't need any low-interest loan; we need a place to bury our cattle.' So I left that draft in my briefcase because it wouldn't have made much sense my saying, 'Well, you guys ought to accept a loan' when they said they didn't want it."

Ball was incredulous that the original proposal failed so miserably. "This program would have kept the affected farmers financially whole, while the courts were determining the ultimate liability. Since all the people were being protected, all the people would have shared in the cost rather than just the farmers, who had done nothing wrong and were the victims of the accident," he said. And so a growing number of farmers continued to get no help from the government.

"The trauma for us didn't even begin, really, until after the quarantine," Halbert recalls. "We couldn't sell the animals, but we couldn't kill them either. There was no burial site yet to dispose of the dead animals. And how do you dispose of seven to eight hundred animals on your own property? The attorneys were telling everyone to keep the sick animals alive for court evidence. So we kept feeding the animals even though we had to dump their milk. But when you have to throw away their products, that takes out-of-pocket money. It's not even like just sitting there, slowly rotting away. It was like dying by being hacked to death. The state totally cut off our ability to make a living without providing due process whatsoever. There was no way to get rid of the animals and there was no way to clean them up. We were caught in a bind. This went on for months and months. So we were going backwards—in double time. It cost a thousand dollars a day to feed the animals. After a couple of months of that ... There seemed no help from anybody, even in terms of getting rid of the animals. Man, at that point I began to understand why people jumped out of windows during the Great Depression. Suddenly the future appeared so uncertain that it was mind-boggling. I've never been under that type of stress. It's hard to describe it. I thought I had a heart condition when I began hyperventilating, breathing in short bursts, and getting tightness of the muscles. My wife began having chest pains and developed a bleeding ulcer. The slowness of the process was excruciating, no matter who you called."

To avoid the bind, then, in which quarantined farmers like Halbert found themselves, other dairymen simply avoided detection of PBB in their animals, which was easy enough. While the half dozen farms that received a massive dose of PBB were immediately tested and quarantined by agriculture officials, most farms were tested only at the request of the farmers themselves. During this time, many farmers sent their sick cows to the slaughterhouse, where the animals ended up as food for humans. State officials concentrated their efforts on testing milk in Michigan's fifty-four dairy plants that pasteurize and package milk from the dairy farms. But since not all farms had been contaminated, the dilution factor—the pooling of contaminated milk with uncontaminated milk—made detection of

PBB less likely. To illustrate, PBB was not detected at any of the dairy plants from June 15, 1974, on, even though significant amounts of PBB in cows' milk were known to have been going into marketing channels via the dairy plants.

At the Halbert farm, the disposal of eight thousand quarts of milk every day soon became yet another problem to cope with. The waste tank in the holding area in no time became full of foul odor from the combination of spoiled milk, wash water and manure. "And neighbors began to complain of the stench when the wind changed," Sandy Halbert recalls. "So Rick decided to haul the waste and milk out, and spread it on the fallow fields. But once the load got bogged down in the field and had to be drained on the spot before it could be pulled loose from the mud." The liquid wastes were allowed to run off, following the contours of the cornfields and disappearing finally into a stand of young corn. "Within a few days, we noticed that the corn in the field had fallen flat, as though someone had driven a steamroller through that part of the field," she said.

Halbert was worried by the ominous sign. Did the lactic acid in the milk take the starch out of the corn? Or was the corn poisoned by PBB? He decided to begin renting a tank truck each day to take the milk to be dumped in an almost inaccessible part of the farm, where there was a stand of scrawny hardwood trees. In less than a week, the leaves on the bushes in the woodlot turned to yellow and wilted. Shortly afterward, Halbert realized his only option was to destroy the entire herd of more than four hundred adult milking cows. And while the arrangements were still being argued in Lansing over how to dispose of the animals and who would foot the bill, Halbert told his work crew that time had come to dry up the cows. Thirty of the highest contaminated cows were sent to the Michigan State University laboratory for research.

"Drying up the cows was not difficult but watching the process was hard for the men," Sandy said, "and they spent as little time as they could around the cows. There was no way of explaining to the animals why their daily routine had changed. At milking times, they hung around the gates of their barns, looking for someone to relieve the pressure of the milk they had produced. For animals who had been producing fifty, sixty, even eighty pounds of milk a day, the absence of the twice-daily relief for the pendulous swollen udders was painful. Once the drying up had been completed, the barns were silent."

Halbert realized the barns would require a thorough cleaning to remove as much of the PBB residues as possible before he could restock his farm—with animals from Iowa and Wisconsin. That meant moving the contaminated cows out of the barns. Halbert decided the best relocation site would be a pasture used as a summertime grazing area for injured cattle. The pasture was made of crumbling deposits of sand, silt and clay, but little grass. He decided to feed the dying and condemned cows extra hay. "It was the least we could do after they had fed us for so many years," Sandy explained.

"Filling the pasture took days, for we could no longer afford to hire a cattle hauler, and each load only added eight cows to a pitiful group milling about in the grassy space," she recalls. "Some of the cows were so weak when they were unloaded that they couldn't stay on their feet. A number of the animals resembled the starving cattle from the drought-stricken Sahel, their hides looking as if they were thrown over their bones. Dozens of them had lost patches of hair on their necks and faces; and the exposed skin resembled elephant hide. There were regular telephone calls from passersby reporting that one of the cows was stuck in the marl; always the same one would wade into the pool for a drink and get stuck in the soft bottom, her legs too weak to pull themselves loose. After several trips to the pasture to pull her out Rick began to wonder whether she had not intuited her ultimate fate and tried to speed the process along.

"We had to do something," Sandy said. "We could not simply sit back and wait for the mess to be sorted out by the insurance companies, bureaucrats and hucksters of false hope." So the men began the arduous cleanup process. Sawdust bedding and even the dirt base had to be removed from each stall. Then pressure washers were used to clean railings, posts and even the concrete feed area. It was mid-August by the time cattle haulers finally arrived to take away the animals to be killed and buried in an isolated state-owned forest in the northern part of Michigan's lower peninsula. When one of the drivers saw the pathetically thin animals plodding slowly up the loading ramp, their ears drooping, their coats dull and coarse, their patches of hair missing to reveal elephantlike skin, he

51

gasped. "My God! What happened to these animals? Is it contagious?" "No," Halbert replied. "You can't catch anything by handling them for this short a time. These cows ate a half a pound of fire retardant in contaminated feed. It's a miracle they're alive at all."

A burial pit for the contaminated animals became available as a result of an unusual piece of legislation. After B. Dale Ball's proposal to slaughter the contaminated cows and pay the farmers for the animals failed to gain support, a substitute bill was adopted and became law on July 2, 1974; it empowered the agriculture director to designate, with the advice of the Department of Natural Resources, a site for the killing and burial of contaminated farm animals. The bill also specified that the state would not be obligated for the destruction and burial costs. The language read, "Nothing in this Act shall in any way obligate the state to reimburse the owner of any livestock or livestock products disposed of under this Act." The effect was that agriculture officials could go to a farm, test its animals and their products for PBB contamination and then place that farm under quarantine until the contaminated animals were removed for destruction. Such a farmer, then, was left to the mercy of Michigan Chemical and Farm Bureau Services, which begrudgingly agreed to pay the cost of the burial operations, to come and take the animals away.

Legislators, Ball recalls, insisted that the disposal costs were "the responsibility of the people who created the accident. I felt that, too. But I felt that when you do something to take a farmer's property or to prevent him from selling it to protect all the citizens, then all the citizens have a responsibility to bear the cost, and not just the innocent victims, which these farmers were. And when you shut off their milk and quarantine their animals to protect you and me and everybody else, then you and I and everybody else ought to share in the cost until you are able to collect the state's money back. That was the basic concept. But Milliken thought it was the responsibility of the chemical company and the feed company, and not the state. The state's responsibility was to protect the public from this stuff in the food supply, which we did by quarantining. But I felt when the state takes a person out of business it has the responsibility to keep them solvent until you can get the guy who is responsible to pay for it. But if you can't, then the public ought to bear the cost, not the individual farmer. I guess my philosophical attitude of what's fair and constitutional maybe is a little different. I think it's unconstitutional to take a person's property to protect the general public without reimbursing him."

If the legislature had followed Ball's advice in the beginning, farmers throughout the state certainly would have been much more cooperative in getting their contaminated animals identified, destroyed and buried—instead of sending them, en masse, to the slaughterhouses for human consumption in order to avoid the economic squeeze farmers like Rick Halbert were in. Actually, Ball did have the authority to order the disposal of contaminated animals; however, as he recalls, "The attorney general said if I did that, in effect, I would be condemning and they [farmers] would go to the court of claims and the state would have to pay for them [the animals]. And the act [passed by the legislature in July 1974] says the state didn't want to pay for them. So I never ordered disposal. We quarantined, and the farmers disposed of the animals voluntarily. So I was caught in a situation where I had the authority to order disposal and was told by the attorney general that if I did that, the state would pay for them; and the state had said they didn't want to pay for them. That was the spot I was in."

But even the passage of a bill establishing a burial site hardly meant an end to Halbert's problems, or to those of hundreds of other Michigan farmers.

"Farmers had lots of animals taken away from them without being paid. Lots of money was involved," Halbert recalls. By then, of course, many farmers had given up hope that the state government would come to their aid. So they sent their animals to the market. The unattractive alternative was to have their animals tested for PBB and, if positive, be quarantined by the Department of Agriculture—and then hope Michigan Chemical and Farm Bureau Services would be willing to reimburse them for lost productions as well as for the cost of replacement herds. "I know a farmer who had a thousand animals that went to the market, and he was getting loads from that feed company every day. But most farmers," Halbert said, "I think genuinely had no idea their cows were loaded with this crap. And the process of trying to recover something from an animal that's lost its productive value as a dairy animal is common."

In any case, then, even after the PBB contamination became public knowledge, the contamination continued to spread, caused unwittingly by the posture of the state govern-

ment, which, in essence, forced the destruction of contaminated animals but provided no relief or compensation to
their owners.

The first of the contaminated animals arrived at the
Kalkaska burial pit only hours after Governor Milliken, on July
2, 1974, signed Public Act 181, which set aside twenty acres of
isolated land in a clearing amid Northern Michigan's jack pine
forest as a mass grave for the PBB-contaminated animals. But
on the third day of operation, the slaughters and burials came
to a sudden halt when a Kalkaska County Circuit Court issued a
restraining order pending an environmental impact statement.
That further postponed the removal of dead and sick animals
from the farms, delaying once more farmers' efforts to start
anew. It wasn't until August 27 that the burials resumed. The
farmers finally had begun to receive some measure of relief.

Yet so much of their suffering could have been alleviated—
perhaps even avoided—if the state Department of Agriculture
from the start had promptly and aggressively sought out the
extent of the problem instead of foot-dragging and withhold-
ing information from the public. Rather than worrying about
how to protect Michigan citizens from a hazardous contaminant
in the state's food supply, the department sought to protect the
agricultural industry by downplaying the potential public
health consequences. The department could have ascertained
the scope of the contamination, removed the contaminated
animals from the market and eliminated much of the problem.
But it didn't. Instead, from the outset it saw itself as the
advocate of the agriculture industry and viewed virtually as
enemies those who said PBB was a potentially serious health
threat to people.

Because the Agriculture Department's attitudes and actions would remain at the center of the acrimonious PBB
controversy for years to come, it is revealing to examine more
closely the department's response to the crisis from the very
beginning.

The department first heard of PBB at 4:30 on Thursday
afternoon, May 2—a full two weeks after Rick Halbert had
called Farm Bureau Services and Michigan Chemical with the
same information immediately after talking to Dr. George Fries
in Beltsville, Maryland. Dr. Fries, however, did not report the
PBB contamination in Michigan until April 24, when he had
performed his own laboratory confirmation of the chemical's

presence in Halbert's feed. Dr. Fries then notified his superiors at the U.S. Department of Agriculture, which in turn passed the information on to the U.S. Food and Drug Administration a day later, on April 25. Yet, the Michigan Department of Agriculture—the agency charged with assuring the safety of the state's food supply— was not told of the problem by the FDA office in Detroit for another seven days. On May 2, at last, John P. Dempster of the FDA office in downtown Detroit spoke on the telephone with Edwin Renkie, administrative assistant to Dr. George L. Whitehead, the deputy agriculture director, in Lansing. Dempster tole Renkie what PBB was and that it had been found in seven dairy herds. Renkie in turn passed the information to his boss a short time later. Dr. Whitehead, a short gray-haired veterinarian who had risen through the ranks of the bureaucracy to become the department's deputy chief in charge of consumer protection, stayed late at his office that spring evening to compose a memo for his boss, B. Dale Ball, to read the first thing in the morning.

"It appears," Dr. Whitehead wrote, "that the economic loss to the dairy industry could be disastrous. Because of the legal implications of this case, we have been very guarded in the release of any information to the outside until we have your decision on what action we will take." But despite its instinctive reaction to keep the PBB contamination under wraps, the department was confounded when the May 8 edition of the *Wall Street Journal* described the Michigan problem in a thirteen-paragraph story that ended by quoting Dr. Whitehead as saying, "I think it's under control." The *Journal* had been tipped off to the story by one of its regular readers, Rick Halbert.

Despite the sobering realization that countless farm animals had been contaminated and that their products had been going to the market for nearly a year, the department waited until May 13—eleven days after it learned about the contamination—to finally issue a press release. The two-and-a-half-page handout said fifteen dairy farms had been quarantined because of PBB contamination, but added that "only a very few" of the state's eight thousand Grade-A farms were involved and "thus there is little need for concern about the public milk supplies." The release further said the state Department of Public Health "is examining the possible effects of the contaminant on human health." Interestingly, the Health Department learned about the PBB problem on May 8, thanks not to any of the federal agencies or the Michigan Department of Agriculture but to the *Wall Street Journal.*

Even more astonishing was a letter agriculture director Ball wrote to Governor Milliken on the same day of the department's May 13 press release. In that letter, Ball made a preposterous and unsubstantiated claim: "We can safely say that the public milk supply is cleaner, safer and more wholesome than at any time in history." The letter was written even as Ball's milk inspectors were still fanning out across the state to collect milk samples for PBB analysis. Curiously, even though the PBB contamination clearly had hit dairy farms the hardest, it took the department's top officers—Ball and Whitehead—four days to notify the dairy division, headed by Ken Van Patten. It took Van Patten's unit nearly another week to gear up to go out into the field to collect milk samples at the state's fifty-four dairy plants. Invoking emergency procedures, fifty milk inspectors scattered across the state, picking up samples and then driving the samples on the same day back to the department's Geagley Laboratory in East Lansing on the campus of Michigan State University. There the proportions of the disaster finally began unfolding: PBB was all over Michigan. Milk analyses of individual farms suspected of having purchased Farm Bureau Services' dairy feed #402 also were positive—and high, ranging from 6 parts per million to forty-nine parts per million. Agriculture officials say it took a week before its inspectors were dispatched to gather milk samples because elaborate planning was required not only for the collection of samples but also for the complex business of devising analytical procedures to measure a chemical familiar to no one but Dr. George Fries.

Finally, on May 17, more than two weeks after it knew about the PBB crisis, the Department of Agriculture convened an all-day meeting attended by more than thirty persons to exchange information about the PBB problem. A list of the attendants is revealing. Present were not only officials from the Food and Drug Administration and the U.S. Department of Agriculture but also officials of Farm Bureau Services and Michigan Chemical, who were accompanied by attorneys. Also on hand at the Geagley Laboratory meeting were industry officials representing the Michigan Milk Producers Association and the Michigan Dairy Foods Council. Interestingly, the state Department of Public Health was represented by only one lower-echelon official, Harold Humphrey, the young epidemiologist.

Ball opened the meeting with a poignant tale. Several years ago, he said, he was attending a dairy meeting in Madison, Wisconsin. "They had a lot of these signs, It's Better with Butter, and so forth," Ball said. "So I thought there would be nothing wrong with the director of agriculture having one of these signs, Milk Drinkers Are Better Off, on his briefcase." Three days later, back in Michigan, Ball wrenched his back in a minor farm mishap, requiring him to use a cane. One day, Ball was walking from his office to the Capitol Building several blocks away in Lansing, holding the cane in one hand and the briefcase with the Milk Drinkers Are Better Off bumper sticker in the other. "Some woman I've never seen before or since looked at me and she said, 'Mister, you'd better get rid of one or the other,' So I got rid of the cane. But I still carry the sign even with our current problem that involves some milk," Ball concluded. "I think that milk is a pretty good product and I hope that out of this we don't do anything to injure the dairy industry."

"Is that false advertising?" someone asked Ball.

"No, that's not false advertising. If it is, nobody can prove it," Ball replied, repeating his hope that the PBB contamination would not have any adverse effect on milk sales. "We believe that the dilution factor—even though there were some large contaminated herds—never did get above the one part per million tolerance that was set by the FDA last Friday," he said.

When the group was meeting, nineteen dairy herds already had been quarantined for PBB contamination. But as George L. Whitehead, the deputy chief in charge of consumer protection, told the meeting, "There's not only milk concerned. But there's also meat and food that has milk added, condensed milk, eggs and dried eggs. I don't know where to stop. It might not just be in cattle, but in feed for chickens or hogs." Dr. Whitehead, a man with a near perpetual frown, then produced a large map of Michigan. Each blue dot on the map represented a quarantined dairy herd, he said. Within a couple of years, more than five hundred blue dots would fill Dr. Whitehead's map. Referring to the PBB analyses performed on some of those nineteen farms, the curly-haired veterinarian said, "I think you'll be quite amazed at some of the levels we've had." Out of thirty-one milk samples tested, the PBB concentrations

57

ranged from 2 to 133.8 parts per million. Three fat samples taken from cows showed PBB levels ranging from .87 part per million to 2,064 parts per million. Ten samples of dairy feed #402 ranged from undetectable to 7,700 parts per million. Rick Halbert's feed contained 2,914 parts per million. One sample of mozzarella cheese, taken from a Port Huron manufacturer, turned up with a high PBB content; so did two other cheese samples from distant parts of Michigan, Onaway and Pinconning. The morning session rambled on, with scientists like Dr. George Fries sharing what knowledge they had of the chemical and similar compounds. The discussions were filled with speculation as to how PBB might be flushed out of animals and how much time might elapse before the milk of contaminated cows might pass the Food and Drug Administration tolerance guideline. After lunch, representatives of Michigan Chemical and Farm Bureau Services spoke reassuringly that the contamination was a onetime affair and that it was over. "The lid is on this problem," said Dr. James McKean, the Farm Bureau Services veterinarian whom Halbert called in the autumn of 1973.

The Friday meeting was nearly over when someone finally asked Harold Humphrey, the cherubic public health epidemiologist, to speak. "Okay, basically the report is short and to the point. I have no results to report," he said. Listening, Dr. George Fries was surprised. He had gotten a call from Michigan officials Thursday afternoon, asking if he could attend the early-morning meeting. Dr. Fries arrived the following morning at the Lansing airport expecting to have to answer questions from a querulous mob of reporters. Not one showed up. And now he was even more surprised to hear the state Public Health Department had not yet gone out to visit farm families who had been exposed to massive amounts of PBB. "... therefore," Humphrey was saying, "the public health concern at this time is focusing on the people that would be most likely to have the highest doses." How long would it be before information was available on the effects of high PBB exposure among such farm families? someone asked. "I would suspect that we should have made the visits in the next seven to ten days," Humphrey said. "I thought, Oh, my God! They should have been out there the next day [after learning about the PBB contamination], giving physical examinations," said Dr. Fries. "I don't know why it took so long."

"We are not as familiar with the territory as the agriculture inspectors are. So it does involve some time in finding where these families live and what not," Humphrey explained. How long will it take to decide if there's nothing wrong? Humphrey was asked. "I don't know," he answered. "I'm hedging a little. Just because we come up with nothing at the moment doesn't necessarily mean that we will never come up with something." It was nearly 4:00 P.M. when the meeting came to a desultory conclusion. Most of the participants took with them copies of the meeting agenda, the heading of which read, "PCC [sic] Feed Contamination Conference." If PBB then was still an unfamiliar chemical to state officials, it wouldn't be long before PBB became a household word throughout the state.

By early August, 149 farms had been quarantined, and it was clear that many farms other than dairy farms had been contaminated by PBB as well. Among the 149 quarantined farms were 22 beef herds, 20 swine herds, 16 sheep herds and 54 chicken farms. Together, the casualty was more than 200,000 animals; the small animals already had been destroyed and disposed of, but more than 2,000 cows still were awaiting the opening of the burial pit in Kalkaska County. Meantime, 290 tons of contaminated feed, 3,000 pounds of butter, 10,000 pounds of cheese and more than 1 million eggs also had to be destroyed. And the dimensions of the poisoning were still growing.

The rest of 1974, Dr. George L. Whitehead recalls, was "extremely critical because everyone was working long hours to resolve a problem with little or no research data and insufficient funding." By the end of October, the Agriculture Department's laboratory division alone had accumulated nearly $50,000 in overtime salaries. "All requests for federal assistance, with the exception of the FDA, were shrugged off. The USDA took the approach that it was not a disease, therefore it was up to the contaminators and the state to handle the problem. Letters to the U.S. Secretary of Agriculture and contacts with other USDA officials were quietly ignored. The U.S. Environmental Protection Agency was not interested because it was not a pesticide, and university research was not begun because they said they had no funding for such research, and some said the problem was already resolved," Dr. Whitehead said. "In short, the research, veterinary and laboratory assistance we needed so desperately during this period was not available, and we continued to do the best we could with department facilities and personnel." But that, as time would show, was woefully inadequate to check the growing spread of PBB, prompting one perceptive farmer to remark, "I think they thought we could just eat the problem away."

# 5
# SEEDS
# OF DOUBT

When stories about the PBB contamination first began appearing in the Michigan press in May of 1974, cancer was very much on the mind of Thomas H. Corbett, a thirty-six-year-old instructor of anesthesiology at the University of Michigan Medical Center in Ann Arbor. A month earlier, Dr. Corbett had, with a great sense of urgency, begun a set of experiments to assess the toxicity of a recently developed inhalation anesthetic called isoflurane that was being tested in humans, with government sanction. He was particularly worried about the Food and Drug Administration's impending approval of isoflurane for widespread use in American operating rooms because the substance had a molecular structure quite similar to two other chemicals that were known to be potent carcinogens in humans; yet, isoflurane had never been tested for its carcinogenicity. And when he began contemplating the nature of the unfolding PBB disaster, Dr. Corbett recalls, "I became concerned about the possible effects of the chemical on human health, realizing that Michigan residents had already consumed Firemaster for over nine months."

The efforts of this unusually public-minded scientist ultimately led to significant reductions in human exposure both to PBB in Michigan and to isoflurane in operating rooms throughout the country.

Tom Corbett grew up in Chicago, where his father worked as a newspaperman with the *Tribune*. Later his family moved to Benton Harbor, a Lake Michigan resort town of sixteen thousand in the southwestern corner of Michigan. He attended the University of Michigan medical school and, in 1968, began a two-year residency in anesthesiology at the University Medical Center. Within weeks, the young physician learned how to administer anesthetics, such as halothane or methoxyflurane.

61

And because all anesthesia machines come equipped with valves to exhaust the gases not inhaled by the patient, Dr. Corbett soon learned to distinguish between halothane's rather disagreeable odor and the pleasant, fruity aroma of methoxyflurane. It wasn't much longer before Beverly Corbett, who was trained as a nurse, also could tell when her husband returned home in the evening which gas he had administered earlier that day. Dr. Corbett at first assumed the smell of halothane and methoxyflurane clung to his body and clothing. Then one night Dr. Corbett, before returning straight home from the hospital, showered and changed his clothes. But it didn't make any difference, as he learned the minute he walked in the house. Beverly knew he had been using methoxyflurane that day. The odor was on his breath. That meant he was inhaling the gases in the operating room, and that the gases were being stored in his body, released over long periods of time.

Troubled by those thoughts, Dr. Corbett a few days later went to the university's medical library and, to his astonishment, found that only two studies had been published on the health experiences of anesthesiologists. Both had been published within the past year. One, a Russian study, found functional disturbances of the central nervous system and that of thirty-one pregnancies in anesthesiologists, eighteen ended in spontaneous abortions, two others resulted in premature deliveries and another produced a child with a congenital malformation. The second study was by scientists at the Northwestern University Medical School who examined the causes of death of 441 anesthesiologists. It found a higher than expected number of deaths due to malignancies of the lymphatic and immunological systems, plus an alarmingly high suicide rate.

The disturbing information left Dr. Corbett torn. He knew he was on to something important. At the same time, he began worrying about his chosen specialty. He was thirty years old and had a young family to support. He decided against abandoning anesthesiology training. Instead, Dr. Corbett devised a Rube Goldberglike solution to reduce his own exposure to the escaping gases in the operating room. Using a simple balloon, he punched a hole in its side and then fitted the punctured side over the relief valve on the machine. Then, using tubes, he connected the neck of the balloon to a suction device on the wall and piped the excess gases outside into the open air. His fellow anesthesiologists, the nurses and the surgeons were bemused. "They all thought I was slightly deranged," Dr. Corbett recalls. "But I was convinced that anesthetic gases would turn out to be an occupational hazard. But of course I had no real proof at that time. All I had was a compelling intuition," he said.

Methodically, over the next year or so, Dr. Corbett collected air samples from operating rooms. He did this during his coffee breaks and at night, since he also held a job as physician at Ann Arbor's Veterans' Administration Hospital. He also had to gain access to, and then learn how to use, a gas chromatograph, the same machine that Rick Halbert knew was needed in his search for the identity of the poison in his feed. By the spring of 1971, Dr. Corbett had demonstrated that operating room personnel were being routinely exposed to high concentrations of nitrous oxide, halothane and methoxyflurane. His alarm was heightened further when he learned, by actually measuring, that both anesthesiologists and their patients were retaining the gases for up to three weeks after exposure. By then, the summer of 1971, Dr. Corbett had become an assistant professor at the University of Michigan and been promoted at the Veterans' Hospital to chief of anesthesiology services. That summer he exposed pregnant rats to concentrations of nitrous oxide in amounts routinely found in operating rooms, finding that such low-level exposure caused embryo deaths in the test animals.

Next he looked into the health histories of female nurse anesthetists in Michigan. Among 525 such women, Dr. Corbett found the incidence of cancer to be three times the rate expected of the general population. Also, the children of nurse anesthetists who worked full time during their pregnancies had birth defects at a rate three times higher than nurse anesthetists who had not worked during their pregnancies.

Dr. Corbett soon began writing articles in professional journals about his findings and called for more research into the long-term consequences of exposure to anesthetic gases. In June 1972 he was named to an ad hoc committee of the American Society of Anesthesiologists that set out to conduct a nationwide survey on the effects of such gases on operating room personnel. Meanwhile, Dr. Corbett resumed his own laboratory investigations of inhalation anesthetics with funds supplied by the Veterans' Administration. By the end of 1973 he found that high concentrations of nitrous oxide and methoxyflurane delayed the skeletal formation of fetuses of pregnant rats. And so his suspicions continued growing that some anesthetic gases may cause cancer.

Soon Dr. Corbett increasingly found himself spending long evenings in medical libraries reading everything he could get his hands on about cancer and chemicals, not unlike the manner in which Rick Halbert, in his farmhouse eighty miles to the west, had set out to learn about chemicals in livestock feed. One such winter night in February of 1974, Dr. Corbett read an article about two chemicals that are extremely similar in structure to many inhalation anesthetics. The article, published in 1968, the year he had begun his residency, said bis-chloromethyl ether and chloromethyl methyl were potent carcinogens when applied to the skin of mice; and it went on to predict that both chemicals are likely to produce cancer in humans. The article's author was Dr. Benjamin L. Van Duuren, a New York University Medical Center scientist who later also would become involved in Michigan's PBB controversy.

When Dr. Corbett finished the article, he didn't realize that Dr. Van Duuren's prediction already had come true—dozens of workers exposed to the two chemicals developed lung cancer. But even without knowing that information, Dr. Corbett was sufficiently alarmed by the similarities of those chemicals to many anesthetic agents. Dr. Corbett called Dr. Van Duuren the following morning and asked if he was aware of the similarities.

"These anesthetics aren't being used in people, are they?" Dr. Van Duuren asked.

"Yes," Dr. Corbett answered.

"Oh, good God!" Dr. Van Duuren said.

The following week Dr. Corbett flew to New York to meet with Dr. Van Duuren, who singled out one anesthetic, isoflurane, to be studied urgently because of its extreme similarity to bis-chloromethyl ether and because the FDA appeared on the verge of approving it for general and unrestricted use. Isoflurane already was being used in clinical trials in seventeen hospitals across the country. "We agreed to work together," Dr. Corbett recalls. "He would advise as I proceeded with the testing. I was a complete novice in carcinogenicity testing." From New York, Dr. Corbett went to the National Cancer Institute in Bethesda, Maryland, just outside Washington, D.C. There, he was astonished to learn that neither isoflurane nor any other inhalation anesthetics had ever been tested for their cancer-causing potentials.

When he returned to Ann Arbor, Dr. Corbett's request for reimbursement for his trip was rejected by the university's department of anesthesiology; he was told he was on a "wild-goose chase." In April, Dr. Corbett began exposing groups of pregnant mice to low levels of isoflurane every other day during the last half of their pregnancy. Then the offspring were exposed to isoflurane every other day for two months. The experiment was funded by the Veterans' Administration. Shortly after the experiment began, Dr. Corbett began reading about the PBB contamination in Michigan.

Meantime, the nationwide survey by the ad hoc committee of the American Society of Anesthesiologists found strong evidence that chronic exposure to anesthetics posed a wide variety of health hazards, expecially for women and their offspring. Female anesthesiologists and anesthetists had twice the risk of spontaneous abortions as did women not exposed to anesthetic gases; and birth defects were twice as likely to occur among their offspring.

Dr. Corbett's isoflurane animal experiments called for groups of mice to be killed and examined at intervals of six, nine and fifteen months. But by the nine-month interval, enough cancers had appeared to strongly indict the substance. Mindful that the findings did not constitute conclusive proof that isoflurane is carcinogenic, he and Dr. Van Duuren never-theless concurred that isoflurane's manufacturer must be noti-fied at once. They also agreed that Dr. Corbett must not wait to begin to "sow some seeds of doubt," as Dr. Corbett put it, in the scientific community that further research must be done, and quickly. Among those who immediately agreed after hearing Dr. Corbett's preliminary mice results was Dr. Irving J. Selikoff, the portly, affable director of the Mount Sinai School of Medicine's famous Environmental Sciences Laboratory in New York City. Dr. Selikoff, whose subsequent controversial involve-ment in Michigan's PBB affair directly led to a marked reduc-tion in further consumer exposure to PBB, called for full-scale laboratory testing of all inhalation anesthetics as well as epi-demiologic studies of operating room personnel.

Isoflurane's manufacturer, predictably, launched an all-out campaign to discredit Dr. Corbett's findings, pointing out its "preliminary nature." But, undaunted, Dr. Corbett continued publicizing his data at forums around the country. In June 1975, at the end of the fifteen-month interval, he killed and examined the remaining mice. Ten out of thirty-seven in the highest exposure group had liver tumors, and five of thirty in a less exposed group also developed liver tumors. The Food and Drug Administration finally agreed to withhold its approval of isoflurane for unrestricted use in operation rooms.

When Dr. Corbett began his isoflurane experiment in the spring of 1974, he also managed to squeeze enough funds out of his Veterans' Administration grant to conduct another feeding study—to test PBB. "I was absolutely flabbergasted that people [in the Michigan health and agriculture departments] were so nonchalant about it."

In late May, Dr. Corbett called Michigan Chemical to obtain a full description and a sample of Firemaster. He was surprised to learn that thorough tests had not been performed to assess PBB's potential to cause birth defects or cancer. "As far as I could determine, no one was planning to perform the now very crucial toxicity studies on Firemaster. Since I had been performing teratogenicity [birth defects] and carcinogenicity studies with inhalation anesthetic agents, I felt obligated to also perform these studies on PBB," Dr. Corbett said. "But I'm an anesthesiologist; I tried getting others at the university involved. I talked to people in pharmacology, in the school of public health, in the medical school; they all should have become involved. But no. Nobody picked up the ball. You wouldn't believe the hesitancy of people. They didn't have the guts to get involved. They said, 'This is too hot an issue; I don't want to get involved.' It was a great disappointment to me. The university should have been right in there fighting. But no, it wasn't."

The PBB contamination took on a different, much more personal meaning for Dr. Corbett in July when he and Beverly took the children to Traverse City to visit his brother, Bill, and his wife. They had rented a house on a farm, and a friend of theirs had given them several chickens as a present. "They were very pleased," Dr. Corbett said, "to be supplied with all the fresh eggs they could eat and took it as a personal affront when I commented that they were the most miserable-looking creatures I had ever seen. They were scrawny, and their feathers were falling out. They looked as if they had been half plucked."

Alarmed, Dr. Corbett asked his brother what the chickens were being fed, adding that PBB also had shown up in chicken feed. His brother telephoned the woman who had given him the chickens. "Sure enough," Dr. Corbett said, "they had been given feed from the Michigan Farm Bureau Services. I advised my brother and his wife not to eat the eggs, at least until I had a chance to have several of them analyzed back in Ann Arbor."

Dr. Corbett took some eggs back with him to the Environmental Research Group laboratory for analysis. The results came back several days later: the eggs were contaminated by PBB. "My sister-in-law finally gave in, and took the chickens to the humane society to be destroyed," Dr. Corbett said. "I soon learned what tremendous odds Rick Halbert had had to overcome to discover the cause of his cows' illness; when I learned that the eggs from my brother and sister-in-law's chickens were contaminated with PBB, I assumed that all the eggs from the original flock of chickens also were contaminated. The woman who owned the flock had been selling eggs to stores around the Traverse City area. Her eggs were undoubtedly more highly contaminated than the ones I had tested because the chickens who had laid the tested eggs had not eaten the contaminated feed for six weeks. The rest of the original flock probably was still eating it. I started calling the Michigan Department of Agriculture in Lansing. An official told me that it was ridiculous—no contaminated feed had been sent to the Traverse City area and the department was not going to check further into the matter. My brother called the Health Department in Traverse City and a Michigan Department of Agriculture representative in his area. Both agencies refused to do anything. After several more calls, I finally gave up in disgust and advised my brother and his wife not to eat eggs. The rest of the population of Traverse City remained at risk by continuing to eat contaminated eggs. I didn't know what else to do."

Shortly after Dr. Corbett returned to Ann Arbor, the samples of Firemaster from Michigan Chemical arrived, and he began feeding the mice PBB in various concentrations. "We fed the experimental group from days seven through eighteen of the nineteen-day pregnancy period. The control group ate regular rodent food without the Firemaster. We also began a preliminary carcinogenicity bioassay with Firemaster—a long-term study that was to last fifteen months. Several of the

67

experimental animals died before the end of the feeding period. We performed autopsies on the animals and found two surprising things—the animals had died from massive gastrointestinal hemorrhages, and they all had greatly enlarged livers." On day eighteen of the pregnancies, both the experimental and control animals were killed. "Autopsies on the experimental animals revealed a continuing pattern of abnormal liver enlargement," Dr. Corbett said. He and his assistants were opening the animals' abdomens, weighing and preserving the fetuses when one of the assistants, a premed student, called out, "Look at this one."

"It's an exencephaly," Dr. Corbett said as everyone gathered around the fetus—its head severely deformed and its brain protruding from its skull. "At least I'm pretty sure it is." Dr. Corbett had never seen an exencephaly before, although he had read about them. He knew the condition could have been due to chance. "But we had never seen this deformity in the hundreds of mice we had examined in previous experiments," he recalled. If it was due to Firemaster, he thought, there ought to be more of them in the remaining fetuses. "Here's another one," the premed student again called out. One exencephaly might be a fluke but two, albeit still not statistically significant, convinced Dr. Corbett he was on to something again. "We ordered more pregnant mice and repeated the experiments, using 100 and 50 parts per million of Firemaster in the food. We also ran additional control groups. We found three more exencephalies in the group fed 100 parts per million."

During this period, Dr. Corbett also took fat samples from three patients—chosen at random—who had died of unrelated causes either at the Veterans' Hospital or at the university hospital during the summer of 1974. None of the three had been farm residents and each had come from a different part of the state. "All three samples had PBB," Dr. Corbett said. "That disturbed me. Three out of three was a pretty high average. It became apparent that Michigan was faced with what was probably the worst single environmental contamination disaster in history, and that this disaster had potential for causing serious acute and long-term diseases in humans, including possibly the production of cancer and birth defects in offspring."

In September 1974, Dr. Corbett learned of a meeting soon to be held at the Michigan Farm Bureau headquarters in

68

Lansing from Dr. Frank Hammer, an analytical chemist at the Environmental Research Group, the Ann Arbor laboratory that had analyzed the chicken eggs and the human fat samples for Dr. Corbett. "Dr. Hammer got me invited to the meeting. Although it turned out he could not attend, I went," Dr. Corbett recalls. "The meeting was attended by members of the Farm Bureau, scientists, attorneys, representatives of Michigan Chemical, insurance companies and the Michigan Department of Agriculture. I listened to the discussion for several hours. The majority of this discussion was aimed at estimating how long it would take for cows above the PBB tolerance level to reduce fat levels to below tolerance concentrations so they could be sold for human consumption. I finally stood up and voiced my concerns for the human population, noting that they were risking the health and welfare of every Michigan resident by allowing them to continue to eat Firemaster-containing livestock products," he said. "The major concern seemed to be the economic loss, which was staggering, and how to get out of this mess as inexpensively as possible. No one mentioned the possible harm to the human population that had been so widely exposed until I raised the question."

Also at the September meeting was a group of farmers. And the meeting adjourned briefly so everyone could step outside and take a look at two contaminated calves one dairyman had brought to the meeting. "They were pitiful-looking animals, small for their ages and covered with scales and sores. The farmer mentioned that he was going to bring another calf that looked even worse, but it died the night before," Dr. Corbett said. Before they left, the farmers expressed concern about selling contaminated products to consumers; many of the farmers had herds with so-called low-level contamination—that is, contaminated in amounts so low that they could be legally sold for human consumption. The owner of one such low-level herd told the gathering that after seeing his cows looking so ill he stopped drinking milk from those cows and began buying milk for his family at the grocery store. Then another farmer, still in his twenties, rose slowly. "We'll do whatever you decide about the animals," he said to Farm Bureau officials, his voice cracking slightly. "I ... I just ... I just want to ... get it over with so we can have a normal life again. It's been so hard on ... it's ..." The young man, tears streaming down his cheeks, sat down, buried his head in his arms and sobbed uncontrollably. After the farmers left, Dr. Corbett showed slides from his experiments, including the birth defects induced by Firemaster. "I stated that certain chemicals that were known to produce birth defects in animals also were carcinogenic in humans, and this possibility must be considered with Firemaster. I restated my position that I did not feel that a tolerance level of one part per million in food for human consumption was safe."

When the meeting ended, one Farm Bureau official approached Dr. Corbett and put his arm around Dr. Corbett's shoulders. "He asked me not to publicize my findings," Dr. Corbett recalls. "He said, 'After all, we don't want to frighten people with these birth defects and things.' I flew off the handle. I told him I'll do anything I want with it, and that the more people I tell, the better. I told him that the Farm Bureau had in no way sponsored my studies and that I would tell anyone who cared to listen." Dr. Corbett did not know the name of the Farm Bureau official. In any event, enough questions had been raised at that meeting apparently to have heightened concerns, particularly at the Michigan Department of Agriculture. The department itself soon convened a meeting on October 9 at its Geagley Laboratory to further discuss the contamination problems, which seemed to keep growing instead of diminishing. "We concluded," recalled Donald R. Isleib, chief deputy agriculture director, "that the PBB-herd health problem was not self-eliminating as we had anticipated." More than forty persons, including Rick Halbert and Dr. Corbett, attended the day-long meeting, which focused particular attention on the continuing health problems among dairy herds that had low levels of PBB contamination. Just before the morning coffee break, Dr. Corbett once more showed his slides and described his experiments with Firemaster. The Food and Drug Administration within a month further lowered the allowable amounts of PBB in food products. "It was gratifying to know that our work had been somewhat instrumental in bringing about this change," Dr. Corbett said. It was shortly after the October 9 meeting that Dr. Corbett called Dr. Irving J. Selikoff, the renowned environmental health scientist who had become familiar with his work on anesthetic gases. He brought Dr. Selikoff up to date on the PBB developments in Michigan and said he was worried because "state officials did not have the expertise to understand the potential dangers of the situation." Dr. Selikoff did not disagree with that assessment. He knew that

70

while state health departments were at home conducting programs such as the immunization of school children, most were ill-equipped and inadequately trained to study the subtle effects of a massive chemical poisoning. "And I informed Dr. Selikoff that his help was urgently needed," Dr. Corbett recalls. Dr. Selikoff dispatched his young and trusted lieutenant, Dr. Henry ("Andy") Anderson, to Michigan to further review the situation with Dr. Corbett. The two of them spent an entire day in Dr. Corbett's office in Ann Arbor talking. "When I got back," recalls Dr. Anderson, "I conferred with and gave Dr. Selikoff my opinion as well as the information given to me. And it seemed there was sufficient interest." Dr. Selikoff then called Dr. Corbett back. "He agreed to bring a team of specialists to Michigan, providing the state would issue an official invitation," Dr. Corbett said. "He suggested I get in touch with the state agencies or with the governor's office." As a federally designated research center, Dr. Selikoff's Environmental Sciences Laboratory would be able to conduct a health study of a broad population at no cost to the state of Michigan.

The first state official the elated Dr. Corbett called was Dr. George L. Whitehead, the agriculture department's deputy chief in charge of the consumer protection bureau. Dr. Whitehead was a logical person to have called because Dr. Corbett had spoken with him throughout the autumn, keeping Dr. Whitehead abreast of the PBB mice experiments he was doing. He related Dr. Selikoff's offer to Dr. Whitehead, explaining the nature of Dr. Selikoff's work.

"You have a telephone," the agriculture official said. "Why don't you call the Health Department?"

"God damn!" Dr. Corbett, incredulous, snapped. "That's your job, buster!"

"Our responsibility is four-legged, not two-legged animals," Dr. Whitehead replied.

"I knew," Dr. Whitehead explained a year and a half later to reporter Stephen Cain of the Detroit *News*, "Selikoff was a sharp guy. He was a physician, and I don't go outside the state getting physicians to come in and do work. That's up to the Health Department." Dr. Whitehead said he "may even have given Dr. Corbett the Health Department's phone number. He made such a big deal out of it. So I told him to call the Health Department. I told him we're not concerned with human health. I didn't want to get involved in that. Hell, nobody

71

wanted to get involved." Closer to the truth, however, is that Dr. Whitehead didn't want Dr. Selikoff to be involved—fearing that such a famous scientist would arrive in Michigan and raise serious questions about the handling of the PBB contamination by state officials. Three days after his conversation with Dr. Corbett, Dr. Whitehead wrote a memo reporting the information to his boss, B. Dale Ball. "It is my opinion that such a study by Dr. Selekoff [sic] could have a very significant impact on this problem. So I thought I would keep you informed." And so the department never took any action on this offer from Dr. Selikoff. "Maybe," said Donald R. Isleib, chief deputy agriculture director, "he [Corbett] felt that he had launched his appeal, and now someone [in the Department of Agriculture] should pass it on. We didn't think it was up to us to pass on the request." Yet Isleib and other agriculture officials would continue making pious statements in public forums proclaiming their "paramount" concern for PBB's potential effects on human health. "We need all of the facts on PBB effects on human health," said agriculture director Ball on April 18, 1975, "if we are to make an informed and reasoned judgment."

By the time Dr. Anderson returned to New York in late October of 1974 and was conferring with Dr. Selikoff about studying the Michigan problem, even top U.S. Food and Drug Administration officials in Washington knew about Dr. Selikoff's interest in studying the human health effects of PBB contamination. But no one acted to bring the noted scientist to Michigan.

After being initially rebuffed by Dr. Whitehead, Dr. Corbett then called Governor Milliken's office. "I was not allowed to speak to the governor personally, but was referred to an aide, Mark Mason," he recalls. Mason was Milliken's staff liaison to the Department of Agriculture. Dr. Corbett in essence repeated the information he had given to Dr. Whitehead. "But I got Mason to promise to discuss this matter with Governor Milliken. Later, the governor said Mason never talked to him about Selikoff," Dr. Corbett said.

Drs. Corbett and Selikoff saw each other in person twice in early 1975 at meetings in New York and in Hollywood, Florida. Both times, Dr. Corbett asked if Dr. Selikoff had received an invitation from state leaders in Michigan. Both times the answer was no. In late March, when he got back from Florida, Dr. Corbett said, "I called back Mark Mason in the governor's office, and received some sort of a reply that they had talked it over and decided it wasn't necessary or something to that effect." Mason, no longer on Governor Milliken's staff, has refused to talk about the controversy.

The state Department of Public Health has steadfastly claimed to this day that it never knew about Dr. Selikoff's offer until it was discovered in late April of 1976 by Edie Clark, an aide to Bobby D. Crim, the Speaker of the Michigan House of Representatives. Yet the department's own internal memos reveal that the highest officers in the department knew about Dr. Selikoff's interest in and desire to conduct studies in Michigan—a mere two days after Dr. Corbett had spoken with the Agriculture Department's Dr. Whitehead. In an October 23, 1974, memo to Dr. Maurice S. Reizen, the director of public health, Dr. John L. Isbister, disease control officer, wrote, "Doctor Sellikoff [sic], a nationally known geneticist, is interested in coming to Michigan to carry out chromosomal studies on those individuals identified as having consumed PBB-contaminated dairy products. You will recall that Doctor Selikoff is a medical researcher associated with Mount Sinai Hospital in New York who has also been involved in the asbestos problems related to Reserve Mining."

Indeed, the Health Department had been advised by knowledgeable experts to contact Dr. Selikoff for help just two months after the PBB contamination was discovered. Dr. B. B. Holder, medical director of the Midland division of the Dow Chemical Company, told Dr. Donald B. Coohon, chief of the Health Department's disease control division, that Dr. Selikoff, "the expert in industrial medicine, may be worth a call." Dr. Holder even gave Dr. Coohon two telephone numbers where Dr. Selikoff could be contacted. But Dr. Coohon passed the information on to three other health officers, Dr. Isbister, Harold Humphrey and Dr. Norman Hayner. Nobody called Dr. Selikoff.

Curiously, it isn't known how the Health Department learned in the first place of Dr. Selikoff's offer, since the department has consistently denied any knowledge of the offer until the spring of 1976, when House Speaker Bobby Crim called the department's officials to his office, demanding to know why Dr. Selikoff's offer never was taken up—especially when all that had been necessary to bring the Selikoff team to Michigan was a mere invitation. "We didn't know anything about it until this meeting," claimed Dr. Reizen. "Crim asked us why we hadn't acted on it. And I said, 'Acted on what? Who? When?' At that point, we thought, Gee, what's wrong with that?"

"Dr. Reizen," recalls Edie Clark, who attended that meeting in her boss's office, "came in to Bobby's office and swore up and down—did everything but cross his heart—that he absolutely had no idea about Selikoff's offer. I never believed Reizen didn't know."

And so no scientifically valid health data on the acute effects of PBB on humans were ever gathered, thus perpetuating the vacuum of information as 9 million people in Michigan continued consuming foods contaminated with PBB while being assured by state officials that it was perfectly safe to do so. "Their ignorance or their stubbornness," Dr. Corbett said of state officials, "perpetuated this mess. They were incompetent boobs. Selikoff would have gone out, defined the problem and cleaned it up."

"It's interesting that the Department of Agriculture has a dual function," he noted later. "One is to promote the Michigan agri-business and the other is to protect the consumers from tainted and unsafe food products. It seems to be a conflict of interest. This agency, even though farmers were complaining that their animals were sick and dying, allowed the sale of these animals and their products for human consumption—both prior to and following the discovery that Firemaster was the causative agent. As a result, millions of Michigan residents now have measurable concentrations of PBB in their bodies."

As the spring of 1975 approached, Dr. Corbett was becoming increasingly disillusioned by the lackadaisical attitude of the state bureaucracy in its handling of the PBB disaster. One March day he was preparing to go to Florida to present the results of his isoflurane study to a meeting of the International Anesthesia Research Society when Clark Hallas, a reporter for the Detroit *News*, called. The PBB controversy had not diminished, even though the Food and Drug Administration four months earlier had imposed stricter PBB tolerance guidelines. A public debate still raged over the inadequacies of those federal tolerance guidelines. And among those who wanted the levels lowered further was Dr. Corbett. By coincidence, when Hallas called, he had some new results from his PBB mice-feeding experiments. And so he invited Hallas out to his office in Ann Arbor. Hallas immediately checked out a company car and drove the forty-five miles to Dr. Corbett's office. And on March 13, Hallas's story ran as the top item on the front page of the Detroit *News*. It began:

> An independent researcher says his studies indicate that the effects on humans of a fire retardant chemical accidentally fed to livestock may be far more serious than state health officials now believe.

The story went on to say that Dr. Corbett's results so far "have caused him to worry that the chemical may result in birth defects and possibly cancer in humans. Wide-ranging birth defects have been reported in the offspring of farm animals exposed to high levels of PBB." Hallas further quoted Dr. Corbett as saying, "The fact that we have been able to produce birth defects in laboratory animals—in some cases with the same levels of PBB that people have eaten—should be a cause for concern." The story also quoted Dr. Corbett as saying, "We're all part of a huge experiment." Dr. Corbett told Hallas that he fed PBB in concentrations of 1,000, 100 and 50 parts per million to pregnant rats and mice. Several animals died from massive gastrointestinal hemorrhage before the end of the eleven-day feeding period. At the 1,000 parts per million level, PBB produced cleft palates in 5 percent of the mice offspring. At 100 parts per million, a protrusion of the brain, exencephaly, resulted in 2 percent of the fetuses. Hallas, as usual, wrote an accurate story, based on what Dr. Corbett had told him. Unfortunately, the headline, while not inaccurate, may have given an erroneous impression. It said:

Human birth defects seen in tainted feed

People who have followed the PBB controversy over the years single out that headline as the one event that contributed the most in scaring the public. About the same time that headline appeared, a twelve-part series entitled "The Poison Puzzle" in the Grand Rapids *Press* revealed how the state's feeble efforts to contain the PBB contamination were failing miserably. The publicity soon drew an uncharacteristic attack directly from the office of Governor William G. Milliken, which issued a "report" characterizing press coverage of PBB as being "filled with rumor, speculation, half-truths and errors of fact." The "report" was the work of an ad hoc "task force" named by the executive office "to coordinate state government action on all phases of PBB—consumer protection, animal health and the human element," according to Mark Mason, the Milliken aide. Curiously, when Paul Bernstein of the Detroit *News* called two state officials listed as members of the task force to elicit further information, he learned that neither knew anything about a task force, much less a report produced by such a task force. Said Dr. George L. Whitehead, "There has never been any task force to my knowledge." The other official, Dr. John Isbister, commented, "I don't know anything about a task force."

But, in any event, the "report" accomplished at least one objective: It silenced Dr. Corbett, if only temporarily. "From that time on, I was quite discouraged, to say the least," he recalls. "I just kept my mouth shut for a while—until I just got to the point where I felt I should speak up again. I imagine it was another six months before I recuperated from that blow." The criticism leveled against him, Dr. Corbett thinks, also may have had an adverse impact on his career progress at the University of Michigan. "It was at a time when I was being considered for promotion," he said. "I was at the level of assistant professor for only three years, which is the minimum time for promotion to associate professor." But because of the public attack he came under, he thinks he was passed over for a promotion. The next year, however, he was promoted—"when," Dr. Corbett recalls, "it seemed that everything I had said previously turned out to be true."

# 6
# RIPPLES

The mercury crisis made itself known in North America in early 1970 when a chemist from the University of Western Ontario discovered that fish taken from Lake St. Clair, located between Ontario Province and the state of Michigan, contained alarmingly high amounts of mercury. Indeed the mercury levels were close to the concentrations found in the fish eaten by residents of the Japanese fishing village of Minamata on the island of Kyushu. In Japan scores of men, women and children developed severe neurological symptoms; many became insane, and others died as a result of mercury poisoning.

And so the Canadian scientist's finding, touching off the discovery of high mercury content in fish and other food stuffs from lakes and rivers throughout Canada and the United States, prompted quick controls on mercury pollution. In many cases, fishing bans were issued for the affected waters. The information also inspired federal regulations on the mercury content of tuna and swordfish, both of which were found to contain extraordinarily high levels of the metallic element.

The discovery of mercury in fish from Lake St. Clair was particularly worrisome to Michigan health officials. The huge lake, virtually in Detroit's backyard, attracted countless fishermen and water sports enthusiasts. The state Department of Public Health in Lansing quickly developed analytical capabilities to detect mercury in human body fluids and fat tissues. And it made its services available to physicians and local public health officers throughout Michigan in evaluation of persons known to have consumed large amounts of fish from Lake St. Clair and several of the Great Lakes nearby. And in the autumn of 1971, the department established a mercury project and $70,000 from the department's annual budget was allocated to get this new project off the ground. Staffed by a biochemist, a laboratory scientist, an environmental sanitarian and a laboratory technician, the mercury project was to have been the forerunner of an environmental epidemiology unit, with the capability to conduct health surveys in the event of toxic substances pollution involving the human population.

Since mercury was but one of a growing list of chemical contaminants in the Great Lakes, the department's mercury project soon was expanded through a federal contract in 1973 to study the relationship between the level of polychlorinated biphenyls—or PCBs, a compound extremely similar in structure to PBBs—in fish and the level in humans who were heavy fish eaters. "The unit was developing in the direction of an environmental epidemiology unit," recalls Dr. Maurice S. Reizen, Michigan's public health director.

In the spring of 1974, however, a Senate House conference committee deleted all the money for the mercury project, whose funding had reached $90,000 in the previous fiscal year. Almost overnight, then, the project ceased to exist, and the small staff was limited to its work fulfilling the federal contract to study PCBs. A few weeks later, Harold Humphrey, the young epidemiologist who was assigned to the mercury project, got a call from Dr. George L. Whitehead of the Department of Agriculture telling him about the PBB contamination. "How's that for irony?" Dr. Reizen, years later, would say. "Well, I guess there's no use being bitter." After Humphrey finished his conversation with Dr. Whitehead, he prepared a memo for Dr. Reizen, noting that, the "health effects of consuming contaminated milk [are] of concern because PBBs are believed to be more toxic than PCBs." Dr. Reizen tried earnestly, but to no avail, to persuade the legislature to restore the funds for the mercury project. "So," he recalls, "we did what we could in an effort to meet what we thought was a significant problem. We borrowed, stole and reassigned scientific and technical people from other programs and made a survey type of investigation of the human health effects of the PBB episode."

From the Department of Agriculture, public health officials obtained a list of farms that had been quarantined, which, at the time, totaled about a hundred; half of them were dairy farms and the other half beef, swine or poultry farms. All were located near Battle Creek in southwestern Michigan or near Fremont, about thirty-five miles north of Grand Rapids, or in

78

the state's Thumb region. These were called epicenters because they were the hardest hit by PBB contamination. "Since it appeared that the heaviest exposure would be those families, we directed our efforts at those farm families," Dr. Reizen recalls. "And the question we asked ourselves was: Are there people who are sick and dying as a result of eating PBB-contaminated meat, milk and dairy products?" On May 31, Dr. Reizen gave the final go ahead— "Okay ... GO!"—to his medical personnel to launch an "initial screening" designed to answer those questions. "We worked literally day and night," recalls Marvin Budd, who helped conduct that study. "We were waking people up in the middle of the night, gathering information. We opened our blood clinics at six in the morning. We just dogged this thing as much as we could. We'd be in a motel room writing up reports, filling out forms until two, three o'clock in the morning! Then we'd open up the blood clinics again at six. This went on from the end of May into July." The department's initial effort screened 217 persons—either from quarantined farms or from families who had purchased foodstuffs directly from the contaminated farms. The screenings consisted of taking brief medical histories going back to 1972, with emphasis on any change in health status since June 1973, the month PBB seeped into the food supply. Blood specimens were analyzed for PBB. The department felt reassured by what it found—or, rather, by what it didn't find.

"Certainly there was no evidence that the people in this study were seriously sick or dying as a result of exposure to PBB," Dr. Reizen said. From this initial search, the Health Department estimated that "over 250 persons" had been exposed to PBB in food on quarantined farms and that "over 500 others" had been exposed after eating foods purchased from these farms. Those estimates fell short by about 9 million. But Dr. Reizen later explained, "Yes, we were continually behind in assessing the situation. But early on our information came from the Department of Agriculture. And our incoming information wasn't that good. But we were at the mercy of the agriculture people."

Although many among the 217 persons in the initial screening reported health problems which coincided with the entry of PBB into the food chain and which required medical attention, Dr. John Isbister, a state disease control officer, concluded, "No consistent clinical pattern of acute toxic illness or chronic effects has emerged during these preliminary investigations."

With that dubious reassurance in hand, the Health Department began designing what it thought—erroneously, as it turned out—would be the definitive investigation of PBB's adverse effects on human health. First, the study, recalls Dr. Reizen, "defined a group of exposed farm families and a group of nonexposed farm families, selected statistically and based on information provided by the Department of Agriculture." The selection of two population groups in the study of a disease pattern is sound science because in order to demonstrate that a group of people exposed to a chemical indeed has suffered ill effects, that group must be compared with an unexposed group, all other variables being equal. Only then can the health differences in the first group be attributed to the chemical. Yet both groups in the state Health Department study turned out to have been contaminated by PBB, thus invalidating its conclusions. This fatal flaw, however, did not immediately come to light; and so the misleading results of the study lured Michigan's 9 million citizens into a false sense of security as they continued eating contaminated food products the state Agriculture Department and the U.S. Food and Drug Administration claimed were absolutely safe and healthy to eat.

This second study's protocol included a more detailed medical history questionnaire than in the inital screening, a full physical examination and the taking of a blood sample for PBB analysis. As he was dispatching interviewers out to the field to recruit subjects for the health survey, Dr. Norman Hayner, a disease control officer, told them they could expect full cooperation from the farmers. "A remarkably small degree of resistance has been encountered in this group of very busy farm families, who are currently planting grain and are concerned about the care and disposal of their contaminated herds," Dr. Hayner said. "It is obvious that quite a few are concerned about their own personal health." But his optimism was quickly shattered. The first group of interviewers were received with hostility at many farms, whose residents had taken part in the earlier initial screening and never again heard a word from the Health Department. Now they were angry and vented their anger at the interviewers who wanted them to participate in yet another health study. "They thought the Public Health [Department] had been too long in becoming concerned and doing something about the problem," recalls Nancy Jeffers Shanks, a department official who supervised the interviewers. She warned her superiors that the successful recruitment of cooperative persons for the second health study "is potentially a real problem." One farmer told a state interviewer, "The state wants us to cooperate with them, but the state won't cooperate with us." Others demanded to know why a second blood sample would be necessary when one already had been taken in the first study. At almost every stop, Health Department interviewers encountered angry farm families demanding to know why reports of laboratory tests and physical examination results had not been forwarded to their personal physicians, as the department had promised. Many families simply refused to take part because, they said, the examinations took too long and that, in the first study, scheduling foul-ups caused prolonged waiting periods.

Eventually the department recruited 298 persons to participate in its long-awaited epidemiologic survey into the "Short-Term Effects of PBB on Human Health," and it began holding clinics in September—four long months after the PBB contamination had become known.

In May 1975, after comparing 165 "exposed" persons from quarantined farms to 133 "control," or nonexposed, persons, the department concluded that PBB did not cause "any identifiable human ailments" because, it said, in essence, that both groups looked about the same in health status.

Dr. Reizen told a press conference, "We are not saying that PBB exposure has caused no ailments—only that we found no consistent pattern of illness or symptoms which occurred excessively in exposed persons and which could, therefore, be attributed to PBB." No doubt, he added, many farm families could be expected to exhibit "some situational stress" from having encountered long, unexplained illness in their livestock and having been faced with quarantines and the destruction of their cattle. In the detailed report, the findings said a number of symptoms turned up in both the "exposed" and the "control" group, such as anxiety, fatigue, headache, severe skin rashes and numbness. But because both groups had "essentially the same frequency of these conditions," the study concluded, PBB could not be the cause.

"After the MDPH [Michigan Department of Public Health] report," recalls Edie Clark, who in the spring of 1975 had begun following the PBB developments as an aide to

House Speaker Crim, "publicity and attention on the issue died down and Dr. Corbett's studies [reported by the Detroit *News* two months earlier] soon faded from public memory." But not for long, however. In June, a toxicologist at the Blodgett Memorial Hospital in Grand Rapids published a critique of the May 1, 1975, study. "It went unnoticed by many at the time, but was later to attract considerable attention among the medical and scientific communities," Clark said.

The toxicologist was Dr. Walter D. Meester, a scientist with impeccable credentials. The holder of both a medical degree and a Ph.D., Dr. Meester was director and clinical toxicologist at the Western Michigan Poison Center, and a member of the department of clinical toxicology at Blodgett Memorial Medical Center, both in Grand Rapids. He was particularly interested in the state Health Department's report because he had been examining PBB-contaminated farm families for a variety of health problems for a year. And it didn't take the scientist long to spot an important fact which had escaped public notice: both groups in the study had been contaminated by PBB. What the study did, then, Dr. Meester said, was to compare one group of contaminated farm families with another group of contaminated farm families—and then, finding almost no difference in the health status of the two groups, concluded that no health problems could be attributed to PBB. "I have come to the conclusion that the data obtained by MDPH does not sufficiently support its conclusions to warrant its publication and/or release in the lay press," Dr. Meester thundered in a paper he wrote entitled, "Critique on the Michigan Department of Public Health Study on the Short-Term Effects of PBB on Health." "The conclusions can very easily be misinterpreted to mean that PBB does not produce any harmful effects on humans who consumed PBB-contaminated food." Then he got down to specifics.

"The comparison between the exposed group and the so-called unexposed control group is completely invalid since more than 70 percent of the subjects in the control group, presumed to be unexposed to PBB, had definite detectable levels of PBB in their blood," Dr. Meester said. He also pointed out that the Health Department study did not consider any symptom significant unless more than ten individuals in either group reported it. This assumption, Dr. Meester said, "precludes any discovery of potentially harmful but real symptoms occurring in a small number of individuals affected by PBB. I feel that some important, although less frequent, symptoms and illnesses may have been missed by the technique utilized by MDPH."

The Health Department also assumed—erroneously—that there should be more ailments and complaints from persons with the highest PBB levels in their blood, Dr. Meester added. "That is not necessarily true," he said. "Blood levels of fat soluble chemicals [such as PBB] are often inconsistent and unpredictable. The assumption that PBB levels in the blood are related to severity of signs and symptoms is a fallacious one." Dr. Meester had a number of other criticisms of the way the state study was conducted and analyzed. "In summary," he wrote, "I feel that the MDPH study on the acute effects of PBB on health was poorly planned, does not conform to the standards of adequate scientific medical and epidemiological evaluation, was incomplete, possibly biased, and does not support the conclusions reached and publicized in the lay press." Dr. Reizen later admitted his department's study was "primitive," but said that despite Dr. Meester's legitimate criticism, "We felt it didn't invalidate our study." Referring to the control group in the Health Department study, which also turned out to have been poisoned, Dr. Reizen said the comparison of the two groups was "analogous to a comparison study of those who smoke two packs of cigarettes a day to those who smoke two cigarettes a day."

The discovery of PBB in the blood of those in the study's control group—that is, people presumed to have been exempt from PBB—was a striking finding because it suggested the extent of the contamination was much broader than previously suspected. Yet, the Health Department failed to disclose the information to the lay public in a meaningful way. Thus more than twelve months would pass before state residents would learn that every man, woman and child in Michigan had been poisoned by PBB. "I would have to agree that state health officials could have handled the public discussion earlier and in a more effective way," said Dr. Clark W. Heath, director of the cancer and birth defects division of the bureau of epidemiology at the world-famous U.S. Center for Disease Control in Atlanta. "When they set up the study during the summer of 1974, there was a strong feeling that this was a limited problem."

Dr. Reizen, asked about his department's study several

years later, said, "This is the best way to illustrate the problem." Holding his open palms about a foot apart, facing one another, he slowly widened the distance as he looked down into the gap. "It's like a stone you throw into a pond. The ripples get bigger and bigger. Each time when we thought we saw the dimensions of the ripple, it got bigger on us."

Dr. Meester's final comment about the state's short-term study was: "The only conclusion the MDPH made with which I am in agreement is that the detection of any long-term effects of PBB exposure must await a long-term study of the problem."

But the Health Department was rebuffed when it sought $1.1 million to begin a five-year long-term study to determine if PBB might cause health problems that did not show up right away, but, rather, might appear after an extended period of time, such as cancer. At about the same time the department was designing its short-term study, it also began planning the long-term study, with the advice of Dr. Heath of the U.S. Center for Disease Control. In early 1975, the department submitted the long-term study's protocol to Governor Milliken's office. But on May 16, two weeks after the department released its reassuring short-term study which virtually exonerated PBB, Gerald H. Miller, Milliken's budget director, turned down the $1.1 million request. "A good deal of effort seems to have been spent to develop a sound study methodology without adequately considering why such a study should be conducted, or fully developing the need-output-impact linkage. This request is therefore recommended for rejection based on inadequate demonstration of benefits to Michigan citizens," Miller wrote. "It is not clear from the request why knowledge of this type will be of benefit to Michigan people.... The impact is totally unclear. How will the knowledge expected to be gained impact upon the health goals of the department and the state?" When the Health Department a week later took its request to the state legislature, it found few sympathetic ears. One lawmaker told Dr. Reizen, "This is a problem for cows—not people."

It took another year before the Michigan Department of Public Health was able to find money to begin its long-term study. The funds—totaling $337,000—came from three federal agencies, the Center for Disease Control, the Food and Drug Administration and the National Cancer Institute. And so in the summer of 1976, more than two years after the PBB contamination was discovered, state health officials began developing a register of four thousand Michigan residents who had been exposed to high levels of PBB and whose health would be followed for an indefinite number of years, perhaps decades. At the same time, another register of two thousand residents from Iowa was to be developed to serve as controls. The control group had to come from out of state because by then it had become quite clear that the population of Michigan had PBB in its blood and also lodged in the fatty tissues, to be stored there probably for life.

The belated interest displayed by the Food and Drug Administration in the health of contaminated Michigan citizens is curious. Unknown to any outside agencies or personnel, the agency several months after the PBB contamination was discovered had conducted its own health survey and found that nearly 40 percent of the persons interviewed had serious medical problems. But the agency merely filed the information away and did not tell anyone about it. "In the summer and fall of 1974, we began to hear reports, mainly through the media, of illnesses being suffered by farm families who had consumed PBB-contaminated food produced on their farms," recalls Sam D. Fine, the Food and Drug Administration's associate commissioner for compliance. He said the agency's inspectors then visited about sixty-five farms that were among the first to be quarantined as well as some of the patients of a Big Rapids, Michigan, osteopathic physician, Dr. David Salvati, who were complaining about symptoms that appeared to have been due to PBB contamination. In all, FDA collected information, including private medical records, on 529 persons.

Dr. Frank Cordle, the FDA medical epidemiologist who ordered the survey, later told the Detroit *Free Press* that he ignored the reports because "I did not consider it a scientific survey. It was just something to satisfy my own curiosity.... We just never saw any importance to it."

Scientific or not, what the FDA inspectors found clearly suggested that something was vastly wrong in the farm community and certainly deserved further investigation. For instance, Albert Vanderwall, a forty-nine-year-old Fremont, Michigan, farmer, said he had been hospitalized for six days in December 1973. Then in March of 1974 he was admitted to Butterworth Hospital in Grand Rapids with a suspected coronary problem. "He is able to get around, but not able to work," the FDA report said. Although heart problem was ruled out, the report added, "Mr. Vanderwall now cannot see to read or drive. He has a loss of energy, has lost thirty pounds over the past nine months, is subject to blackout spells and has been since December 1973." Vanderwall's farm was quarantined after a chicken was found to have been highly contaminated with PBB. Also in Fremont, one of the hardest hit areas, dairywoman Nancy Rottier told FDA inspectors she had begun suffering from migraine headaches, usually three to four times a week, for the last five months. Her farm was quarantined after milk containing 15.1 parts per million PBB was discovered. Then her headaches disappeared, since she stopped drinking her own cows' milk. A subsequent physical examination by her own doctor found Mrs. Rottier "entirely normal." In Newaygo, just a few miles southeast of Fremont, fifty-year-old Ethel Johnson told FDA officials she began experiencing unusual fatigue in the fall of 1973 and "just couldn't seem to make a recovery." She became abnormally nervous and began losing weight. A thorough physical examination turned up nothing. Almost every night, she said, she had to get up three or four times to urinate. Her husband advised her to drink more milk. She did. But her problems worsened. Her ankle and feet then began swelling. After a week's hospitalization in Fremont, doctors were unable to come up with an explanation for her ailments. They told her to go home and "relax." But the swelling continued, and her hands and feet often throbbed at night. Another doctor told her the swelling probably was caused by her circulation, "which wasn't the best." Before long, Mrs. Johnson was experiencing dizziness and a lack of coordination, often staggering, as if intoxicated, when walking and missing her mouth when eating. Her problems began improving after April 1974 when she stopped drinking milk because of the publicity about sick dairy animals, she said. Her husband, Melvin, told the FDA inspector he also had coordination problems that set in during the winter of 1973. He spilled coffee frequently, tripped and stumbled often and had fallen in the barn numerous times. Like his wife, Johnson also missed his mouth when eating. An ophthalmological examination found nothing wrong with his sight. Occasionally he also had sharp stomach pains that felt as if he were "stabbed with a knife," Johnson said. He said he thought his problems were due to advancing age. Johnson was fifty-two. Tests later revealed that the Johnsons' milk had contained 11.2 parts PBB per million, an extremely high dose.

Similar symptoms but with varying degrees of severity were reported by nearly 40 percent of the 529 persons interviewed by the Food and Drug Administration. Yet the information went nowhere but a metal filing cabinet in agency's office in southwest Washington.

Dr. Cordle, the FDA epidemiologist, said he read all the reports but saw nothing unusual in them. "'I'm tired. I ache.'— that's the kind of thing doctors hear every day," he told Kathy Warbelow of the Detroit *Free Press* "Those are very common complaints. We never did any analysis because then someone would ask you to draw conclusions, and you can't get conclusions out of this sort of thing." Dr. Cordle added, "We did nothing with it because that information is part of an inspection. First of all, FDA has no authority to follow up health problems. We had no mechanism."

"That FDA health survey just created another element of mistrust," said Marvin Budd, a state health officer. "And it added a lot of confusion. Many people didn't fully know the difference between the state Health Department and the FDA . To them we were all the same—'the government.' The people probably were expecting help. But they never heard from the FDA again. We never did."

More than three years after the Food and Drug Administration conducted its survey and then stashed the reams of data it collected in a filing cabinet, the agency was chastised by U.S. Representative John E. Moss, the California Democrat who was chairman of the House subcommittee on oversight and investigations. The FDA then claimed it indeed had forwarded its medical findings to the Michigan Department of Public Health. But the department says it never received any such information. In any case, the FDA's Dr. Cordle said he saw no need for the agency to have acted further at the time since the state Health Department had begun its own medical investigation. As it turned out, that was the flawed short-term study that concluded, "PBB has not been shown to be the cause of any identifiable human ailments."

Despite the flawed conclusions of the state Health Department's short-term study, and despite the Food and Drug Administration's volumes of evidence implicating PBB in widespread human illness, officials of both agencies for years to come would obstinately claim that there was no evidence PBB might be harmful to humans. As proof, typically, Dr. Reizen would make public statements that he knew of women with extremely high concentrations of PBB who had given birth to healthy children, who in turn were growing up to be quite normal. That certainly may have been the case; yet both Dr. Reizen and the FDA would sit on information involving the unexpected deaths of people whose bodies were loaded with PBB. One such case involved an otherwise healthy six-month-old infant named Sarah Robinett of Dexter, Michigan, a community of 1,700 just west of Ann Arbor. Her death was attributed to viral pneumonia. But later findings certainly raised the question that her natural immune system may have been damaged severely by PBB.

Dr. George L. Whitehead, deputy agriculture director in charge of consumer protection, learned of the death of Sarah Elizabeth Robinett on October 21, 1974, when he got a telephone call from Calvin Kittendorf. Kittendorf was employed as a driver to transport contaminated animals from farms throughout Michigan to the burial pit in Kalkaska County. Earlier that day, Kittendorf had gone out to the farm of William J. Robinett to pick up two stunted steers, one sow and two goats for destruction. When he arrived on the farm, Kittendorf learned from Margaret Robinett that it was funeral day. Her six-month-old granddaughter had died suddenly three days earlier. She told Kittendorf she thought the child's death had been caused by the mother's heavy consumption of milk that turned out to have been contaminated by PBB. Dr. Whitehead then notified Harold Humphrey, the Health Department epidemiologist. But the department displayed little if any interest. An autopsy performed by the Washtenaw County medical examiner revealed very little, except that the infant's lungs were "heavy," suggesting pneumonia as a possible cause of death. On October 24, six days after the baby's sudden death, Judith A. Putz, a Food and Drug Administration investigator, stopped at the Robinett farm and was surprised to learn that "no one from the state had visited the family." Yet after her own visit, both Humphrey and another state medical official, Dr. Norman Hayner, would pump her for information about the death of Sarah Robinett. "I responded with the data that I had accumulated," investigator Putz recalls. The Robinetts' family physician had told her that the baby appeared entirely normal. During her visit to the farm, she said she saw dogs with great patches of hair missing. The family members told her that a Farm Bureau Services representative from the Dexter Co-op had advised them not to eat their chicken but that the eggs from the chicken were safe to eat. They followed his advice. Next, Putz visited Dr. Wallace R. Kemp, the family physician. He told her that Sarah Robinett had been born on April 16, 1974, weighing eight pounds, thirteen ounces, and went home from the hospital four days later. *Elaine Robinett's pregnancy was full term and the birth was normal, Dr. Kemp said. Four weeks later, he weighed the baby during a checkup; all was normal and her weight had increased to nine pounds, thirteen ounces. A little over three months later, he gave the baby her first shots. Margaret Robinett, the child's sixty-two-year-old grandmother, told Putz that at the August 26 appointment with Dr. Kemp, the infant's right eye was checked because of what appeared to be a growth above the eye, between the nose and eyebrow. She remembered the doctor saying it was a cyst, although Dr. Kemp later said he had no record of having checked for any growth above the baby's right eye. In any case, on October 16, two days before Sarah Robinett suddenly died, Elaine Robinett recalls, the baby's left eye got red and that she was "crabbier then usual." The next day, Mrs. Robinett said her baby's entire left eye was red and that she would not eat and began running a high fever, accompanied by heavy perspiration. Elaine Robinett called Dr. Kemp and described her child's symptoms to him over the telephone. He prescribed an ophthalmic ointment for her eye. Before dawn on October 18, Elaine Robinett checked Sarah and found her sleeping soundly. To her relief, the baby's fever apparently had broken. When she checked Sarah again at 7:30, she found her child blue in the face and her fingers curled. After a few frantic moments of artificial resuscitation, she called Dr. Kemp. He arrived a short time later and assumed the baby was dead, "although she was warm yet, but starting to stiffen out."

*Interestingly, subsequent analysis of the birth weights of nearly three hundred Michigan children with presumed PBB exposure born between 1973 and 1977 shows that those born in 1974 had the least mean weight. That year, of course, is the logical year for such an effect to show up—since most 1973 babies were born before PBB actually got into the food supply some time in the summer of 1973. Furthermore, then, the 1975 babies should be the second most affected group. They were. These are the mean birth weights by year: 1973, 124.88 ounces; 1974, 116.45 ounces; 1975, 122.89 ounces; 1976, 127.07 ounces; and 1977, 127.30 ounces.

William Robinett, Sarah's twenty-seven-year-old father, was a full-time laborer. But he also worked part time for a nearby dairy farmer; for his work there, Robinett was paid in animal feed instead of money. Robinett's own animals were used only to meet the food needs of his family, which consisted of his sixty-two-year-old mother and eighty-six-year-old grandmother, his wife's fifteen-year-old brother and their own daughters, ages three years and twenty months. It turned out that the dairyman for whom Robinett worked part time had bought feed from March through May 29, 1974, from the Dexter Co-op, a Michigan Farm Bureau Services feed outlet. On May 29, he told Robinett to stop using the feed. Coincidentally, also starting in March, Elaine Robinett, about eight months pregnant, began drinking four to five cups of hot chocolate each day. Shortly afterward, she began feeling excessively tired. And so she began drinking more milk. After Sarah was born, Elaine Robinett breast-fed her for the first month and then put her on infant formula. Mrs. Robinett said she felt no adverse effects from having consumed so much PBB-contaminated milk other than fatigue, which she attributed to "having three children so close [to one another]." She also said no other family members suffered any deleterious health effects, although her grandmother began suddenly experiencing breath shortness after March 1, about the time the family's milk supply had first become contaminated. During much of this period, the entire family together consumed about four dozen eggs a week—which also turned out to have been contaminated.

Analyses on the fat and liver tissue samples taken from Sarah Robinett showed astronomical amounts of PBB. In her fat tissue, the reading was 4,400 parts per billion; in her liver tissue, the reading was 3,860 parts per billion. (In contrast, a cow in Michigan today with more than 20 parts per billion PBB is slaughtered and buried to prevent human contamination.) One sample of goat milk, which the Robinetts drank, showed 7,300 parts per billion; and a cow's milk sample showed 50,400 parts per billion. Yet, Sarah Robinett never drank any cow or goat milk. Nor did she eat any eggs. Her only exposure to the toxic chemical had been while in her mother's womb and then through her mother's breast milk for one month. The child was buried in St. Patrick's Cemetery in Whitmore Lake, just north of Dexter.

# 7
# ENEMIES OF THE PEOPLE

Veterinarian Susan Jacoby's telephone was ringing off the hook in early August of 1973 when she returned from a rare six-week vacation. Dr. Jacoby has an animal practice based in Constantine, a small southwestern Michigan town of 1,700 near the Indiana border. The first call she answered came from one of the best dairy farmers she had known in thirty years of veterinary practice. His cows began developing numerous health problems while she was away. "So I went through my records in previous years, and I had made an average of three, four calls a month out to that farm over the years," Dr. Jacoby recalls. When she arrived, the farmer told her that a cow had simply "gone down" and then died three days later. It was the tenth cow that had died mysteriously while Dr. Jacoby was vacationing. "Oh, I hope it has changed now," she told him. But the deaths mounted. In the rest of that month, Dr. Jacoby made nine more visits to the farm. Then she called the Michigan Department of Agriculture for help. "They have a diagnostic team, and we looked through the herd, and the symptoms had been intractable milk fevers, metritis [uterine infection] that we had a lot of trouble curing, a lot of foot trouble and very atypical pneumonia in calves," she said. The Agriculture Department veterinarians took one look and diagnosed the problem as "fat cow syndrome"; they did not even bother to take one blood or tissue sample for laboratory analysis. The team said the cows had been overfed carbohydrates and advised the farmer to feed his cows hay but not corn or grain. But there was no improvement. Some of the cows indeed had appeared too fat, but Dr. Jacoby "had a feeling that it was more from toxic conditions than overfeeding. But it was only a theory; I'm only a practicing veterinarian, not a research scientist." The summer of 1973 was not the first time she had seen worrisome health problems in

91

farm animals that were misdiagnosed by Michigan Agriculture Department "experts." Shortly after she graduated from veterinary school in Havana, Cuba, and arrived in Michigan, Dr. Jacoby almost immediately diagnosed an unusual disease in hogs known as erysipelas. "I was new in practice. So I called the department and they said, 'There is no erysipelas in Michigan.'" But she finally ignored the Agriculture Department's reassurances and administered antiserums to contain the outbreak. "Well," she recalls, "I knew there was erysipelas in Michigan. But they didn't know it yet." Dr. Jacoby was right. There indeed was an erysipelas outbreak in 1948, and numerous others in Michigan since then. "The department is sometimes too far removed from what's actually happening. It takes too long to get what is happening at the grass roots to the knowledge of the bureaucracy."

And so in 1973, Dr. Jacoby was not entirely satisfied with the state veterinarians' instant diagnosis of fat cow syndrome. She began performing postmortems, or autopsies, on the dead cows. What she found strengthened her conviction that the cause of the animal health problems was some toxic substance rather than a vague syndrome due to overfeeding. "When I got all these dead cows cut open, I found signs in the liver of fatty degeneration. Now that can come from a lot of things; it is not from overfeeding, if at all, because toxic materials will affect the liver cells and make them accumulate fat and then they cannot digest the fat the way they should," she said. Despite her postmortem findings, Dr. Jacoby said nothing. "I'm only supposed to report infectious diseases that I diagnose. I'm not supposed to report anything that I don't know. There is no provision that I have to report anything I don't know." So Dr. Jacoby and the farmer struggled along. But the problems continued, and got even worse. The cows began getting skinnier. They developed abscesses, hair loss and elongated hooves. Cows that had no apparent difficulty calving would suddenly die afterward instead of getting up. Nothing seemed to respond to treatment. Finally spring of 1974 came around and PBB was identified in a few dairy herds.

"So I told the farmer, 'Maybe we should test for PBB.' He said, 'Well, I don't know. I've never fed magnesium oxide. And maybe I shouldn't test. Maybe that just gets me into more trouble.' So I had to talk him into testing for PBB," Dr. Jacoby recalls. "So we tested for PBB, and he had low levels of PBB. But I had to insist on it. Nobody came to say, 'We'd better test all of the herds.' The Michigan Department of Agriculture was not only very slow initiating research into the cause of livestock problems, but did not effectively contain the spread of the contamination or protect the consumer—and particularly the livestock owner."

The PBB levels found in the cows of Dr. Jacoby's client were well under the level that would have resulted in quarantine. "So he was not put under quarantine, and we just kept struggling along," she recalls. Then the young heifers that came along began looking very sick, and some died. Laboratory tests on a fat sample taken from one dead heifer showed above quarantine levels. The farm finally was quarantined. The farmer never bought feed containing magnesium oxide, but did purchase other feeds from Farm Bureau Services. "So that's why he got a low contamination, but very possibly over quite a long period of time," Dr. Jacoby said. "That's one of the difficulties in tracing the PBB down. It went over such a long time that we don't know where, when and how much they [the cows] got."

Dr. Jacoby's experience was rare only because she had called the Michigan Department of Agriculture for assistance. Countless other veterinarians all over the state also were seeing similar animal health problems, but they did nothing—with the exception of perhaps three others, including, of course, the late Dr. Ted Jackson, Rick Halbert's veterinarian. If more veterinarians had complained to the state Agriculture Department, an early warning signal might have been sounded. But there was—and is—no such reporting system or network. "There should be legislation to require a veterinarian to report something he is having trouble diagnosing," says B. Dale Ball, the Michigan agriculture director. "In the past, the veterinarian has had to report a contagious disease but not a difficult diagnosis. The law should be amended to require a veterinarian to report a situation that he can't figure out, whether he thinks it's a contamination, a disease or just something he can't identify."

"There is no system to feed up information to some point at the federal or state level," Rick Halbert added. "I would have thought that veterinarians and farmers would have been concerned or been alarmed at certain symptoms they were seeing in some animals. Apparently the veterinarians just didn't catch on."

One who did, of course, was Dr. Jackson. At a December 1973 national bovine veterinarians conference in Fort Worth, Texas, Ted and Lois Jackson ran into many other Michigan animal doctors. "Most of them had just written off the problems they were seeing," recalls Mrs. Jackson. "They said, economically, they couldn't spend much time trying to solve the problems they saw. But by then Ted realized how widespread the problem must be. Of course at that time we didn't know yet it was PBB. But Ted knew it was something unusual."

After they returned home, Dr. Jackson worked harder than ever, trying to unravel the strange illness that had struck so many Michigan herds. Eventually, of course, he succeeded. But his untimely death a mere year after PBB was discovered deprived him of much of the public recognition that later went only to Rick Halbert for having solved the mystery. For many years afterward, Halbert continued receiving publicity as the dairy farmer who solved the PBB contamination; yet Ted Jackson's name was almost never mentioned, a fact that eventually made Lois Jackson chafe. "Rick is a brash, ambitious young man," she said. "He never mentioned Ted." Yet when the *Journal of the American Veterinary Medical Association* in September 1974 published an article about the Halbert herd, she said, the article carried both Jackson's and Halbert's by-lines. "Rick didn't have a thing to do with it," Mrs. Jackson recalls. "He just brought his records. Ted and I wrote it. And we only had to rewrite it once." Even today, written requests for reprints of that article still arrive—from all over the world—at Lois Jackson's cheerful yellow house on a hilltop in Battle Creek near Kalamazoo College, where she is a librarian. Yet, probably very few people in Michigan are even aware of the role Dr. Jackson played in discovering PBB. In describing how the PBB mix-up occurred, for instance, the Detroit *Free Press* repeatedly told of Halbert's efforts but merely referred to Dr. Jackson as "a Battle Creek area veterinarian." More than two years later, Lois Jackson was reading the May 10, 1976, issue of *Time* magazine when she came across yet another account of the PBB episode. In it, Halbert was cited, but, again, her deceased husband was not. She wrote *Time* a letter, suggesting to the editors that "You should do your homework more." She never got a reply.

94

Ted Jackson died on May 14, 1975. That summer he had been scheduled to address the American Veterinary Medical Association annual meeting in Los Angeles. Instead, his speech was read to the convention. Finally in January 1978, Dr. Jackson was honored posthumously by his alma mater, Michigan State University's veterinary school. On that winter day, Lois Jackson drove the fifty miles from her home to East Lansing where, at the university's Kellogg Center, she accepted for her husband the coveted Alumni Award plaque. The belated honor took Lois Jackson by surprise, partly because her husband had been unsparingly critical of the establishment's reluctance and inability to help solve the PBB problem, including Michigan State University. "The state never moved in on this; it was hoping it'd go away," Dr. Jackson had said. "And Michigan State University—it has some of the best people in the world. But they were so intertwined with teaching that they couldn't be broken loose to get into the field and follow through on a problem the size of the PBB one."

If Ted Jackson had lived longer, he most likely would have played a central role in exposing the policies of the government and the Farm Bureau Services that allowed the PBB contamination to continue even after its discovery. Instead, that burden fell on the broad shoulders of a stocky red-haired veterinarian 135 miles to the north by the name of Alpha ("just like in the Bible") Clark, Jr.

But to all who knew him, he was simply Doc Clark, an unassuming and easygoing but hardworking man with simple tastes. His favorite leisure activities, in fact, were spotting deer at night and, when not working during the day, watching healthy animals graze in the rolling expanse of north central Michigan, where he grew up and decided to settle down with his pretty bride, Marlene, after obtaining his degree in 1958 from Michigan State University. "I wouldn't trade the view I have out my window for a million bucks," he is fond of saying.

But starting in late 1973, Doc Clark suddenly had less and less time to admire grazing animals or to "shine" deer. Too many of his clients were calling to report health problems among their cattle. Dr. Clark's Tri-County Veterinary Clinic is located just outside McBain, a community of five hundred in Missaukee County, on Route 66 where the two-lane highway takes an abrupt ninety-degree turn to the west heading into town. Although Dr. Clark spends the hour from one to two

95

each afternoon in his clinic treating household pets, most of his clients are dairy farmers, many of whom live in the neighboring counties of Mecosta and Osceola. So that normally requires the animal doctor's spending a huge chunk of his time merely getting from one farm to another, depending on where the calls come from. But 1974 proved to be the busiest year of his life, as he put almost a hundred thousand miles on his white-and-rust-colored, station-wagon–sized El Camino pickup truck, which held his tools and medicine.

The animal health problems began in late 1973 when many cows suddenly became extremely difficult to breed; others failed to respond to normal treatment after developing routine infections. Early into 1974, a growing number of Dr. Clark's 150 or so clients began calling more and more often to report problems: lots of abortions, physical degeneration after calving, digestive problems. And on and on. Dr. Clark began performing postmortems, and many enlarged livers turned up—"some were like pumpkin pies," he recalled with a grimace, as he closed his hand into a fist. By spring, many cows became lame. Yet Dr. Clark was helpless. He had no idea what was causing all those problems. Having exhausted his veterinary repertoire and being still unable to cure the animals, Dr. Clark nearly considered quitting his practice. "I knew something was wrong, but I didn't know what." In May, on a television news broadcast, he learned that some livestock in southwestern Michigan had been contaminated by a chemical known as PBB. It was the first time he had heard the strange name. But soon he put it out of his mind, especially after the local feed co-op assured farmers in the area that none of the contaminated feed had reached north central Michigan. And besides, now that spring had arrived many of the health problems likely would abate, Dr. Clark thought, since cows normally are more prone to infections and other illnesses in the winter, due partly to their being confined in barns for so long. Once they could start grazing outdoors again, things would return to normal. But the problems only got worse. "I never had a spring like 1974," Dr. Clark, forty-three, recalls.

He was a depressed man when he arrived at the farm of Jake Kamphouse in late May. They discussed the problems that were still going around. Could it be bad feed—perhaps containing that chemical PBB? Dr. Clark wondered out loud. Why, no, Kamphouse replied, producing a May 17 letter he had received from the Falmouth-McBain-Merritt Cooperative. The letter, addressed to "All concerned dairy farmers," said the co-op has "NEVER handled this number [#402] feed. We appreciate your patronage and intend to continue giving you good service with a good feed." The one-page letter added, "The feed plant at Battle Creek is producing '100%' clean feed now and has been for some time." A similarly worded letter was sent by Donald A. Shepard, manager of Farm Bureau Services' feed department, to the organization's eighty-seven dealer outlets around the state for distribution.

Farm Bureau Services made its claim that all its feeds were "100% clean" after yet another cleanup effort at its giant feed plant in Climax, near Battle Creek. What the letters conveniently neglected to mention, however, was the reason why another cleanup was even necessary: the discovery that feeds being produced at the plant continued to be contaminated by PBB residues that clung tenaciously to the mixing equipment. The claim by the Falmouth-McBain-Merritt co-op that it "NEVER" handled contaminated feed also turned out to be wishful thinking, as tests later showed.

Doc Clark, after reading the letter Kamphouse had shown him, dismissed the idea that many of the animal problems in his clients' herds might be caused by this exotic chemical. He had no reason not to believe the letter. Yet the health problems among the cattle persisted into the summer. Garry Zuiderveen's herd in Falmouth, which had an annual average of fifteen thousand pounds of milk per cow, now was down to under twelve thousand pounds. His nephew, Kenneth Zuiderveen, just down the road, was experiencing an 85 percent calf mortality rate, in addition to similar losses in milk production. Jim and Mary Van Haitsma had to cull six of their highest milk producers after they suddenly stopped making milk. Whereas two calves had died in 1971 and again in 1972, and three in 1973, seventeen calves had died in 1974—by spring. The annual per-cow milk output dropped from sixteen thousand pounds in 1972 to a rate below fourteen thousand pounds. Yet neither the Zuiderveens nor the Van Haitsmas had bought the dairy #402 feed that Rick Halbert liked to use. In October 1973, they did buy a 55 percent protein dairy supplement from the local co-op to use as a top dressing in parlor feed. The cows, however, refused to eat it. The co-op then took back the feed and mixed it with shelled corn and some other ingredients, and returned it to the farmers. The cows eventually ate the stuff, Jim Van Haitsma recalls, "but it took them an hour to eat what they normally would eat in ten minutes."

In August, Dr. Clark went to judge a livestock show at the Newaygo County Fair in Fremont, a dairy community about two hours' drive southwest of McBain and one of the areas then thought to be among the hardest hit by the PBB contamination. Judging such a show was great fun for an animal lover like Alpha Clark. And while there, he chatted with some of the area's dairymen about PBB, and a few took him out to their farms to show him what PBB could do to once robust animals. "When I left Fremont, I knew what was wrong. And I was scared to death. I said nothing for six weeks, except to Marlene," Dr. Clark recalls. He was still pondering the chilling similarities between the PBB-contaminated cows in Newaygo County and the sick cows in his own area when a distraught dairyman called him. "Three of Clarence Martin's cows were down in their free stalls, couldn't get up. The whole herd was stiff and lame," Dr. Clark recalls. He was able to get them on their feet again, but they failed to improve otherwise. In mid-September, Dr. Clark heard that PBB had been found in James Kohler's dairy herd in Cadillac, only about fifteen miles west of McBain. When he learned that Kohler had bought his feed from Saginaw in the eastern part of Michigan and not from Battle Creek in the southwest, he became frightened. Could PBB perhaps have contaminated the feeds purchased by farmers all over the state, including in Missaukee, Osceola and Mecosta counties? Dr. Clark decided to learn for himself. In the meantime, another of Dr. Clark's clients, Harvey Winkle, had sent two cows he suspected of PBB poisoning to Michigan State University's animal health diagnostic laboratory to be sacrificed for studies. But only one of the animals actually had to be killed. The other dropped dead upon arrival. Analyses later showed both had significant levels of PBB. "Now I know PBB was in our area," Dr. Clark said at the time.

He began systematically collecting milk samples from bulk tanks to be analyzed for PBB. Five out of the first six samples had detectable amounts of the chemical. And so, after all this time, the angry veterinarian fumed, PBB indeed had poisoned farm animals in areas much larger than the public was led to believe by Farm Bureau Services and the Michigan Department of Agriculture. Next Dr. Clark began regularly taking fat samples from cows for PBB analysis. Because the chemical tends to concentrate in fat, tissue analysis is a better indicator of PBB presence than milk analysis. A fat biopsy involves a relatively minor surgical incision near the base of the tail in order to remove a chunk of fat. Dr. Clark had never performed a fat biopsy before, and the first time he did it took almost an hour. But before long he mastered the technique and learned to perform the operation in a matter of minutes. By now, Dr. Clark and many of his client dairymen had become extremely suspicious of the farm co-op and the Agriculture Department. So they did more than just send these fat tissues to the state laboratory for PBB analysis. They also split each sample in two, and sent the split sample to private laboratories for independent analysis. Although results of such sensitive chemical analyses indeed can vary slightly from laboratory to laboratory—and even from technician to technician—the private laboratories' results invariably came back reporting higher PBB levels than the Department of Agriculture laboratory. "In some cases, the deviation was dramatic, differing by up to ten times higher than the state results," according to Edie Clark, a special assistant on PBB affairs to the Speaker of the Michigan House of Representatives, Bobby D. Crim. In other instances, the private laboratories detected PBB in samples that the Department of Agriculture said were free of PBB. Among the private laboratories used by Dr. Clark and his clients were the Wisconsin Alumni Research Foundation in Madison, Wisconsin, and the Environmental Research Group in Ann Arbor, Michigan.

"I seen Dr. [Charles] Cole [of the Agriculture Department] on television the other night," said a farmer from Sturgis, "and he said their tests was the same as these other [private laboratory] tests. But I have several tests at home to show that where it was tested in WARF it showed problems—which was on the same cattle which would not show at the Michigan state [Department of Agriculture]. So I think there's a little crooked work going on some place." Another farmer, from Sears, added, "We tested thirty-two cows. We sent in every sample into the state. The first two showed traces. After that we never showed another trace. Then we sent the same samples to WARF: fourteen of them showed traces." (Such discrepancies continued for years. As late as 1976, for instance, Falmouth dairyman Roy Tacoma sent split samples from ten cows to the state laboratory and to WARF. The state found PBB in six of the samples; WARF discovered PBB in nine. And in one case, the cow could have been sold for meat based on the state result but not on the WARF result.)

Interestingly, the Wisconsin laboratory as a standard practice forwarded the results of its analyses to the Department of Agriculture in Lansing. Yet the department ignored the results even when they showed a cow to be contaminated at levels above the federal tolerance guideline—meaning that the entire herd from which such a cow tissue had come should be quarantined. The department told Edie Clark it did nothing because it considered such samples "unofficial" unless collected by a licensed veterinarian. "Still," Clark wrote later in a report, "whether or not an 'official' sample was ever collected was usually up to the farmer. In many cases, whether or not a farm was ever quarantined was voluntary and up to the farmer." Even Donald R. Isleib, chief deputy agriculture director, had to admit that such was the case. "It is impossible to identify every herd which might have ingested Farm Bureau feed," he said. The Department of Agriculture's refusal even to follow up on WARF's test results illuminated yet another major inconsistency in the department's handling of the disaster. "Although the Wisconsin lab reports were not considered good enough to impose a quarantine," said Edie Clark, "the same information was considered good enough by the department to release animals from quarantine." This dichotomous government policy, however, did not make Farm Bureau Services unhappy since the upshot minimized the farm co-op's liability by keeping down the number of animals quarantined and, ultimately, slaughtered.

By the spring of 1975, Dr. Clark had become a bitter and disillusioned man. A lifelong conservative Republican, he had "thought it was the worst thing in the world when the kids demonstrated against the government" during the years of U.S. involvement in Southeast Asia; now he was convinced of a deliberate government effort to cover up the extent of the contamination in order to protect the Michigan Farm Bureau, an influential interest group in Michigan, especially with the Republican party, led by Governor Milliken. In late April, when Dr. Clark was interviewed by a central Michigan television station, he openly expressed this belief. "I called it a cover-up. I implicated Milliken, Farm Bureau, the Food and Drug Administration, the Michigan Department of Agriculture all in the

cover-up. And I talked about my concern for human health."
Before the month was out, a sympathetic state veterinarian told
Dr. Clark, "MDA is out after your ass." Dr. Clark, taken aback,
didn't know what to make of the remark or its meaning, and the
state veterinarian did not elaborate. He was more concerned
with finding ways to restore the health of his clients' animals,
which he and the farmers now realized had been poisoned by
PBB. Obviously, they didn't consider going to the Agriculture
Department for help. Rather, Dr. Clark contacted a scientist at
Purdue University in Indiana, Farrell Robinson, who agreed to
conduct some experiments using a total of eighteen cows. And
in late July and early August, Dr. Clark arranged to have the
cows transported to Lafayette, Indiana.

In mid-December, Doc and Marlene Clark drove to
Lafayette to meet with Dr. Robinson to discuss the Indiana
scientist's work. The most interesting information Dr. Clark
learned was that federal investigators had been around to see
Dr. Robinson, asking questions about him. Later Frank Spies,
the U.S. attorney for the western district of Michigan, confirmed that Dr. Clark was under investigation for possible
violation of interstate shipment laws involving the transportation of livestock "without proper documentation." Spies said the
fact that the cows may have had PBB was not a factor in the
investigation. Dr. Clark was stunned, for he had obtained
permission to ship the cattle to Purdue over the telephone from
Dr. Charles H. Cole, chief assistant state veterinarian. But now
agriculture director B. Dale Ball said no one had given such
permission. Moreover, the Agriculture Department began
threatening to take away Dr. Clark's license. But Dr. Clark filed a
counter suit, charging a conspiracy to violate his civil rights.
The fiasco finally ended in May 1976 when Spies said Dr. Clark
would not be prosecuted. "Even if we could prove a violation,
and there is some question, prosecution was not warranted,"
Spies said. Dr. Robinson's studies at Purdue showed that many
of the sick animals' symptoms were "probably due to PBB."

Like Dr. Tom Corbett, the Ann Arbor anesthesiologist,
Alpha S. Clark, Jr., was a resilient fellow, and he continued
trying to warn the public that the PBB contamination still had
not been effectively contained—due largely to a "cover-up" by
Farm Bureau Services and the Agriculture Department. But
few people were interested. Watergate was over, and Jerry Ford,
a native Michiganian, had ushered in a new era of good

101

feelings. Indeed, despite the intermittent press coverage, most people in Michigan—even a full year after PBB had been discovered in their food supply—didn't really know what the PBB fuss was all about; and most of those who did know assumed that it was largely a farm problem that had been taken care of by the government. Thus the life of Alpha Clark took on an uncanny resemblance to that of Dr. Stockmann, the fictitious physician in Ibsen's *An Enemy of the People*. In that drama, the doctor discovers the water of the health spa for which the town is famous to be dangerously contaminated. Alarmed, Dr. Stockmann attempts to publicize his discovery of the health hazard. But instead of receiving public accolades from his fellow townspeople for having performed a public service, he is denounced by the establishment, for whom the news is highly inopportune, as the real-life doctor would learn years later, in a painful, humiliating way.

But if Dr. Clark's attacks on Farm Bureau Services were largely ignored, and perhaps a bit stridently delivered, they also confirmed the suspicions about the co-op harbored by the late Ted F. Jackson.

After the contamination became known, the farm co-op, in attempting to allay public fears, announced that it had begun a "massive recall" of the suspected #402 feed even before PBB was identified. That recall, according to Donald R. Armstrong, executive vice-president of Farm Bureau Services, was initiated in mid-January, right after the second set of mice-feeding experiments done by Dr. Gatzmeyer of the Department of Agriculture and four months before PBB was discovered. Ken Jones, the feed company's risk manager, said only five or six farmers in Michigan had purchased the contaminated #402 feed and that "with the exception of a very few pounds, we got it all back." But when the Detroit *Free Press* checked the veracity of Jones's claim it found evidence to the contrary. Five out of six farmers told the *Free Press* they never heard of a recall.

Farm Bureau Services also said it made a second massive recall in the spring of 1974, after the mix-up came to light. This recall, Jones said, included all Farm Bureau Services feeds that had called for magnesium oxide as an ingredient. "Every farmer in the state [who had purchased such feeds] should have been contacted," Jones said. "And we think we did as good a job as humanly possible." Yet when the *Free Press* checked with fifteen such farmers, eleven said they were never contacted in the second "massive" recall. Some of the eleven, in fact, got letters assuring them that the feed company's products now were "100% clean." One farmer, Keith Johnson of Newaygo, for instance, told the reporters that his contaminated feed was not recalled even after his farm was quarantined. Johnson finally buried the feed on his own land. When *Free Press* reporters Kathy Warbelow and Ellen Grzech confronted Jones with such discrepancies, he replied, "What can I say?"

As a result of its two "massive" recalls, Farm Bureau Services eventually recovered 45 tons of the contaminated dairy feed #402. But between March and December of 1973, the company had made 535 tons of it. Also, the distribution of the contaminated feed was prolonged by the Food and Drug Administration because it did not follow its customary procedure involving the recall of a livestock feed contaminated by toxic chemicals. Ordinarily, in such cases, the agency would issue a Class I recall, accompanied by enough publicity to attract "concentrated news media coverage." But in the PBB episode the agency merely took Farm Bureau Services' word that two "massive" recalls already had been initiated and were nearly completed, admits Sam D. Fine, the FDA's associate commissioner for compliance. And so he said he considered it "doubtful that further publicity would serve any useful purpose" and decided the agency should not issue any press releases at all about the recall.

If Farm Bureau Services' recall attempts were less than effective, its efforts to clean up its Climax feed plant produced even unhappier results. Because of its electrostatic properties, PBB adheres tenaciously to solids such as metals, soils and concrete—just about everything it came in contact with. Each time the chemical was mixed into feed and moved through the production system at the feed plant, traces of PBB clung to metal surfaces from which the chemical would be slowly taken up by subsequent feeds. Thus from the time PBB was first mixed into livestock feed in the summer of 1973, all subsequent feeds—whether or not their formulas called for magnesium oxide as an ingredient—became contaminated with PBB. Feeds that called for magnesium oxide were contaminated directly by the substitution of Firemaster FF-1 for the prescribed magnesium oxide; and feeds that followed such a mix would pick up PBB residues as they went through the same equipment. And so countless amounts of feed were contaminated and distributed all over Michigan. Yet, this secondary, or cross-contamination did not stop with the discovery of the PBB-magnesium oxide mix-up, since Farm Bureau Services failed to anticipate such a phenomenon until subsequent feed analyses showed that feeds continued to be contaminated by PBB. Even with such information in hand, however, the company merely undertook another cleanup and then, without immediately knowing that effort's efficacy, sent out letters assuring customers such as Jake Kamphouse that its feed was now "100% clean."

As a result of such a dubious policy, for instance, feed analyzed at the McBain co-op as late as September of 1974—four months after PBB was identified as the contaminant—would reveal high concentrations of the chemical. One particular feed, known as #410, which Rick Halbert also had analyzed, contained as much PBB as 1.1 parts per million. "That feed," said Dr. Clark, "was maybe the most used Farm Bureau Services feed by dairymen in Michigan. It was sold up and down the state. Once I knew that, I knew everyone in Michigan was polluted."

The likelihood of sustained PBB cross-contamination at the Farm Bureau Services plant also was not appreciated by the U.S. Food and Drug Administration, which certainly had previous knowledge of this phenomenon at the facility involving another substance. As early as December 1971, shortly after the plant opened, an FDA inspection found that nonmedicated feeds were being cross-contaminated with medicated feeds containing DES, or diethylstilbestrol. The problem: inadequate cleaning of equipment between batches of different medicated and nonmedicated feeds. As a result, Farm Bureau Services closed its plant to clean all processing equipment, including the storage bins that held DES feeds. It also flushed three to six tons of soy meal through the system after the medicated feed mix in order to pick up DES residues. The soy meal then was stored in a special bin until the next time the DES feed was to be mixed. The only trouble with this procedure was that it was inadequate. An FDA follow-up inspection on February 25, 1972, revealed that nonmedicated feeds were still being contaminated by DES. In May 1974, the federal regulatory agency visited the feed plant again for a three-day inspection after the PBB mix-up was discovered and found numerous shortcomings. These included inadequate measures to avoid cross-contamination of nonmedicated feeds with medicated feeds, a significant build-up of residue materials in various pieces of equipment, open bags of antibiotics and other unlabeled bags of ingredients being stored in the raw materials storage area, and discrepancies in drug records. More than eight months later, on the last day of January 1975, Farm Bureau Services officers met with the FDA at an informal hearing to discuss the problems found during the 1974 inspection. Farm Bureau Services pleaded with the agency for leniency and forgiveness, saying that it hoped that the FDA would not prosecute someone "just for the sake of prosecution." One co-op official said his company had "suffered enough," referring to the PBB disaster. Farm Bureau Services got off the hook. Two months later, the Food and Drug Administration conducted several follow-up inspections at the plant and again found numerous "deviations," such as the lack of manufacturing instructions on master formula records for medicated feeds, no production formula records for each specific batch of medicated feed and no records to show the performance of each step in the process of making animal feeds. In plain view of government inspectors, metal cans holding drug components and other feed additives were labeled only on their removable lids. The FDA inspection report also noted, "The feed conveying system between different pieces of equipment was not designed to prevent low level contamination of feeds."

And so despite such federal government inpections that might have sounded the alert for the cross-contamination of PBB, the feed company was allowed to continue doing business as usual.

The supreme irony is that Farm Bureau Services itself became a direct victim of the cross-contamination phenomenon. On May 6, Rick Halbert, disregarding Dr. Jackson's advice, returned most of his contaminated dairy #402 feed to the feed company. In order to bag it, Farm Bureau Services ran the feed through its entire system at its plant in Climax. To avoid the cross-contamination effect, plant workers ran a load of flush material through the entire system after Halbert's feed was processed. That same day, Farm Bureau Services, which operates an egg marketing division, decided to provide all the feed for its three hundred thousand chickens from its own feed plant rather than from sources in localities around the state where the chickens are kept. A load of urea then was run through the system after the flush material presumably had picked up the PBB residues that clung to the equipment from Halbert's feed. Soon it became apparent that such flushing did no good, for all three hundred thousand chickens became heavily contaminated and had to be destroyed. The bagging of other returned dairy #402 feed in this same manner undoubtedly intensified the cross-contamination effect.

Interestingly, the state Department of Agriculture never ordered Farm Bureau Services to clean up its facility. When FDA inspectors finally raised the possibility of cross-contamination involving PBB residues, one Farm Bureau Services plant official replied that the Michigan Department of Agriculture had been analyzing feeds for PBB contamination but that no "violative" samples turned up. That meant, of course, PBB indeed was showing up and cross-contaminating feeds that the plant produced for quite some time after the original mix-up was discovered. But it is not known how some "violative" feeds ended up being sold instead of destroyed. Yet sold they were, as Alpha Clark learned when feed at the McBain co-op as late as September of 1974 was contaminated at more than twenty times the legal limit.

Farm Bureau Services' first major cleanup attempt occurred during Mother's Day weekend in early May of 1974, when men used powerful air hoses to blow away PBB residues that clung to metal surfaces. Ironically, this effort backfired because during the hosing the plant's giant circulation fans were on, so that PBB residues were picked up by the air currents and carried to other places throughout the plant. And nobody even thought to clean those areas for months.

It was right after this "cleanup" that the feed company sent out letters, such as the one farmer Jake Kamphouse showed to his veterinarian, Dr. Clark, claiming that all its feeds were now "100% clean." But on May 23, a week after such letters were mailed, Farm Bureau Services got results back on feeds that were collected and analyzed for PBB after its Mother's Day weekend effort. Feeds taken from fifty-seven out of sixty-one bins were still contaminated, and at levels ranging from 100 to 800 parts per billion. (The Food and Drug Administration did not establish a PBB tolerance guideline for feed until late June, when it banned feed with more than 300 parts per billion. In November, the agency reduced the level to 50 parts per billion. Nearly two years later, the Michigan legislature dropped the level still further to 10 parts per billion.) Five days after Farm Bureau Services got the feed results back, its executive vice-

106

president, Donald R. Armstrong, telephoned B. Dale Ball, director of the Michigan Department of Agriculture. The ensuing conversation, which later came to light, reinforced the suspicions of many people, including Alpha Clark, that the two organizations were engaged in a cover-up. Ball was out of his office on the afternoon of May 28 when Armstrong called. But when he returned that evening, he found a message on his desk to call Armstrong. And so he called Armstrong at home. They discussed the continuing contamination of feeds coming out of the company's plant in Climax, and how its customers might react if they discovered they were still buying contaminated feeds the co-op claimed were "100% clean." When asked about the conversation several years later, Armstong at first denied that it had even taken place. But his memory improved when his own notes from that conversation were produced by lawyers representing a farmer suing the company for selling him such contaminated feeds. Armstrong's notes from the 8:45 P.M. discussion included this passage: "Discuss last Thursday [May 23] problem—indicated customers could come back on department and us if they knew we produced feeds after knowing we had contamination in equipment." But Ball had a different version of that conversation. "I told him if he did something like that [sell PBB contaminated feeds while saying they were "100% clean"] he'd be liable for prosecution, and we would look bad and that it was a bad thing to do from the standpoint of the Farm Bureau and the Department of Agriculture. I advised him not to do it," Ball recalls. But Armstrong apparently did not heed Ball's advice. The company's risk manager, Ken Jones, later admitted when asked if the company indeed had knowingly sold contaminated feed while telling its customers otherwise: "We knew there was contamination there. But we went ahead and shipped it. Right."

Shortly after his night-time telephone conversation with Ball, Armstrong composed an eight-page "Current Position Statement" sent to local Farm Bureau presidents throughout the state. Referring to another cleanup attempt, which took place over the long Memorial Day weekend, the statement said, "All feeds have been tested and given a clean bill of health by the Michigan Department of Agriculture.... Since the total cleanup operation has been completed and certified by the MDA, all feeds now manufactured at Battle Creek [meaning Climax] are completely clean." Armstrong's wishful thinking once more was shattered when results came back on feed

107

samples showing PBB at levels up to 310 parts per billion. The samples had been collected not only at its main feed plant but also at Farm Bureau co-ops around the state. Among the highly contaminated feeds was dairy #410 from six different locations, including Dexter, where the family of Sarah Robinett lives.

And on June 28, a month after his conversation with Armstrong, Ball's department released a four-page PBB "fact sheet," telling the public that "MDA and FBS [Farm Bureau Services] are monitoring PBB levels in current lots of feed. Both feel that no further significant contamination is occurring." And the co-op never withdrew or even modified any of its reassuring letters to farmers all over Michigan. Indeed the company cleaned its plant at least ten times in 1974 and each time sent out such reassuring letters afterward. Not once did the company explain why so many cleanup efforts were necessary in the first place. The cleanup efforts involved the dismantling of some equipment, and even replacing certain parts, or scraping off encrustations. Often the process involved sandblasting, steam cleaning and industrial vacuuming. But nothing seemed to work. Storage bins seldom were emptied or cleaned entirely before new feed batches were mixed; thus new clean feeds became contaminated by remnants of previous contaminated batches that remained in the bins. PBB was found in elevators, mixers, grinders, mills, carts, buckets, scoops, troughs, mangers, bunks and other feed-handling equipment as well as in the bins themselves. The stuff was everywhere and no amount of cleaning seemed to get rid of it.

And so the company kept selling contaminated feeds to unsuspecting farmers. The farmers fed the stuff to their animals. And the animals passed the PBB on to consumers— but not before the chemical had contaminated everything it touched along the way before coming to rest in human blood and fatty tissues, there to remain forever. In this manner, PBB became so pervasive and widespread in the Michigan environment that the Food and Drug Administration eventually was forced to admit that PBB somehow had become an "unavoidable" contaminant in the food supply of at least 9 million citizens.

Ultimately, the Michigan Department of Agriculture, by testing feed samples from nearly three hundred outlets that handled Farm Bureau Services products, managed to track down nine hundred tons of contaminated feed. At such outlets, PBB was found not only in feed and the equipment but also in the beams and even on the loading docks. The nine hundred tons of feed were destroyed, but it is unknown how much contaminated feed escaped confiscation and, instead, were eaten by farm animals. In all, forty-five hundred Michigan farmers are known to have purchased Farm Bureau Services feeds during the critical years. But that figure does not represent the unknown number of additional farmers who bought feeds on a cash-and-carry basis, a procedure that did not have the benefit of invoices. Also unknown is the quantity of Farm Bureau Services' franchised products—ultimately sold without obvious Farm Bureau Services identification—that contained PBB as a result of cross-contamination. These products include Manna Mate, a special feed for young calves containing a mixture of corn, oats and molasses; and Aureomycin Crumbles, an antibiotic mixed with alfalfa meal sold by American Cyanamid of New Jersey, among the country's biggest chemical manufacturers.

Among the many Michigan farmers who used Aureomycin Crumbles was Tom Butler, a tall balding man of forty-two who had farmed in Gregory, near Ann Arbor, since high school. He used the medicated feed occasionally to correct minor sinus infections and lung congestion problems in some of his adult sixty cows. Shortly after he used the Crumbles in the fall of 1974, Butler noticed that many of the cows suddenly became highly irritable. Then the milk production began dropping significantly, followed by many other symptoms: curled hooves, infections that did not respond to treatment, breeding problems, emaciation, hair loss and death. Soon Butler, his wife and four teenage children began suffering health problems as well. But Michigan State University dairy scientists first told Butler and his brother-in-law, Ron Thomas, who owned an adjoining farm, that the animal problems were caused by low protein silage; later they said excessive iodine in the feed was the cause. When Butler and Thomas finally had a fat sample from one of their cows tested, a "low level" of PBB— 50 parts per billion—showed up. But they were told by state officials that such a level was nothing to be concerned about. "We were peasants and they're the experts. So we never thought of questioning them," Butler recalls. It wasn't until early 1976 that Butler, while reading several back issues of the *Michigan Farmer* magazine, was struck by the similarities between his ailing herd and those of other farmers who also had "low level" PBB contamination. Butler and Thomas together began speaking out at public forums, warning about the dangers of even small amounts of PBB. But as Richard Lehnert, editor of *Michigan Farmer*, wrote in an article about Butler and Thomas, "For families who claim adverse health effects from their exposure to PBB, probably the most devastating 'symptom' they face is the loss of their credibility. Officials at public agencies who are supposed to help them walk away in disbelief." A year later, only Thomas continued speaking out. "I'm done testifying at hearings. If they want to eat poison, let them eat it," a disgusted Butler said. "I don't blame Farm Bureau Services and never have. It was an accident. But I can't accept what these agencies have done and how they've treated us. The kids all learned 'God Bless America' at this table. This is contrary to everything we've tried to imbed in our kids."

Just before PBB struck, Butler, who owned 370 acres and rented another 130, bought 440 acres of land in Michigan's upper peninsula community of Carney, near the Wisconsin border. He hoped to move eventually to Carney because of the encroaching civilization from Ann Arbor to the southeast and from Lansing to the northwest. "Things were going so well for us. We were even thinking about buying an airplane so we could make the trip to the U.P. [upper peninsula] easier while we got the farm ready there. We really had the world by the tail," Butler said. Then PBB poisoned his farm. "The kids were getting bigger and yet we were getting less done. I really knew something was wrong when Sean, who had been looking forward all year to playing football, decided not to. He just couldn't run," Butler said. One morning Butler approached his fourteen-year-old son from behind, grabbed him by the shoulders, spun him around and asked, "What's wrong with you? Are you on dope or something?" Tests later showed that Sean's fatty tissues contained 590 parts per billion of the chemical. Butler himself had 410 parts per billion in his tissues. And in March 1976, he was turned down for additional life insurance coverage by the Harvest Life Insurance Company in Cleveland because of the PBB in his body. An internal company memorandum said, "Unfortunately the above case was declined at this time due to findings of bromide ingestion from which the applicant is having numerous present problems (including severe fatigue to the point of disability). We will, however, be happy to reconsider in one year when the permanent effects can be evaluated."

# 8
# A QUESTION OF HOW MUCH

The struggle of living things against cancer is as old as time, yet our awareness of the causes of cancer has been slow to develop. As early as the first century A.D., Pliny the Elder, touring the Roman provinces, confirmed reports by the first-century Greek geographer Strabo that slaves who wove asbestos into treasured robes for priests and burial garments for the nobility were suffering from a strange and acute form of lung disease; nearly two thousand years later, society learned a label for the ailment: asbestosis, an irreversible, lung-scarring disease that often is fatal. But for centuries the medical specialty we now call occupational health remained a mundane and esoteric field few scientists chose.

During the Italian Renaissance, however, Bernardino Ramazzini, a professor of medicine at the University of Parma, began a systematic study of occupational diseases. In 1692, Professor Ramazzini, nearly sixty years old, was snooping around the sixty-foot wells near Modena trying to find clues to explain that city's frequent typhus epidemics. He stumbled upon a worker who was nearly frenetic as he cleaned out the municipal cesspool. "No one who has not tried it can imagine what it costs to stay more than four hours in this place. It is the same thing as being struck blind," the worker told Ramazzini. When the workman finished his chore and came up from the cesspool pit, the professor was taken back by his bloodshot eyes. Ramazzini asked him whether cleaners of privies used any remedy. "They go back at once to their homes, as I shall presently do," the worker replied, "shut themselves in a dark room, stay there for a day and bathe their eyes now and then with lukewarm water; by this means they are able to relieve the pain somewhat." The professor's uncharted excursion into the sewers of Modena led to eight years of studying forty-two

111

work-related diseases. In 1700, *The Diseases of Workers,* his work, was published in several languages. But it gained almost no attention.

Seventy-five years later in London, a physician named Percivall Pott discovered what probably was the first clinical evidence of a work-related cancer. After studying the high incidence of cancer among chimneysweeps, Dr. Pott declared that their scrotal cancers were caused by soot. A giant step had been taken to increase awareness that external or environmental agents could cause malignancies. Dr. Pott had found that many chimneysweeps, often as little boys when they first were lowered into their soot-filled workplaces, would develop scrotal cancers even before they reached age thirty. At the time, however, Dr. Pott was unable to furnish the "proof" that today's scientists would demand. And so for the next century there was little further recognition that chemicals in the environment could cause cancer after repeated contact. To be sure, a high prevalence of skin cancer would be detected among arsenic workers exposed to fumes in copper smelters and tin foundries in Cornwall and Wales; and it also would be noticed that workers in the cobalt mines of Saxony and the pitchblende mines of Bohemia suffered a high rate of lung disease, later identified as cancer. Yet these were seen as aberrations— perhaps as phenomena of the pre-Industrial Age, before the blossoming of industries whose products and by-products would invade the environment of every living thing—and even things as yet unborn.

And so it was not until the Industrial Revolution that hazardous working conditions began gaining public attention, perhaps because the deplorable working conditions now had come to involve many more people as masses of laborers congregated in factory towns all across Europe and the United States. Starting in the last quarter of the nineteenth century, then, the notion began taking hold that cancers are traceable to the age of industry. Each step toward modernization, each piece of technological wonder that advanced civilization seemed to come at the cost of workers' lives and well-being. By the turn of the twentieth century, a half dozen sources of industrial carcinogens, or cancer-causing substances, became known. Civilization had entered a new era in which man, alone of all forms of life, learned to create cancer-producing substances. Later, another notion took hold: The unwitting introduction of such

112

carcinogens into the environment would threaten all living organisms.

To prevent or minimize exposure of human populations to carcinogens, then, scientists must use laboratory animal experiments to predict a substance's potential to cause human cancers or other illnesses. However, until recent years, control or regulation of a substance (such as asbestos) was not instituted until human evidence developed, such as the scrotal cancers Dr. Pott saw among chimney workers. And that clearly is an unacceptable means of assessing public health risks. The critical question, then, is whether or not tests of substances using laboratory animals predict accurately for man. The answer is yes, although it is still being disputed obstinately by scientists working for the petrochemical industries. After all, animals are our last line of defense against invisible man-made carcinogens and other toxic chemicals. "Basic biological processes of those molecular, cellular, tissue and organ functions that control life are strikingly similar from one mammalian species to another," says Dr. David P. Rall, director of the National Institute of Environmental Health Sciences. As he and others point out, every chemical known to cause cancer in humans, with possibly two exceptions, also causes cancer in animals. It also is important to note that numerous agents (such as 4-aminobiphenyl, diethylstilbestrol, mustard gas, vinyl chloride, bis-chloromethyl ether and aflatoxin) were first shown to be carcinogenic in laboratory animals before tragic evidence developed later to demonstrate that they also cause cancer in man. "The scientific community—and the downstream lawyers and politicians—are beginning to believe that animals tests do predict for carcinogenicity in man," says Dr. Rall, who has extensive experience in comparative pharmacology, cancer chemotherapy, pesticide toxicology and drug research. "The only alternative to animal testing today is human testing—allow the chemical on the market and await the results," adds Gus Speth, a member of the U.S. Council on Environmental Quality and chairman of President Carter's toxic substances strategy committee. "That's been the pattern to date, and the drawbacks are serious," Speth writes. "It typically takes cancer from fifteen to forty years to show up after exposure. By the time the carcinogen has been positively identified, many thousands may have already contracted cancer." Speth and others deplore the popular perception—fueled by industry spokesmen—that "any chemical in massive doses will cause cancer in test animals." "This is flatly false," Speth says. "The ability to cause cancer is a relatively rare phenomenon exhibited by only a small portion of the many hundreds of thousands of chemicals. To date, less than twenty percent of over six thousand suspect chemicals have been found to cause cancer. Most chemicals are not even suspect."

The reasons for using large doses in testing a chemical are practical and economic ones—but with scientific validity. A two-year study involving six hundred animals costs between $150,000 and $300,000. So there are economic restrictions as to the number of rodents used. Thus the scientist must exaggerate the dose in order to produce enough cancers to lend statistical relevance to a chemical's effect upon the small population of test animals. "If low doses were used on a six-hundred-animal population," Speth said, "a carcinogenic effect that could cause thousands of cancers in a population of two hundred million could go entirely undetected in the test."

Is it proper and scientifically valid to extrapolate laboratory results on test animals to man? Again the answer is yes. Almost all known human carcinogens are carcinogenic in laboratory animals, says Dr. Rall. "And for at least six carcinogens with quantative human exposure data, the doses causing cancer in man and in the most sensitive laboratory animals are reasonably close."

Indeed man may have even more sensitivity than laboratory animals to certain substances. In an experimental analysis of the subchronic toxicity of about twenty cancer chemotherapeutic agents in laboratory animals and in man, according to Dr. Rall, the results suggest that "man may be up to ten times more sensitive than the typical small laboratory animals." Small animals tend to metabolize and excrete foreign substances, such as an organic chemical, more quickly than do larger mammals. Thus, higher body burdens of a chemical would develop in man over the years than in laboratory animals in the customary two-year experimental period. And since chemically induced cancers are believed to originate in one or a few cells, it should be remembered that man has hundreds of times more susceptible cells than a mouse or a rat. Arsenic, for instance, is associated with both skin and lung cancer in humans; yet it has not produced cancer in laboratory animals. "Thus there is clear historical evidence that if there is strong evidence that a chemical is carcinogenic in appropriate laboratory animal test

114

systems it must be treated as if it were carcinogenic in man," Dr. Rall asserts. "Laboratory animals do predict for human animals."

Laboratory experiments now are under way at the National Cancer Institute to ascertain the carcinogenicity of PBB. It simply is not known if PBB is a cancer-causing chemical because such tests have not been done before. Yet more than 9 million people in Michigan and perhaps elsewhere now carry the chemical in their blood, fatty tissues and bone marrow. Indeed if PBB turns out not to be carcinogenic, it would be the first chemical in a family known as halogenated aromatic hydrocarbons to be tested that is not a cancer-causing agent.

And so the real test tube is the state of Michigan, whose 9 million citizens unwittingly have become the guinea pigs in a ghastly and vast experiment into the effects of a toxic chemical on human beings. "What happened in Michigan is a natural experiment—a paradigm of environmental contamination," says Dr. Irving J. Selikoff, director of the Environmental Sciences Laboratory in New York City, which now is studying the effects of the disaster. "Since PBB was made for a limited time, in only one place, and the contamination seems still essentially limited to Michigan, we will have the opportunity to properly research the effects of a pollutant, comparing what happened to exposed people and to those who were not exposed." Dr. Maurice S. Reizen, Michigan's public health director, admits, "Yes, the people of Michigan are the guinea pigs. Who really knows what happens when PBB breaks down in the body? I don't. The jury is still out. The state has begun a long-term study, but those results won't be known for fifteen to twenty years. I'll give you my phone number."

But preliminary evidence from the laboratories already suggests that PBB indeed is a carcinogen. Dr. Renate D. Kimbrough, a well-known toxicologist at the U.S. Center for Disease Control, has found liver tumors that appear to be malignant in a small group of young rats exposed to a single dose of PBB. But the rats were sacrificed after fourteen months of life in order to get a quick picture about the potential carcinogenicity of PBB. Had the animals been allowed to live for the full twenty-four months, Dr. Kimbrough believes, the tumors would have become cancerous. It was largely Dr. Kimbrough's preliminary findings that prompted the National Cancer Institute to undertake a full-fledged PBB car-

115

cinogenicity test. But those results will not be known until late 1980 or perhaps early 1981. That study will use mice, which are considered more sensitive than rats to chemicals such as PBB, according to Dr. Arthur C. Upton, director of the National Cancer Institute (who happens to be a native of Michigan, although he left the state in 1951).

Millions of contaminated persons in Michigan have been struck, understandably, by the absence of any dramatic, sudden or even unusual symptoms or changes in their health. Yet the knowledge that PBB virtually does not leave the human body once it has entered can hardly be a comforting thought. Farmer Rick Halbert, for instance, has 6,200 parts per billion PBB in his fatty tissues, but he has experienced no medical problems over the years except a minor coordination problem with his left hand. Yet he is acutely aware of the chemical lurking in his body and admits to feeling "a little hot under the collar perhaps, but otherwise all right.... I basically feel all right—or at least I perceive that I do. This whole subject gets me sort of turning inside, you might say. It's a very emotionally disturbing issue, frankly."

Once the chemical enters the human body, it takes up residence forever; and there it accumulates. This process began in the summer of 1973 and continues today, since, for instance, milk from contaminated cows is still being diluted with clean milk and then sold to the public. The PBB intake, then, becomes a cumulative affair. Lodged in the body's fatty tissues, PBB could strike quickly when those reserves of fat are drawn upon, perhaps during times of stress. This is why the Food and Drug Administration has advised obese persons who are highly contaminated to avoid losing weight. But the fatty tissues not only serve as a place for the deposition of fat (which makes up 18 percent of human body weight); they also have many other vital functions with which the stored PBB may interfere. Fats are distributed in organs and tissues throughout the entire body, including in cell membranes; thus fat-soluble chemicals such as PBB are even stored in individual cells, where they are in a position to interfere with the most vital and necessary functions of oxidation and energy production and, perhaps as a result, to cause cells to become cancerous.

One of the most significant consequences of PBB, like its chemical relatives, may be its effect on the human liver, a marvelous and probably the body's most extraordinary organ.

The liver has no equal because of its versatility and the indispensable nature of its functions. And because it oversees so many important activities, even the slightest damage may bring unhappy results. The largest internal organ in vertebrates, the liver is a dark red gland that provides bile for the digestion of fats. The liver also stores iron, copper and many vitamins, and produces proteins essential for blood clotting. Its activities are so numerous that it generates a tremendous amount of heat, making it important in internal heat production. The liver is deeply involved in the metabolism of all the principal foodstuffs. It stores sugar in the form of glycogen and then releases it in carefully measured quantities as glucose to keep the blood sugar at a normal level; it maintains cholesterol at its proper level in the blood plasma; it inactivates the male and female hormones when they reach excessive levels. Without a properly functioning liver, then, the body may become defenseless against a countless variety of both man-made and naturally occurring poisons in the environment. Indeed in 1977, Dr. Selikoff's research team discovered grossly incompetent immune mechanisms of numerous Michigan farm residents highly contaminated by PBB. A year later, in a study of the state's general population, the New York scientists turned up an unexpected frequency of abnormal liver function tests that indicate the presence of liver disease. Thus an inability to resist diseases, including cancer, now is a worrisome prospect facing millions of people contaminated by PBB.

Cancer is a unique disease, considering its irreversibility, long latency period and unrestrained growth of cells. And the baffling question of what happens after the human body is exposed to a low level of chemical carcinogen is one of the most vexing that confronts modern society and its designated regulatory agencies, such as the Food and Drug Administration. The central question, in essence, is: If cancer is unique, then are the man-made agents that cause it also unique? In other words, are chemical carcinogens governed by the same rules that govern the metabolism of other foreign (but noncarcinogenic) substances? Or are they metabolized in such a way as to lead directly to a malignant tumor? Is there a "safe" level of exposure to a carcinogen? Toxicologists know that the human body is capable of coping with small amounts of poison. So they try to find a level at which the human defense system is swamped, or overloaded, leaving the body unprotected. This is

117

the so-called threshold level. Although the conservative view is that such thresholds do not exist for carcinogens, *Science* magazine, the respected weekly publication of the American Association for the Advancement of Science, believes that "an increasing number of scientists now argue that complex metabolic routes can minimize the danger from many carcinogens and that thesholds or no-effect levels can be observed in many cases." Such thinking, however, is worrisome to scientists such as Gus Speth of the Council on Environmental Quality. "We know that exceedingly small amounts of chemicals can cause cancer," he says. "Indeed, there is scientific uncertainty today on whether 'no effect' or safe exposure levels even exist for carcinogens. Despite this difference of opinion, there is broad agreement on this: So far, we have no scientific basis for setting a safe threshold dose for a carcinogen. Until such a scientific basis is demonstrated, if we have to make a mistake we should make a mistake in the direction of protecting public health. And that means we assume, for the present, that there is no safe level for a carcinogen. In a matter so grave as cancer, makers of social policy cannot wait for our scientists to give us the precision we would prefer in regulating hazardous chemicals. Until we have precise methods for determining chemical safety, prudence must prevail; we must regard suspect chemicals, indicted on the imperfect evidence of animal tests, guilty until proved innocent," Speth wrote in an Op-Ed page essay in *The New York Times* in 1978.

For all the talk about cancer, we still know abysmally little about this dreaded group of diseases, especially what happens within a cell to change its orderly multiplication into a process of wild and uncontrolled proliferation we call cancer. But theories about the causes and origins of cancer abound. One of the most cogent—and relevant in modern society—is that advanced by Professor Otto Warburg, a German biochemist at the Max Planck Institute of Cell Biology who had devoted his life to the complex process of oxidation within the cell. Professor Warburg believes that a chemical carcinogen acts by destroying the respiration of normal cells, thus depriving them of energy. This damage may result from even minute doses, especially if often repeated. The effect, once achieved, is irreversible. He thinks that the cells that survive the initial onslaught of a chemical then struggle to compensate for the loss of energy. Since a living cell, like a flame, burns fuel in

118

order to produce the energy on which life depends, its sudden inability to continue the energy-producing cycle results in a primitive and far less efficient energy-producing method called fermentation. This struggle for survival, the theory goes, continues through subsequent cell divisions so that all descendant cells acquire this abnormal and irreversible method of respiration. Eventually, Professor Warburg says, these aberrant cells reach the point where fermentation is able to produce more energy than respiration. At this point, cancer cells may be said to have developed from normal cells. His theory is intriguing because, for one thing, it would explain the long latency period of cancer. It also would explain why repeated but low doses of a carcinogen are more dangerous under some circumstances than a single large dose. Whereas the single massive dose may kill cells outright, small but repeated doses may allow some cells to survive, though in a damaged condition. It is these surviving cells that turn cancerous. This theory explains why there is no "safe" dose of any carcinogen.

Yet the Food and Drug Administration routinely sets "safe" limits of human exposure to many toxic chemicals, including suspected carcinogens such as PBB. But when the government establishes such a "tolerance" level for an environmental pollutant in our foods, it is, in effect, authorizing public exposure to a dangerous and perhaps cancer-causing substance. To do otherwise—that is, to totally eliminate foods containing that substance—would be too costly and dislocating for industry, the reasoning goes. The paradox, however, is that the public is further penalized by government taxes to maintain a policy designed to assure that it does not get a lethal dose. Of course, in the end, the consumer gets it both ways, the taxes and the poison. This is precisely what happened in Michigan. One can only hope that it will not take a large-scale human tragedy, predicted for Michigan by some scientists, to resolve the debate over "safe" levels of suspected carcinogens.

The FDA was notified of the PBB contamination by April 25, 1974, and it immediately took the attitude that the chemical was an "avoidable" contaminant, meaning that it never should have gotten into the food supply, says Dr. Albert C. Kolbye, Jr., associate director for sciences of the agency's bureau of foods. "Therefore," he continued, "there could be no justification for sanctioning any PBBs found in foods." Yet it took until May 10, more than two weeks, for the FDA to come up with a tolerance

119

level of 1 part per million for milk and milk products. Anything below that level was allowed for sale. Another nineteen days elapsed before the agency set a tolerance level of .3 part per million for animal feed and .1 part per million for eggs. Two more weeks would go by before the FDA set a tolerance level of 1 part per million for meat, and this was done only after the U.S. Department of Agriculture made a formal request.

One part in a million sounds like a minute amount. And so it is. But chemicals can be so potent that such a seemingly infinitesimal amount as 1 part per million—or even part per billion—can do damage by bringing about vast biological changes in the body. And some of the early samples of contaminated milk and meats in Michigan contained hundreds and even thousands of parts PBB per million. Interestingly, the FDA's tolerance level was decided upon not on any basis of concern for public safety but on the agency's laboratory capability to detect and then confirm the presence of PBB. In other words, the tolerance level was a result of inadequate knowledge and scientific shortcomings. In early November, the FDA reduced the PBB tolerance levels (to .3 part per million for milk and meat, and .05 part per million for eggs) "based on the development of improved analytical methods and a comprehensive review of the available toxicology data," Dr. Kolbye recalls. But for six months, 9 million people were exposed to potentially dangerous levels of PBB simply because of scientific shortcomings and research that had not been done. The Michigan episode, then, highlights the problem that no practical field method of analysis exists for many toxic chemicals until long after they have escaped from their intended channels to pollute the environment.

But Dr. Kolbye is certain that time will prove the FDA's PBB guidelines provided a more than adequate margin of safety. "In my estimation, the PBB problem will go down in history the same as the cranberry scare," says Dr. Kolbye, who also holds a law degree in addition to his medical degree. (Shortly before Thanksgiving of 1959, President Eisenhower's secretary of Health, Education and Welfare, Arthur Flemming, announced that shipments of cranberries from Oregon and Washington had been contaminated by a weed killer, aminotriazole, in possibly harmful amounts. And he recommended that cranberries from those two states be taken off the market because aminotriazole caused laboratory test animals to develop thyroid cancer. A seemingly reasonable recommendation. But it left shoppers no way of telling whether their Thanksgiving cranberries originated in Oregon or, say, New Jersey. Then just three days before Thanksgiving Day, Flemming announced that government scientists had developed a technique to certify cranberry batches as either containing or not containing aminotriazole. But by then most Americans had opted to do without cranberries with their holiday turkeys. But for months afterward, cranberry growers throughout the nation suffered sales declines. Among them was the family of Al Kolbye. "It almost ruined us financially," he says, recalling his youthful days as the field foreman on his family's cranberry farm in southern New Jersey. Dr. Kolbye thinks the Food and Drug Administration properly stood its ground in the years after 1974 as Michigan consumers clamored for further reductions in the PBB tolerance level. "People were panicking, raising hell. There was a convergence of the whole spectrum of human fears, perceptions and concerns," Dr. Kolbye recalls. "We're a cancerphobic country and the fear of cancer can almost be a political force. People in Michigan would be remarkably lean if the FDA had followed the recommendations of certain politicians and scientists in Michigan," he said, meaning that almost all foods probably would have been banned if a zero tolerance level had been adopted, as many in Michigan demanded.

But a state legislative study published in March 1978 disagreed with Dr. Kolbye's contention. The study said if the federal agency had imposed a zero tolerance level immediately back in the spring of 1974 all the contaminated animals could have been identified and destroyed, and the chemical eliminated from human food channels. The study was authored by Edie Clark, the legislative aide to Speaker of the House Bobby D. Crim, who had become an authority on PBB matters. She wrote:

> It is important to understand that there was never really any need to establish a tolerance guideline for PBB. PBB was an identifiable and containable substance which could have been eliminated completely from the food chain, and the Michigan Department of Agriculture is and was at that time legally empowered to quarantine farms based on suspicion. Michigan residents had been exposed to high levels of PBB for about one year before it was identified. There was no need for them to be exposed to any more.

Instead of quarantining all known contaminated animals, the FDA recommended a tolerance guideline and the state adopted it, in spite of the fact that there was no information about what the health effects might be or what the average body burden of Michigan residents was already. The decision to establish a tolerance guideline appears as if economic considerations were taking precedence over public health considerations. The bureaucrats were taking a not-very-well-calculated risk.

Interestingly, the dialogue in Michigan's protracted debate over the PBB tolerance levels conveys the impression that PBB was the only chemical in the state's environment. But, of course, the vexing problem of environmental pollution is immensely complicated by the reality that humans—unlike laboratory animals living in rigidly controlled conditions—are never exposed to only one chemical. As Dr. Rall, director of the National Institute of Environmental Health Sciences, put it, "The issue is not simply one of threshold or no threshold. The issue is adding a new carcinogen to the present pool of carcinogens." Even if it were demonstrated that a "safe" threshold level did indeed exist for an animal, Dr. Rall says, don't forget that that mouse or rat doesn't smoke, doesn't breathe hydrocarbons or sulfur oxides from fossil fuels, doesn't take medicine, doesn't drink alcohol, doesn't eat bacon, smoked salmon or well-done hamburgers. Indeed mathematical models developed by scientists at the National Institute of Environmental Health Sciences in North Carolina suggest that each additonal exposure to carcinogens, no matter how small, will contribute to the total carcinogenic effect. Such chemicals when released into the environment do not remain segregated.

"We talk about [tolerance] levels as if a single exposure is what happens," frets Dr. Selikoff. "But here in the real world we have a cumulative effect. And in our regulatory thinking, we haven't even addressed this question yet. This is a vast, huge and important question. We're entering a new phase of environmental history," he declares. Such cumulative or synergistic effects of more than one carcinogen have been clearly demonstrated by Dr. Selikoff, whose mammoth studies among asbestos workers proved the substance to be a powerful human carcinogen. Dr. Selikoff found that a smoker exposed to asbestos is thirty times more likely to develop lung cancer than a nonsmoker who also has been exposed to the substance—and ninety times more likely than a nonexposed nonsmoker.

Thus we as a civilization must become more concerned about the cumulative effects of not just one toxic substance but the delayed and combined effects of a sea of invisible chemicals that threatens to engulf our planet. Society traditionally has been most impressed by diseases that have quick and obvious manifestations. Yet some of our worst enemies are turning out to be those that set in unobtrusively. Perhaps the most sobering thought of all is the realization that, with chemical carcinogens, our fate could be sealed twenty years or more before even the appearance of the first symptom.

# 9
# NO ACTS OF GOD

For dozens of Michigan farmers who found themselves banned from the market as spring turned to summer in 1974, the first ray of hope appeared with the approach of the July Fourth holiday. On Tuesday before the long weekend began, Governor Milliken signed Public Act 181, which provided state-owned land for a mass burial pit in which to dispose the quarantined animals. Such a pit meant that, at last, farmers could get rid of their now valueless cows, clean up their farms and start anew. But the law also specified that the state would not be obligated for any costs connected with the disposal of the contaminated animals. Farm Bureau Services finally signed an agreement with the state, taking responsibility for burying the animals. The arrangement also called for the co-op to lease the land from the state and hire private contractors to carry out the pit's operations. The state provided Agriculture Department personnel to supervise the killing and burying of animals, with Farm Bureau Services reimbursing the state for the services of its personnel.

The pit went into full operation within hours after Milliken signed the act on July 2. That day and the next, 116 cows were "euthanized" and buried before the work was halted for the holiday weekend. But before the operation could resume the following week, the local Kalkaska County Commission had obtained a restraining order that stopped any further work. Once more the farmers were quickly back in the same no-win position they had been in from the very beginning of the PBB disaster. Their first major setback was when the governor and then the state legislature rejected proposals by the Agriculture Department that the state condemn and bury the quarantined animals, compensate the farmers for such losses and then sue Michigan Chemical and Farm Bureau Services to recover all

124

those costs. The state nevertheless had gone out and quarantined contaminated farms—barring a farmer from removing his animals or their products from the farm. But unlike Rick Halbert, most farmers did not have the extra land to hold the quarantined animals in some out-of-the-way location while they cleaned up the barns before restocking, even if they had the money to do so. At the same time, attorneys were telling the farmers to keep feeding their animals, which represented evidence in claims and lawsuits against the companies involved—even though the cows' milk then had to be dumped. "Farmers were simply shut off from their markets and stuck with useless animals," recalls Halbert. "This went on for months."

And so after month after month of steady negative cash flow, Halbert recalls, "most farmers who were faced with this impossible ruinous situation agreed to have their animals destroyed. The total loss of everything they had worked for for generations was madness; but living with the constant drain on their emotional and economic resources was an even more insane condition."

The government's hands-off policy not only failed to help the affected farmers but also greatly prolonged and even intensified public exposure to PBB. The reason is because other farmers, realizing their animals were contaminated but seeing the inequities of the government's policy, simply eluded the PBB testing program. And that was easy to do. "The number of quarantines rose very slowly," Halbert points out. "If you look at the history of this case in terms of the numbers of farms quarantined over time, the first quarantine was May 10, 1974. By the end of the summer, by August 1974, there were only about forty farms quarantined. That was forty in about a three-month period, and since then, it's increased over ten times that number. Good heavens, even in August 1977 they found a [highly contaminated] farm in the Thumb area." But by the same token, there were many other farmers who, confronted by physical signs that their animals were contaminated, wanted desperately to have their herds tested. They felt that without a quarantine they had little or no chance for a just compensation settlement from the companies involved. But Agriculture Department officials were too busy and took quite a long time before visiting such farms. And so in the meantime those farmers continued selling the milk produced by their

125

animals; and when the cows stopped producing altogether, they were sent to the slaughterhouses. "When you have animals that are not producing," Halbert explains, "and this was happening all over the state, farmers would send them to the market; this is what you'd call culling cows. There were literally thousands of animals going to the butchershop. Some of these animals were loaded with PBB." Among such animals, for instance, were those owned by Lee Heming, a dairyman from McBain. He suspected PBB as the cause of many of his herd's health problems as soon as he heard about the contamination in the spring of 1974. But the local Farm Bureau co-op told him, "We don't have to worry about it because we didn't have any PBB up here." But Heming's animals continued getting sicker, aborting, losing their hair and failing to respond to treatments after developing infections. Finally he called the Department of Agriculture and, in October, Heming's farm was quarantined for high PBB contamination. "They didn't come to us," Heming said later. "The farmer had to go to them. That's the strange part—they didn't seek the PBB out."

And during this time, a second round of PBB contamination began, again undetected until much later. When many of the animals on untested farms began dying, they were hauled to rendering plants, a standard dairy practice. There they were ground up, processed and then turned back into animal feed—recycled. These products then were sold to many unsuspecting farmers who had escaped the original PBB contamination via Farm Bureau Services feeds; also not exempt this time were pet owners. And so the contamination continued to ripple through the environment.

"Farmers all over the state were trying desperately to figure out if they had good cows or bad cows," recalls Halbert. "The government should have sent a team to Michigan, day and night, for a week or two weeks, and figured out what happened and cleaned it up. Instead, it took years just to find out who got the contaminated feed. And since PBB was recycled by secondary contamination as new feeds picked up PBB while going through Farm Bureau Services equipment, the contamination went on and on and on and on. At the slaughterhouses, animals were coming in from everywhere." Many of these animals were dubbed "leaners," meaning cows that could stand up only when packed in hauling trucks tightly enough to lean on one another to keep from falling down. Once they reached the slaughterhouses, these cows were converted into hamburger meat. There was no way for state officials to keep all the farmers from selling such contaminated cows for human consumption—even when the animals were visibly sick. With tens of thousands head of cattle butchered each month at slaughterhouses all over Michigan, anything more than a spot check here and there was impossible.

Yet the Michigan public had been lured into a false sense of security by the façade of government actions to solve the disaster, reinforced by the Department of Agriculture's constant reassurances that the contamination was well under control. Soon the summer of 1974 arrived, and hundreds of thousands of vacationers from all over the Midwest and other parts of the country came to Michigan to fish in its many lakes and camp in the scenic parks along the state's 2,300-mile stretch of shoreline. But they took home with them not only pleasant memories of a glorious Michigan summer but also a dose of PBB as well.

Even when the long-awaited animal burial operation was stopped after only two days, there was little public sympathy for or even awareness of the farmers' plight. "The initial reaction in the political arena was that the PBB contamination was 'only a farmers' problem'" recalls Halbert. "The state seemed to have the ability to totally cut off your ability to make a living without providing any due process whatsoever or any way out. There was no way to get rid of the animals. There was no way to clean up the animals. Farmers were caught in a bind. Every situation, every rule was against you. You couldn't get rid of the animals. And on most farms, the animals represent about twenty to fifty percent of a farmer's total investment. You just don't 'get rid' of that investment and then go down to the bank to ask for more money. It doesn' work that way. It just wasn't a situation that we could ameliorate. You just can't take a productive part of society and just throw them in the wastebasket, you know. Michigan Chemical and Farm Bureau were fighting each other; farmers were out in left field trying to fend for themselves; they had absolutely nobody helping them. The state government viewed it as though it was a problem for the Farm Bureau and Michigan Chemical, and their insurance companies were pointing fingers at each other, saying, 'No, it's your problem.' That went on for months. The farmers were caught in a third-party dispute."

When the Milliken administration finally sought federal assistance, Washington had only disheartening news. There are all kinds of financial assistance programs for victims of natural disasters or infectious diseases, but not for a man-made chemical catastrophe. "The [federal] Disaster Relief Act of 1974 does not cover families affected by PBB," said Dr. John Dempsey, director of Michigan's Department of Social Services. "In my opinion, such indemnification or assistance should be possible under that act," he said. "However, the federal authorities tell us it is not now possible. So as presently written, the act does not provide for indemnification to farmers whose livestock or crops must be destroyed because of chemical contamination. In order to make the benefits of the act available to farmers affected by PBB contamination, the law needs to be changed. Whether the cause of human error or natural phenomena, the effect is the same; and the assistance to each should also be the same," Dr. Dempsey said.

"There is no reason why chemical assaults on us cannot be handled with the same swiftness and skill we have come to expect in dealing with infectious diseases or natural disasters," Rick Halbert adds. "In 1976, there was an outbreak of swine cholera in New Jersey. The U.S. Department of Agriculture sent in teams of veterinarians. There were a hundred or so. There was overnight quarantine of premises, cleaning them, finding out where the problem was, where it wasn't, and establishment of a baseline. This was never done in Michigan by anyone. The whole problem troubles me greatly. Our system of government can at times be very insensitive to the extreme needs of its citizens. People affected were not deadbeats or loafers. But politicians in Lansing and Washington, it seemed, could care less. If a hundred thousand gallons of fuel oil is spilled, the National Guard is called out and emergencies are declared to save a few ducks. I just don't understand . . ."

But if federal aid was nonexistent, state assistance programs were not in much better shape. "Our experience through contact with families affected by PBB has revealed that welfare programs cannot effectively meet the problems resulting from chemical contamination of farmstock," according to Dr. Dempsey. In essence, the farm families did not qualify for welfare bacause they owned too much property—land, equipment, animals and other assets. It made no difference that such property was contaminated and much of it rendered valueless. The Michigan Department of Agriculture, where farmers traditionally go for aid, also did not offer much help. "Unlike cases where animal disease is involved," director B. Dale Ball said,

128

"the state had no legal power to pay indemnity to the farmers so quarantined, or to otherwise assist them through this financial hardship. In cases of communicable animal diseases, such as tuberculosis or hog cholera, the state may quarantine and condemn the affected animals and pay indemnities to the owners. However, since PBB is a 'man-made' contaminant and not a disease, we had no legal authority to authorize indemnity payments."

And so the affected farmer was left alone to the mercy of Farm Bureau Service and Michigan Chemical, the two companies responsible for the disaster in the first place, as he demanded compensation for his contaminated animals and lost production.

Meanwhile, there seemed no end to the legal wrangling over the safety of the animal burial pit; and after three weeks, Ball announced that his department would reluctantly offer advice to quarantined farmers who wanted to bury their animals on their own land rather than wait indefinitely for the court case to be resolved. "I don't see how farmers can be expected to continue feeding and milking nonproductive cows indefinitely, dumping the milk and going deeper into debt," Ball said. "I want to emphasize that this decision was made very reluctantly, since I do not believe this is the best method of disposing of the animals, considering all of the environmental laws involved. However, I feel there is no alternative since farmers are faced with the necessity of disposing of possibly five thousand affected animals." Ball recommended that farmers contemplating burial of animals on their own land consult guidelines issued by the solid waste division of the Department of Natural Resources.

On July 25, the state court of appeals in Grand Rapids remanded the case back to the Kalkaska County Circuit Court for immediate trial. But Circuit Judge David F. Walsh, who on July 9 had upheld the original restraining order, then disqualified himself. Finally the state supreme court administrator appointed Judge Charles A. Wickens of the nineteenth circuit to hear the case.

Farm Bureau Services, meantime, began to lease "holding" sites where animals destined for destruction could be held until the burial site became available. "This was done to minimize farmers' losses and to assist them to get back into business as soon as possible," said Kenneth G. McIntyre, attorney for Farm

Bureau Services. But by early August, with still no resolution of the burial pit question in sight, Ball wrote to the quarantined farm owners suggesting that they "may be able to qualify for direct financial payment and also food stamps." He added, "I realize that this suggestion may be distasteful to some persons, and hope that you will accept this as only a suggestion, given in a spirit of desire to help you in any way during this serious problem." Enclosed with his letter was a list of county social services offices and the assorted information applicants would need when applying for welfare. But in the next three years, no more than 30 out of more than 540 farms "with major difficulties" even approached the Department of Social Services to seek help, according to Dr. Dempsey. "The PBB-affected families have, for the most part, been successful farmers whose standard of living is well above the public assistance standard. They do not generally need or want public assistance which can only help provide food, shelter and minimum personal needs." What such families truly needed, he said, was "help to replace their lost livestock and feed, to make the payments on their machinery and equipment and to meet the expenses of continuing farming operations until their income from operations is restored. In some instances, they may also need sustenance but are reluctant to apply for welfare because of their feelings of pride and independence."

On August 21, Judge Wickens spent all day hearing testimony about the burial pit and reviewing an environmental impact statement provided by the Department of Natural Resources. Then he dissolved the restraining order, saying the state had presented "a battery of experts I must admit I am impressed with," adding: "I feel sorry for all parties involved in this case." Farm Bureau Services had diffused some of the local opposition by hiring local residents for many of the tangential jobs on the site, including a community private police agency to maintain security. The site itself was a fifteen-acre clearing amid a north central Michigan's jack pine state forest near the community of Kalkaska, about twenty-five miles east of Traverse City. The site was selected by the Department of Natural Resources because of its remoteness and distance from human inhabitants, and its distance from surface water and depth of ground water tables. Six days later, the burial pit was back in full swing.

The animals arrived in all hours of the day and night. In small groups, cows, sheep, chickens and hogs were ushered into holding areas, where they were separated by ownership. Not far from the holding areas heavy bulldozers scooped out long fifteen-foot-deep trenches. As the animals one by one went through the "kill chutes," they were injected with a muscle relaxant which instantly immobilized and suffocated them by paralyzing the muscles of their diaphragms. "After they went down, they were shot [in the head with a rifle]. Then they were loaded onto a wagon and carried on skids down to a trench," recalls John W. Youngs, sales manager of Farm Bureau Services hardware department at Kalkaska. There the cows were lifted airborne by the jaws of a log-handling machine and then dropped into the trenches, where their abdominal cavities were slashed open to allow gases to escape in order to prevent bloating. The large animals were laid side by side in a single layer; the smaller animals were stacked on top of one another up to three feet high. Each night, the carcasses were covered by sand to within a yard of ground level and topped by a foot of bentonite, an absorptive clay mineral, and then sealed with topsoil. "This operation started at six A.M. and might have continued until eight or nine at night," Youngs recalls. The animals that arrived after dark were unloaded and kept in the holding pens until morning when the "euthanizations" resumed. Often the animals arrived in such heavy volume that workers such as Youngs resorted to using paint to mark the animals "so that we could identify them by owners as they went through the kill chutes."

The Department of Natural Resources, in its environmental impact statement, had estimated that the Kalkaska burial site would operate for no more than three months, since, according to agriculture director Ball, perhaps no more than five thousand head of cattle needed to be destroyed and buried. But, as Dr. Howard Tanner, director of the department later said, "the site accepted far more cattle than we were ever led to believe initially." By November, almost twice that number were already buried in the trenches of Kalkaska, which some had begun calling Animal Auschwitz.

Then early on the morning of November 4, Donald R. Isleib, chief deputy director of the Michigan Department of Agriculture, got a telephone call from the Food and Drug

131

Administration's John Wessel in Washington. Wessel, scientific coordinator to the agency's commissioner for compliance, said the FDA as of that day was further reducing the PBB tolerance guideline levels. Isleib immediately realized the import of that action: countless more farm animals, which previously tested below the 1 part per million level, now would have to be destroyed and buried. When it learned of the reductions, Michigan Chemical threatened to challenge that action in court and immediately withdrew from its participation with Farm Bureau Services in footing the cost of operating the Kalkaska burial pit.

Back in the spring of 1974, when the two companies realized the problems that confronted them as a result of the mix-up, both encountered difficulties with their respective insurance carriers in having payments to farmers started without a definite showing of liability, according to persons involved in those discussions. "We finally were able to get the carriers to proceed with a claim settlement on a fifty-fifty basis and to settle the liability question at a later date," Donald Armstrong, Farm Bureau Services' executive vice-president, recalls. "This procedure is a rare one for insurance carriers and reflects the concern that Farm Bureau Services had for the farmers involved." The feed company paid for the burial costs out of its own assets and directed its insurance carriers to use all of their funds to settle farmers' claims. Eventually the insurers went along and even tried to expedite matters by setting up a central office in Lansing, the state capital. Still, things proceeded at a slower than hoped for pace. While most of Farm Bureau Services' insurance was underwritten by two major companies, various amounts of that were subcontracted to other, so-called secondary, carriers. For instance, the feed company's first $250,000 of coverage was carried by Fireman's Fund and the next $5 million by Auto-Owners. Michigan Chemical's first $1 million coverage was carried by Travelers Insurance and the next $2 million by Lloyd's of London and the next $10 million by Aetna Insurance. Such arrangements, while a customary practice in the insurance business, tended to interfere with the payment of claims because no single one of the secondary carriers was willing to pay until assured that all would be required to do so, recalls Daniel J. Demlow, the state insurance commissioner.

Even before the FDA's revised guidelines were issued on November 4, there was a delay in claims settlement when Farm

Bureau Services in mid-October had to sue one of its own carriers, New Hampshire Insurance, which in 1974 took over the company's $5 million coverage from Auto-Owners. New Hampshire Insurance claimed its own investigation showed that Farm Bureau Services had received the Firemaster in 1973—before the 1974 coverage went into effect. But the feed company prevailed.

Farm Bureau Services swallowed hard when the Food and Drug Administration reduced the PBB tolerance levels, but begrudgingly agreed to continue footing the cost of burying new animals that now would violate the tougher federal standards. Even when Michigan Chemical refused to go along, Armstrong recalls, "we offered to acquire holding pen areas to permit Michigan Chemical to hold quarantined animals pending its challenge of the new FDA guidelines, and in that way free farmers of the burden of maintaining such animals." But this offer was rejected, causing Farm Bureau Services to reassess its position: if Michigan Chemical's challenge proved successful, the co-op would face the prospect of having to justify the necessity of destroying animals long-since buried. So the feed company asked the state Agriculture Department to exercise its discretion by ordering the disposal of quarantined animals. But the department refused, still worried that such action would make the state liable for claims later. The upshot was that the disposal operation at Kalkaska once more came to an eerie standstill. By then, Farm Bureau Services and Michigan Chemical had paid $10 million in property damage claims filed by farmers. It was estimated that the new regulations would necessitate the slaughter of five thousand more cattle.

The impasse dragged on into the new year. In mid-January, Governor Milliken called his executive secretary and trusted advisor, William N. Hettiger, into his office. Hettiger was known and feared in Lansing as "Milliken's Haldeman," the man the governor relied on for the tough assignments. Hettiger was the quintessence of a political operative, with his elegant and intimately expansive demeanor and his pastel-colored dress shirts with "Bill" stitched on the French cuffs. The governor had just won reelection two months earlier and Hettiger, having already served as Bill Milliken's director of the Department of Administration and then as his executive secretary, had only days left before he was to leave government service to set up his own lobbying firm in the state capital.

Hettiger, thus, was understandably reluctant when Milliken asked if he would serve as a third-party mediator and call all the insurance companies to a meeting with the purpose of creating another settlement fund. Hettiger knew such an undertaking could not be accomplished overnight. He didn't want to do it. "The governor can make you feel like you're trampling on the flag if you didn't perform some public service," Hettiger said later, with mock sheepishness. He agreed to take the assignment. On January 20, Milliken called a meeting of the companies in Grand Rapids. Presiding was U.S. District Court Judge Noel Fox. Hettiger was accompanied by Demlow. They met in the imposing courtroom Judge Fox normally used to hear cases.

In the judge's chambers just before the meeting began, Fox said he hoped that Demlow and Hettiger could persuade the insurance companies to agree to a new settlement fund without the court's having to find guilt or innocence. Hettiger also learned then why his boss had insisted that he take this assignment. Judge Fox had called the governor and requested Hettiger by name. When the three emerged from the judge's chambers into the courtroom, Hettiger was struck by the number of people in the room. "There were tons of lawyers there. It was a shock," he recalls. All the representatives at the meeting had full authority to commit their companies to the creation of a new settlement fund. Fox, Demlow and Hettiger sat down on the judge's bench, and, looking down, Fox called the meeting to order. "Then he just got up and walked out!" Hettiger recalled years later, laughing. "And there Dan and I were, facing this crowd of lawyers. The first thing I did was to ask everybody to separate themselves so I could tell who was who." The talks went on for more than two weeks without any substantive progress. Finally Hettiger decided it was time to get down to serious business. The companies had stubbornly refused to put up the $15.5 million Hettiger insisted on. One morning in mid-February Hettiger and Demlow showed up for the meeting with a calculated gamble. "I acted mad at the lawyers and told them if they didn't agree [to the $15.5 millions figure] I'd use every ounce of influence I had with the governor to get him to declare a state of emergency. Then I got up and stormed out. Demlow then threatened to revoke the licenses of every company in the room that did business in Michigan. Then he walked out after me. We knew it probably never would've stood up in court; but they didn't know it. And even if they did know, they must've known how long it'd take going through the courts to challenge the revocations. But Dan and I never even got as far as the elevator. They all came running after us," Hettiger said much later, shaking with laughter and satisfaction. Details of the settlement package were quickly worked out, and Hettiger left government service. "We had met the main needs as we knew it at the time," he recalls. "Nobody then even said anything about human health. There was no press [coverage] in Grand Rapids, but I got a lot of personal satisfaction."

With the creation of a new settlement fund, workers at Kalkaska resumed their grim task. But in the time that had elapsed, some farmers got tired of waiting for Farm Bureau Services to pick up their condemned animals and, instead, sent their sick cows—perhaps across the state line—to slaughterhouses and their dead ones to rendering plants to be recycled not only as livestock feed and pet food but also as tallow to be used in soap, margarine, candles and lubricants. When the claims settlement process resumed, it was immediately clear that the companies had become more niggardly with their money now that many more farmers were filing claims as a result of the stricter federal PBB standards.

"Farmers had lots of animals taken away from them, without being paid. There was lots of money involved," recalls Halbert. "That's when the scope of the problem began to hit print. Some farmers called the media, saying everyone in Michigan was eating PBB. There was a lot of posturing—I don't know what the motives were, but some people took the tack of saying they were tired and described various health problems they said were due to PBB." The press jumped on the story, if only briefly. Splashed across the front pages of many papers, for example, was a picture of a state senator standing with a pile of seventy dead cows, followed by such headlines as "Charlevoix Area Dairy Farmer, Wife, Live in Fear of Effects of PBB," "Study Needed of People," "Tainted Sheep to Be Sold for Food," "Illness Plagues PBB Exposed Families Exposed to Poison Feed," "Liver Damage Found in 15 Who Ate Tainted Products" and "More Ills Traced to Bad Feed." The Grand Rapids *Press* followed with a twelve-part series called "PBB—the Poison Puzzle." The Detroit *News* reported on the work of Dr. Corbett in Ann Arbor. Reacting to the sudden deluge of

135

publicity that had aroused considerable public alarm, Governor Milliken placed an urgent call to Dr. Alexander M. Schmidt, commissioner of the Food and Drug Administration. "The situation in Michigan is deteriorating," Milliken told Dr. Schmidt, and suggested that the agency make a public statement. "He didn't suggest the content of the statement—just that, if we could make a statement, it was time to do so in order to prevent the development of a panic situation in the state," recalls Dr. Schmidt. The agency responded later that day with an "advisory" stating that foods which met the FDA's standards were safe for human consumption. "But this release," recalls a bitter Alan L. Hoeting, then deputy regional director of the FDA's office in Detroit, "generated headlines such as 'Whitewash Is Denied As State Probes Effects of Tainted Food' and 'Tainted Food Is Safe, FDA Reports.'" And so despite the assurances of both federal and state governments, signs began appearing in grocery stores and restaurants all around Michigan telling customers that their products were from out of state. And in western Michigan, the heart of the dairy industry, thirteen meat packers began refusing to accept meat containing any PBB at all—even traces that the government said were harmless. "Our purpose is to restore the confidence of the consumer in Michigan of beef," explained Orie VanderBoon, operator of the Ada Beef Company in the Grand Rapids suburb of Ada. "It's obvious that consumers aren't convinced that such meat is safe. I personally don't feel that any evidence has been presented that it isn't, but that isn't the point," VanderBoon said. "It's a shame. The farmer is getting the brunt of this thing. But it's going to be worse if we don't win back the confidence of the consumer." That same week, Meijer's, one of the state's major supermarket chains, announced it had "invoked additional safeguards to protect its customers." The measure, according to Harvey Lemmen, president and general manager of Meijer's, was the supermarket's own testing program to assure that the Michigan meats it bought were only from "noncontaminated" herds. A similar program for milk and eggs also was adopted. Six days before the Meijer's press conference, Hoeting of the FDA in Detroit got wind of the imminent bombshell from the Michigan Farm Bureau and called Meijer's executive officers in Grand Rapids. He spoke with Harold Hans, vice-president of merchandising, but was unable to persuade the supermarket chain to change its mind.

136

Hans said Meijer's decided on its own testing program after randomly testing ten meat samples from its shelves and finding PBB in all ten.

Action such as Meijer's, of course, merely reflected the public's growing doubts about official reassurances that foods with traces of PBB were harmless. But if several Farm Bureau Services employees shared those worries, their concern was overtaken by other considerations. On at least three occasions, the co-op's employees, including David Moody, who worked at the Kalkaska site, diverted cattle destined to be buried there for their own use. The first time was in early September 1974, shortly after Judge Wickens had cleared the way for the pit to resume full operation, when Moody drove two black angus steers to the Strauss Meat and Packing House in the town of Weidman to be butchered. Then the meat was divided among Ken Jones, Wayne Playford, Clyde Springer, Ann VanDyk, Whalen Fox and Moody, all employees of Farm Bureau Services. They each reimbursed Moody for the processing costs and his expenses, including gas money for delivering the butchered meat. The second "diversion" took place in June 1975 involving a condemned Holstein dairy cow, again taken by Moody to the Strauss Meat and Packing House for butchering. Perhaps emboldened by their earlier successes, on the third occasion in August 1975, Moody and friends had six cows processed and then distributed. On this occasion, John Youngs, who was responsible for building the holding pens and kill chutes at the Kalkaska pit, got in on the deal. Moody obtained half of one cow and gave a portion of it to his friends in Detroit, charging them only for the processing costs.

In August 1975, the $15.5 million settlement pool negotiated by Hettiger and Demlow six months earlier ran out, and that fall Governor Milliken called another round of negotiations. "After lengthy and extreme negotiations," recalls Armstrong, the Farm Bureau Services boss, the feed company reached an out-of-court settlement with Michigan Chemical, whom it had sued for $200 million in connection with the shipment of Firemaster instead of Nutrimaster. The settlement was reached in January of 1976 for $19.6 million. "Farm Bureau Services gave up its right to make claim against Michigan Chemical for Farm Bureau Services' own losses forever in exchange for which Michigan Chemical and its carriers agreed to fund a new settlement fund from which the remaining claimants were to be paid," Armstrong said. "We were by far the largest single PBB claimant."

The settlement of the $200 million suit once more raised the hopes of affected farmers across Michigan. With the approach of spring, their thoughts were turning to the spring-time ritual of crop planting, and that requires huge sums of money. But a random survey of fifty-four farmers by *Michigan Farmer* magazine revealed that only sixteen had been able to reach a settlement with the insurers of Farm Bureau Services and Michigan Chemical. The magazine further asked those who had reached settlements if they thought they had gotten a fair shake. One farmer responded, "I don't think anything would be fair in a case like this. But it was enough to keep us going." Melvin Molineaux of Coopersville said, "We were paid what the cattle are worth now [after being contaminated by PBB] rather than what they were worth before." He also said he did not receive compensation for milk production. Stuart Cochran of Three Rivers, who lost his entire herd of two hundred, was more bitter about the way he had been treated. He told *Michigan Farmer*, "The insurance companies threatened that 'If you don't settle, your claim will go to the bottom of the pile.' I lost practically a life's work, and I was treated like I was at fault. The insurance adjusters jumped all over us, and didn't believe the number of cattle we had. And we had receipts!"

One of the first Michigan lawmakers to get into the PBB fray was a plain-speaking cash crop farmer from St. Charles named Donald J. Albosta, who was cochairman of the House Agriculture Committee. Albosta in the spring of 1975 proposed that all Michigan meats be labeled as such. The proposal generated uproarious opposition from the food industry, and Albosta's proposal was amended to direct the Department of Agriculture to hold a public hearing on the question of whether the state should impose even stricter PBB tolerance levels than the federal standards allowed. The hearing was held at the cavernous National Guard Armory in Lansing on May 29. Earlier that month, the state Department of Public Health had released its short-term study, and because its findings seemed to exonerate PBB, agriculture officials had hoped to hold its public hearing closer on the heels of the health report, since they violently opposed any further reductions in the tolerance levels. But the hearing had to be delayed until the twenty-ninth to accomodate Dr. Albert C. Kolbye, the Food and Drug

Administration's associate director for sciences in the bureau of foods. Kolbye is a physician, an epidemiologist, an attorney and an assistant surgeon general of the United States; and, like the state Agriculture Department, he strongly opposed further lowering the PBB guidlines. The delay to accommodate Dr. Kolbye did not displease the Michigan Farm Bureau, which had begun applying heavy pressure on state agriculture officials to stonewall the Albosta effort. (The delay is significant because one year later another such hearing was hastily arranged and held during the absence of leading scientific voice supporting a drastic reduction of the PBB standards.) Dr. Kolbye began his testimony by reiterating the Michigan Health Department findings that "no human disease has been identified as a direct result of polybrominated biphenyl contamination." However, he did issue a set of warnings to persons who had been highly exposed to PBB products, such as farm families who butchered their own animals for meat and drank their own cows' milk. "When such people are identified, the following areas of concern should be explored by their physicians. Patients should be observed for any indication of alteration in liver function. Patients should be observed for any alterations in the immune mechanism. Mothers should receive cautions about breast-feeding infants. Patients should be advised to avoid all weight reduction programs unless under the guidance of a physician." Dr. Kolbye concluded by saying that he was "confident" the existing federal standards provided the necessary margin for human safety. But a mere three years later, a University of Wisconsin pathologist, Dr. James R. Allen, produced alarming results after feeding rhesus monkeys a diet containing PBB at levels the FDA to this day maintains are safe.

The Michigan Department of Agriculture's other star witness at its May 29 hearing was Dr. Reizen, the state health director. He described the findings of his department and then concluded, "Just as living cells tend to adapt to these environmental changes [such as PBB poisoning], man will have to learn to live with a degree of contamination which represents the best level of control he can reasonably achieve. In conclusion, having no evidence that PBB contamination of meat and dairy products at levels much higher than the current FDA-established levels produced illness in humans, the Department of Public Health supports the current levels as being realistic and very much within an acceptable margin of safety for humans."

139

Virtually the only scientific witness to favor a reduction of the PBB standards was Dr. Walter D. Meester, the Grand Rapids toxicologist, who brought the most sense as well as the best science to the forum, even though, at the time, he had not yet had the opportunity to fully review the state Health Department's short-term study. He said he did not agree with the "zero tolerance" concept, an idea championed by some, including Albosta, that would bar food products with even an iota of PBB present. "I don't quite agree with this 'any detectable amount' because, with increased sophistication of our [detection] methods, it may be that we can pick up such tremendously small amounts of PBB in the future that we wouldn't be able to eat anything because all foods will be shown to contain such small quantities of PBBs that we would all starve to death." But he did favor a 300-fold reduction of the federal tolerance. "Of course," Dr. Meester added, "this might be subject in the future to change if it is shown that even .01 can cause any serious hazards or any health problems in the future."

The director of the Western Michigan Poison Center continued, "What evidence do you have that continued exposure to very low levels will not cause a buildup in the human body? It is very hard to get rid of . . . . And just like many other toxic agents that I deal with, some people react violently to a very low level, whereas someone else is able to tolerate a relatively high level."

In the audience pondering Dr. Meester's remarks about individual variability to a toxic substance was farmer Harley Hinkley. Later he walked up to the microphone and said he was wondering "if this here PBB would work just like whiskey in some men. Some men can drink a whole pint and others can't drink nothing." B. Dale Ball, the hearing's presiding officer, snapped gruffily, "I think the crowd knows the answer to that." But Dr. George Fries, the U.S. Agriculture Department scientist who identified PBB in Halbert's feed, took the question more seriously. "The answer is yes; there is individual variability and susceptibility to any toxic compound in any species."

Yet the concept proved a difficult one for some to grasp, and others simply refused to buy it. Larry Crandall, a thirty-three-year-old dairyman and a neighbor of Halbert's, for instance, testified that he and his family, including a seven-year-old daughter and a four-year-old son, all ate highly contaminated meat unknowingly but still feel fine. Crandall said a fat biopsy revealed he had a PBB content of 3.0 parts per million. "Again," he said, "I felt as well as possible under the circumstances this past year; by this I'm referring to the great emotional drain and psychological blow resulting from the disruption of our farm business and destruction of a lifetime of dairy progress." Crandall concluded, "Our family has shown no health problems and we have no qualms about eating or drinking products that fall under the existing guidelines."

Larry Crandall had become something of a spokesman for some farm families who maintained that they were perfectly healthy despite, in many cases, extremely high PBB body levels. They were adamantly opposed to any further tampering with the PBB standards in foods. Many of them, already back in business, realized that a further reduction in standards would require the destruction of their replacement herds, which now had been contaminated by PBB residues still in the farm environment. Another such spokesman was dairyman D. Blaine Johnson of Hesperia, north of Grand Rapids. "We drink lots of milk, ate nearly a whole cow," Johson testified at the May 29 hearing. But everyone in his family, including four children ages three to thirteen, feels fine, he said. "Most of us were gnawing on meat from 100 to 2,500 parts per million in the fat for over a year's time. This thing could have been a human health disaster for us farmers involved. But, by the grace of God, it doesn't look like anyone has been really hurt." His wife, Adela, added later in a private conversation, "There can't be anything to it. Well, do you see anything wrong with us? Now, I'm not saying there won't ever be, but . . . I really feel our lives are in God's hands—PBB or whatever. What good does it do for us to know about it? Maybe it's better we don't know about it. You can't uneat it." Halbert, who also was at the hearing, commented, "It is surprising that farm families have not had an epidemic of illness, considering their exposure. But thank God for small favors."

The last person to speak at the May 29 hearing was Garry Zuiderveen of Falmouth. "If anyone here has any doubt as to what can happen to animals, look at the cattle outside in the trailer. We have animals on display from four farms, all at below the .3 part per million tolerance level," he said. "Heaven help us if the same thing happens with humans that has happened to the animals on four farms." The hearing then was adjourned by Ball, as everyone awaited a decision to be made in July at the meeting of the Agriculture Commission, the policy-setting body of the Agriculture Department.

"The hearing was as phony as a three-dollar bill," Don Albosta charged in the meantime. He was incensed, for one thing, because Ball refused at the hearing to let him read into the record a letter from Dr. David T. Salvati, a Big Rapids physician who, like Dr. Meester, had been treating a number of families from contaminated farms. Ball had termed the letter hearsay evidence, even though, Albosta noted, Ball himself had stated the hearing was to concern itself only with human health. Yet Ball had allowed extended time to scientific witnesses who testified that PBB does not seem to harm animals except in extraordinary amounts. One such witness was Dr. H. Dwight Mercer, a veterinarian with the Food and Drug Administration's bureau of veterinary medicine. In March, Dr. Mercer headed a "low-level herd survey," whose results, incidentally, were released on May 5, a mere three days after the badly flawed and misleading state Health Department study was announced. The herd survey results, not surprisingly, were equally reassuring. After examining sixteen contaminated herds and fifteen control herds presumed to be uncontaminated, the study concluded: "There were no herd health problems observed that could be attributed to the presence of low levels of PBBs." However, the entire FDA team, including five veterinarians, had spent only one day actually observing all thirty-one herds in the study. Dr. Mercer admitted to Lester O. Brown, a congressional investigator, that the group had "only a few days to plan and accomplish the study," and that that was why in the course of six days they only spent one day examining the animals. The rest of that time was devoted to collecting and reviewing records, as well as gathering blood, urine and feed samples. "Dr. Mercer told me that the way FDA determined that the herds were or were not exposed was by questioning the farmers about whether they had purchased contaminated feed," recalls Brown. "At the time of the survey, Farm Bureau Services had not informed some of the farmers in the control group that the feed they had been buying was indeed contaminated," wrote Brown, a staff member of the House subcommittee on oversight and investigations, after conducting a probe of the federal government's involvement in the Michigan disaster. Analyses of

142

feed gathered by the FDA team later showed that some of the control, or presumably unexposed, herds in the study had eaten feed with as much or more PBB than the contaminated herds. In fact, two of the control farms in the study later were quarantined for high PBB contamination. One such farm belonged to St. Joseph County dairyman Dale Hackenberg, who owned three hundred head of cattle. "I was one of the herds that was supposed to be a control herd that wasn't supposed to have any PBB," he recalls. "And what's so funny is, three days after they come out and did all this biopsy on the animals, I was quarantined. . . . The lowest one I had was .02 part per million, and the highest was 1.4 parts per million."

And so the FDA herd survey team had committed the same blunder that the Michigan Department of Public Health made in its human health study. By comparing two like groups, the FDA, seeing not much difference in health symptoms or milk production changes, concluded, therefore, that PBB could not be implicated. The team reached that conclusion even though the contaminated group in 1974 had a sharply higher calf mortality rate (19.28 percent) than the control group (11.1 percent). The contaminated group also had run up higher veterinarian bills in all three years examined (1972–74) than the control group. Finally, both groups had shown declines in milk production. Yet such data were not deemed "statistically significant" by the FDA. Investigator Brown noted later that the study also did not "properly reflect the true population of dairy cows in Michigan because it included a high percentage of Guernseys, when most of the Michigan dairy cow herds are made up of Holsteins." But at the May 29 public hearing, no one challenged Dr. Mercer.

It is important to note that the Food and Drug Administration has never said that its PBB standards have anything to do at all with the health or illness of farm animals contaminated by it.

"The FDA tolerance guideline of .3 part per million for PBB in meat and milk eventually touched off a heated controversy unparalleled in Michigan agriculture," says a state legislative study published in March of 1978. "This number, what it represented, and the way in which it was used is largely responsible for widespread economic devastation on Michigan farms today." The study was written by Edie Clark, the PBB assistant to the Speaker of the House.

143

"The problem was compounded by the defendants, Michigan Farm Bureau and Michigan Chemical Company, who adopted the .3 part per million tolerance guideline as the cutoff point for financial restitution. Unless the farm had been quarantined, the farmer was not considered eligible for financial restitution." Yet, Clark wrote, "the tolerance guideline was never established as an indication of animal health. It meant that if a hamburger, for example, were contaminated at .29 part per million, it would be considered satisfactory for human consumption. It did not indicate that the animal from which that hamburger was derived was healthy. In fact, many farmers who were contaminated but never quarantined suffered appalling losses. They were below the tolerance guideline, and so were not considered eligible for reimbursement from the defendants. They could, however, legally market milk and meat originating from animals which were obviously ill and, in some cases, barely able to stand. Many farmers found dead and dying animals in the field every morning, and most calves died within days of birth."

The federal PBB standards not only were established arbitrarily but also were enforced in a capricious manner, says Clark. "The Michigan Department of Agriculture contends that if all animals had been tested in time, all of them would probably have been found to be over the tolerance guideline. However, it was years before some of of these animals were tested, and during that period of time the cows were excreting PBB through the milk. The PBB may have ravaged the cows' physical condition, but by the time a veterinarian collected a tissue sample from the animals, the PBB level had dropped below the guideline. So the animal remained unquarantined." A good illustration of this phenomenon is contained in a study, ironically, by the Michigan Department of Agriculture. In the spring of 1975, the department sent one of its veterinarians, Dr. Duaine Deming, to seventy-two quarantined farms to see if a way could be found to lift the quarantines from those farms. Even though the seventy-two farms had been quarantined in the first place because samples of either milk or fat tissue had violated the federal standards, Dr. Deming discovered that only sixteen now had even a detectable level of PBB in milk. And of those sixteen, only three were still above the tolerance level. Yet the animal health problems had been extraordinary: 73 percent of the farmers reported sterility problems, 64 percent reported drastic milk production declines, some by as much as 50 percent; 63 percent reported retarded growths and 57 percent reported excessive calf mortality. Still other problems included abortions, physical degeneration, abnormal hoof growths. And so the study clearly demonstrates that PBB, if not caught in the act, can ravage farm animals and yet slip away without a trace. Even Dr. Kolbye of the Food and Drug Administration later conceded, "Some cattle with low residue levels may be survivors of the earlier, much higher level of PBB contamination. Even though they may have legal PBB residues at the present time, it'd seem reasonable to expect that their health status might deteriorate in the future with consequent weight loss, remobilization of PBB residues, possibly leading to PBB levels which exceed the present guideline."

The Department of Agriculture enforced the federal tolerance guidelines in two basic ways. One was to collect bulk milk samples from dairy distributors; the other was to wait for a farmer to voluntarily send a fat sample to the department's Geagley Laboratory for analysis. If a bulk milk sample, for instance, contained PBB above .3 part per million, then the department would determine which dairy farms had contributed milk to this bulk tank. Presumably, by tracing the sample backward, the department would eventually discover the origin of the PBB tainted milk. The problem was that a dairy distributor's tanks can contain milk from dozens of farms, making it extremely difficult for the Agriculture Department to trace backward to find the violative milk supplier. Besides, milk from such a heavily contaminated herd in most cases became so diluted, or watered down, when comingled with noncontaminated milk that countless contaminated herds never were discovered.

"In still other instances," added Clark, "private dairymen would add cows to a herd that was milking over the tolerance guideline in order to dilute the PBB factor below the 'actionable' level. This was, in some cases, done with the knowledge of department officials." One such farmer was Blaine Johnson of Hesperia. After he learned that the milk in his bulk tank contained as much as 22 parts per million of the chemical, he did some individual milk tests in order to isolate and then remove the cows with the highest PBB levels. Then he replaced them with "clean" cows, and added the new milk to those produced by the low PBB cows. It worked. The bulk milk's PBB

145

content fell just within the government level for milk. So he was able to resume selling his milk. To this day, the Department of Agriculture has taken the position that even if a cow's meat exceeds the government standard, she may be milked—so long as the milk in the bulk tank is below the tolerance level. In other words, the milk from cows whose meat is deemed unsafe to eat was—and still is—being sold to people.

In safeguarding the public food supply from excessive PBB contamination, the reliance on analyses of milk—and, occasionally, fat tissue—samples had major shortcomings that were never publicized, according to Edie Clark. "In fact," she said, "a PBB analysis conducted on a cow is actually no indication of how much PBB the animal was exposed to, or of how much damage may have been done. Too many other variables—such as length of time since exposure, diet, distribution through the body and perhaps even genetic predisposition—enter into the picture for a tissue analysis to be considered an accurate reflection of anything." Even the more reliable tissue analysis is only an accurate measure of how much PBB is in one area, not in the whole cow. According to Clark, sixteen such samples were taken from one cow and every one showed varying amounts of PBB, ranging from high above the legal standard to barely detectable. And the more commonly used test, milk analysis, "is a totally inadequate method" for determining a cow's PBB body burden, she added. Too many factors enter into play to affect the level of PBB in milk, even from day to day, she said; these variables include how much exercise the animal has had, what stress it might have endured recently and even the condition of housing. "Still," Clark wrote in her 1978 report, "the Department [of Agriculture] used milk analyses, on a regular basis, to release animals from quarantine. And even then, not all animals from contaminated farms were tested. Most probably were not."

Because of the inadequate tests and the questionable procedures used to lift quarantines, farmers—many unknowingly—continued selling PBB-contaminated products to unsuspecting consumers. One such dairyman who finally got suspicious was Bill Oeverman of Tustin in Osceola County, just south of Cadillac. After the Department of Agriculture lifted his quarantine—without doing any sample testing—he asked Dr. Alpha Clark to extract fat tissues for PBB analysis from a group of cows enroute to the slaughterhouse. The animals looked miserable, Dr. Clark recalls. In fact, one of them dropped dead on its way up the gangplank to the truck bed. When the laboratory reports came back, two of the animals had PBB exceeding the tolerance level. But, of course, by then the animals had been sold—and probably eaten as hamburger meat by innocent consumers. "We had wanted to shoot our animals," said Ada Oeverman. "But Farm Bureau said they were low tolerance, so that we could sell them. We had no choice. So we put them on the market. This one particular cow we kept back, and we sent two tests in. She came back 'nondetectable' each time, but we knew she had PBB." Mrs. Oeverman said a state Agriculture Department veterinarian told her and her husband that a nondetectable reading meant the cow had no PBB. "So then we sent her to Purdue University and they found out there that, well, she had PBB. They found it in her bone marrow." After the Oevermans' herd was quarantined in November 1974, the Agriculture Department told them that if they would kill a single highly contaminated cow, the quarantine would be lifted. Oeverman refused, but when that particular cow died anyway, on a Friday, the quarantine was lifted the following Monday. Later when the Oevermans continued seeing problems with their other cows, Ken Jones of Farm Bureau Services came out to their farm and told them, "You're starving them with malnutrition." Doc Clark, who was there that day, angrily retorted, "No, it is not a deficiency. It's PBB." Jones insisted, "No. You need a dietician." Bill Oeverman told Jones, "What I need is a mortician. We've got eighty-six dead cattle lying there."

Even when the Agriculture Department was presented with irrefutable proof that a farm had been contaminated, it did its best to minimize the potential liability to Farm Bureau Services. "Typically," says Edie Clark, "a farmer may have sent a sample in for analysis. If the sample was considered 'official,' and it was over the tolerance guideline, then the farm would be quarantined—but only for the specie of animal from which the sample was derived. In other words, a dairy-and-swine farm may be quarantined only for dairy or only for swine." Too, the imposition of a quarantine did not assure that contaminated food products were kept off the market. The Agriculture Department even gave some farmers forewarning that they were about to be quarantined. The response of the farmers is not hard to guess. They were faced with two alternatives: sell

147

their animals immediately and get a decent return, or wait for the prohibition notice to arrive in a day or two, lose those animals—their livelihoods, really—and then get in line to sue Farm Bureau Services and Michigan Chemical, hoping for a fair settlement. Dr. Donald A. Isleib, chief deputy agriculture director, explained his department's seemingly incongruous policy by saying that two divisions within the department were involved, the animal health division, which imposes quarantines, and the dairy division, which revokes milk shippers' permits. Often, news of an impending quarantine would reach the farmer via the animal health division before the actual revocation of a farmer's shipping permit arrived from the dairy division. And if the farmer in the meantime decided to unload all his soon-to-be valueless animals on the market before the notice arrived, he did so legally, if not, perhaps, with a clear conscience.

It turns out that Agriculture Department officials often used the telephone not only to warn farmers of impending quarantines but also to release low-level PBB cows from a quarantined herd so a farmer could sell those animals. One such incident took place in January of 1976 when thirty-seven cows from a quarantined farm were sent not to the Kalkaska burial pit but to the slaughterhouse in Coldwater, Michigan. Bill and Bonnie Hughston, who have a farm adjoining Doc Clark's, own a truck operation, among other things; and their drivers delivered thousands of contaminated animals to Kalkaska. In late January, the Hughstons got a call from Farm Bureau Services, requesting that they have some animals picked up at the farm of Jim Fish, who owned a Guernsey herd in Hickory Corners, just a few miles west of Rick Halbert's farm. "Well, we sent these three trucks down there," recalls Bonnie Hughston, a pretty and gregarious woman who once was a trick rodeo rider. "Then we got a call from Dr. [Marvin] Wastell of Farm Bureau Services. He said, 'Load the cattle and then I'll tell you where to go with them.' This sounded rather odd to us because we knew how to get to Kalkaska. We didn't need to be told where to go." Dr. Wastell said seventeen of the cows should be sent to Kalkaska, and two to Michigan State University for research. But when he told the Hughstons where the remaining thirty-seven cows should go, they refused to go along. "Our trucks just sat there. We said, 'Well, we have to know when our trucks pull

148

out of there, because our driver is waiting to know,'" Mrs. Hughston continued. "And he said 'Well, these are to go to LaPorte, Indiana, for slaughter.' It was a quarantined herd! We knew that Doc Clark had been accused of taking cattle for research into Indiana. So we were a little upset that we were just to load cattle to go to Indiana." Bill Hughston called Dr. Wastell in Lansing and told him, "I can't go without some type of papers. This is different than going to the pit." Dr. Wastell told Hughston, a lanky, reserved man, to call Dr. Duaine Deming, a Department of Agriculture veterinarian. "You call Dr. Deming, and he'll okay it," Dr. Wastell said. Hughston became extremely skeptical and was still pondering the unexpected turn of events when Dr. Wastell again called, urging him to telephone Dr. Deming. When he finally did, Dr. Deming told him, "Yeah, go ahead. It's okay." But Hughston still refused. "I'm not moving them to Indiana without papers," he said. "I'm not going to move a truck until I have proof." Next, Dr. Wastell called him back, saying, "I've okayed it. Get those trucks a-moving." Hughston still refused, and brusquely told Dr. Wastell, "These are going to Indiana. I want an okay from Indiana because that's how Doc Clark got into trouble—by taking them to Purdue for research [even after getting verbal permission from the Michigan Department of Agriculture]." Back and forth the long-distance calls continued. "Our driver, he's sitting there all this time. He keeps calling us to ask, 'What am I supposed to do?' We told him, 'Don't take those cattle anywhere until we tell you.' So this went on from early morning until it got late at night," recalls Bonnie Hughston. Finally, Bill Hughston told Dr. Wastell, "I'm sorry, but I have a family to support. I have five boys and I can't afford to have my trucks tied up."

"Well, we'll stand behind you," Dr. Wastell said. "Farm Bureau is behind you. If you get into trouble, we'll back you up." But Hughston was not persuaded.

The day-long standoff finally reached an end when Dr. Wastell told Hughston to have his driver haul the thirty-seven cows to a packinghouse in Coldwater, a city in south central Michigan near the Indiana border. When Hughston called Dr. Deming, the veterinarian assured him, "Yes, it's okay to take them."

"But they're quarantined," Hughston replied sharply.

"We'll temporarily lift the quarantine," Dr. Deming said.

149

Hughston reluctantly instructed his driver to take the cows to Coldwater. Two days later, the Hughstons received a letter from the Department of Agriculture releasing the thirty-seven cows from quarantine. It came in a Farm Bureau Services envelope.

"The ultimate consequence of the Agriculture Department's procedures was to limit the liability incurred by Michigan Farm Bureau, although there is no known existing information to indicate that this was done intentionally," concluded Edie Clark in her 1978 report to the House Speaker.

As for monitoring the human food channels for PBB, the state Agriculture Department conducted periodic "market basket surveys" of what it said were representative cross sections of foods available to Michigan's consumers. Typically, it would find—and dutifully report—that only 1 and 2 percent of the samples tested contained PBB. But what the department did not disclose was that Michigan is a beef-deficient state—meaning that 70 percent of its beef is imported. Thus, such market basket surveys included mostly non-Michigan beef products which the department knew would be free of PBB. "In fact," according to Rick Halbert, "the major danger was always that of beef animals. If I might say so, there was never any systematic or direct regulatory attempt to find the beef animals when the quarantines initially came down on May 10. Basically I think the philosophy of the agencies was that it was too difficult at that point in time to run around doing biopsies on these individual beef animals; so they concentrated on dairy farms where you could dip out of the bulk tank and immediately know whether there is a problem or not in terms of milk supply. The beef animals went to market, and many of them for months on end were not looked at because nobody had the personnel. You had just a couple of [analytical] machines in the whole state of Michigan working on the problem, running out these tests. There were samples backed up for months, three or four months in some cases. As a result, this problem spread like cancer because no one is out there bringing it under control quickly."

As many as 100,000 heavily contaminated animals may have gone to the market just in the nine to twelve months that PBB was in the food chain before the accident was discovered. In a typical year, Michigan's nine thousand dairy farmers cull about 24 percent of a total of 450,000 adult milking cows.

150

"And," according to Halbert, "based on the percent of farms that had significant levels, perhaps five or ten thousand went to market that were quite high and perhaps a thousand animals went to market that were astronomically high." The Agriculture Department did not even begin its market basket surveys to monitor the human food supply until January 1975, nine months after the catastrophe had come to light. Even so, the meats that were checked were not kept out of the supermarket counters. Rather, they were sold before the test results returned. "There's no such thing as perfect law enforcement," said agriculture director Ball, comparing his department's PBB monitoring efforts to that of a policeman who once stopped him for speeding but failed to catch other speeders. But, Halbert recalls with bitterness, "There was never a general alert put out to farmers saying: 'The feed you got may be contaminated' and 'Don't eat any animals or their products until they've been checked out.' Not even to this day." Ball says he never saw the need to warn each and every farmer in Michigan about PBB. "We assume farmers can read the papers. I can't mail something to every farmer in the state. He can test the same as we can if he's concerned."

Such an unfeeling attitude permeated the Department of Agriculture from top to bottom, and it produced tragic results all across the state. Bob Wellman, a onetime Barry County "Young Farmer of the Year," and his wife, Margaret, bought their dream 860-acre farm and stocked it with two hundred and fifty healthy Holstein cows in Hastings just about the time the shipment of Firemaster arrived at Farm Bureau Services' feed plant. Their herd's milk production began dropping late that summer. By Christmas, nearly thirty calves had died. "If I can raise four kids, I certainly can raise calves," a resolute Margaret Wellman told herself. One day she finally stood helpless in the barn, sobbing. The calves continued to die. "There was nothing I could do, and nothing the vet could do either." After the PBB contamination became known, Margaret suspected PBB as the cause of their problems. "I kept trying to tell Bob that it was PBB. Our cows looked just like the ones with PBB poisoning I saw on television—overgrown hooves, sores, skin problems, swollen joints. I went to the Farm Bureau in Hastings but they told me PBB wasn't in the feed we were buying."

The herd's milk production continued falling. In the fall of 1974, Margaret finally persuaded her husband to test their cows for PBB. They found PBB. Although the contamination levels were below the federal tolerance guidelines, the cows remained sick and, by now, nearly 90 percent of the calves were dying. And many of the adult cows now were quite ill. Some became lethargic and stiff-legged. Others developed open sores; and many got infections that would not heal. Eventually more than forty cows died. And, as at the Halbert farm, rats and mice suddenly disappeared. And all but one of the seventeen cats and their litters died. Yet, because no animal on the farm had tested at above the .3 part per million tolerance level, the Wellmans continued selling the animals and their products, even though they had decided to stop eating their own produce after a side of beef from their freezer showed .25 part per million PBB. And since late 1973, the Wellman family has been plagued by lethargy, stomach problems and many other inexplicable ailments. "Our sixteen-year-old daughter is so tired all the time that the other day she was crying with sheer exhaustion," Margaret Wellman said in 1976. A son's finger and toe began to swell painfully for no apparent reason. Mrs. Wellman, who, at age thirty-four, had never had menstrual problems, underwent a hysterectomy because of excessive bleeding, and then was put on tranquilizers. Bob Wellman developed a strange lump in his back. He also became too tired to handle the farm chores alone, so he hired a man and his thirteen-year-old son to help him. The teenager soon became irritable and lethargic, and later was hospitalized several times. But doctors could find no explanation for his symptoms. The boy's father developed swollen knees and other arthritislike symptoms that forced him to quit the farm work. "It's like we suddenly went from age thirty to sixty," said Margaret Wellman.

Even though they themselves had stopped consuming their own produce, the Wellmans faced a terrible dilemma: either sell the cows and their milk for human consumption or face financial ruin. They sent the sick animals to the market. "It's been on my conscience ever since," Bob Wellman said.

At its July meeting in Traverse City, the Agriculture Commission decided that no evidence had been presented at the May 29 public hearing in Lansing to justify a reduction of the federal PBB tolerance levels. And for a time, it appeared that the issue might at last begin to fade, since the decision had come shortly after the state study that found that no human health problems seemed to be caused by PBB and the federal study that found that low levels of PBB did not seem to harm farm animals.

But beginning in the winter of 1975, a series of jolting events would rock the entire state population out of its complacency and, for the first time, PBB became a household name throughout Michigan.

# 10

# A SAD STATE

The bloody carnage began on a foul morning in November
of 1975. The sleet was being driven by winds of up to fifty miles
an hour as friends and neighbors of Al and Hilda Green
gathered on their 250-acre farm in Lake County in north
central Michigan for the massacre. Earlier Green used an earth
mover to dig a trench 15 feet deep into the ground and
measuring 100 feet by 50 feet. And now as the 108 cows and
calves were being ushered into their mass grave, members of
the news media, including Jane Haradine of the Grand Rapids
Press, were struck by the ghastly appearance of the animals.
They were bony, many without udders; some walked stiffly,
their joints creaking, their hooves curled grotesquely out of
shape, their skins running with open abscesses. Haradine was
especially taken aback when she saw animals with protruding
bones.

Soon after the shootings began, it became apparent that
the slaughter would be even more difficult than anticipated.
Rifles jammed. Cows escaped out of one end of the ditch and
had to be rounded up. The sleet made aiming difficult and
many animals had to be shot repeatedly before they died.

Green himself stayed home during the shootings. "Al loves
these animals. It's too much for him to see them killed," his
white-haired wife, Hilda, told reporters. Green had driven the
animals to the trench and then simply walked away silently.
"We're doing this for you people," Green, inside his home, told
reporters, many of whom were from metropolitan areas such as
Grand Rapids and Detroit. "I could sell these cattle on the open
market today and they'd be in the supermarket tomorrow. But
these are sick animals and they should be kept off the market,"
Green said. He said the animals were sick and were producing
milk at only 10 percent of their previous levels. "I won't eat

them or drink their milk, and I don't want you to," said the crew-cut, fifty-eight-year-old dairyman. "It was a hard decision to make. I'm bankrupt." Green hoped the publicity now would help "clean up this damn mess and be done with it." At one time, he and Hilda had more than two hundred cows, Green said. But since May of 1974 the animals had gone "steadily down, down, down," with many of them simply dying. He had asked the Agriculture Department to quarantine his herd, but it refused after only a few out of seventy-five tissue and milk samples turned up positive, and those were at "trace" levels well within the established federal standards.

After they were turned away by the Department of Agriculture, the Greens approached Farm Bureau Services. But the co-op refused to accept animals for burial that did not exceed the federal PBB standards. It was then that the Greens decided to destroy their sick animals. Many other farmers were pretty much in the same boat. Their cows were obviously sick and contaminated but, because PBB analyses showed "legal" amounts of PBB, they were not quarantined. And yet, some were finding it increasingly difficult to market their produce. Leonard Rehkopf, for instance, a dairyman about sixty miles north of Grand Rapids, found himself "shut off" by the dairy where he was selling his milk after his name appeared on a list of producers with contaminated herds. The situation worsened when retail outlets—grocery stores and restaurants—around the state began publicly shunning Michigan products as well. When Rehkopf called the Department of Agriculture for help, he got nothing but apologies. Kenneth Van Patten, the dairy division chief, told him, "I know of nothing that we can do." Rehkopf finally went out and shot his remaining twenty-six cows, and then moved his family out of Michigan. They felt the state just "wasn't cleaning up this mess," said Mrs. Rehkopf, twenty-three, whose first child died after six weeks in 1973. "So we figured it was best to get as far away from Michigan as we could." They moved to Brewster, Washington.

The shooting of sick defenseless cows shocked not only Michigan's general public but the entire nation as well, since the slaughters were broadcast on network television news. But no one found those acts more revolting than other farmers in Michigan. "I don't see how in the name of God they can justify that!" said Adela Johnson, the dairywoman from Hesperia. Among those at the farm of Al and Hilda Green on that dreary

November 10 morning was Dr. Alpha Clark, the McBain veterinarian. When the shooting began, he could not stomach the scene. And so he left. "I felt very badly. My job is to save these animals, not shoot them. I couldn't stand it. I'm not accustomed to killing cows," Dr. Clark recalls. He sat in his El Camino and wept.

When the killing stopped, a somber Garry Zuiderveen, the Falmouth dairyman, put away his rifle and remarked, "No way could I do this to my cattle." Later that month, Zuiderveen shot eighty-seven of his cows. And they, too, could have been sold legally. Zuiderveen's herd had been quarantined on the basis of readings from a single animal, which died shortly after the quarantine notice arrived at Zuiderveen's farm. Then Farm Bureau Services refused to accept Zuiderveen's cattle for burial, as it had done previously and routinely with other quarantined herds. "Because our viewings of his cattle do not suggest the necessity of destruction, we have refused to play any role in their destruction," said the farm co-op's attorney, Kenneth G. McIntyre. Yet, when three state veterinarians inspected Zuiderveen's animals just a few months earlier, they saw an entirely different picture which convinced all three of them that the entire herd was severely contaminated by PBB. Moreover, two of the inspectors, Drs. Duaine Deming and Frank Carter, further recommended that the quarantine on Zuiderveen's farm not be lifted, and their boss, Dr. John F. Quinn, chief of the animal health division of the Agriculture Department, agreed after he read the reports filed by the three veterinarians.

Many of Zuiderveen's 200-odd animals began "going down" in the spring of 1974. For the next year and a half, nearly every other calf died just a few months after birth. And in 1974, he had to cull twenty-four cows, an extremely high amount for the number of milking cows he had, about seventy-seven. The three state veterinarians reported seeing "very dramatic" retarded growth among the calves that survived, and abnormal hooves in the adult cows. Milk production was down dramatically and 30 percent of the cows were sterile, again an extraordinarily high number. (In normal practice, dairy farmers stop milking their cows after the seventh month of pregnancy in order not to deprive the yet-unborn calf of any nourishment in the final two months before birth. Cows also have a nine-month gestation period. But after calving, the cows go right back on

156

the milk line and, a short time later, are bred once again. Calves, then, represent a dairy farmer's future, and they are bred for the first time around two years of age.) Dr. Charles C. Cole, one of the state veterinarians, reported "a lack of growth was evident in all ages" among Zuiderveen's herd, and said animals fifteen to seventeen months of age were no larger than normal animals that were six months old. "It is my opinion these animals would not make a good replacement stock," Dr. Deming agreed. He also was struck by "a slowness or reluctance to move on the part of the animals."

Cows are terribly shy creatures, despite their enormous hulk. And when strangers approach they often turn and retreat. But many of Zuiderveen's animals simply did not move when the three veterinarians approached. For one thing, many of them were down and unable to get up on their hind legs. Others, Dr. Cole noted, "just stood, almost like in a trance." There seemed to be minimal contamination in the adult animals but a much higher degree in the young stock. Dr. Deming concluded in his report, "It is my opinion from the history and observations that there is general contamination in this herd in all groups of animals," adding that it "would not be in the interest of consumer protection" to lift the quarantine from the Zuiderveen herd. Yet Farm Bureau Services refused to accept Zuiderveen's quarantined animals for burial in the Kalkaska burial pit. So he, too, went to the Department of Agriculture for help. But, like the others, Zuiderveen was turned away. "If we were to require Farm Bureau Services to accept the Zuiderveen animals at Kalkaska," explained Dr. Isleib, the chief deputy agriculture director, "Farm Bureau Services could reasonably assign responsibility for that decision—and its costs—to the Michigan Department of Agriculture." In late November, Zuiderveen was burying nineteen more dead calves one day when he realized he had but one alternative.

"We worked here over a year before we even knew what it was," said Zuiderveen in a personal account that was repeated with only slight variations by countless other farmers. Zuiderveen's experience sheds light on why it took nearly a year before such a widespread public health hazard was identified. "We were afraid to tell our neighbors. At first the problems weren't really that abnormal, except that they wouldn't respond to treatments. Farmers, see, are very proud people. So many of us didn't tell others about our own problems because that might

157

reflect on bad management practices." Halbert agreed, saying, "Farmers might say, 'I lost a cow.' But he wouldn't say, 'I'm losing twenty to thirty percent of my calves.' That'd show incompetence. And there's also some amount of stoicism involved." By January 1975, Zuiderveen said, "I realized something was dreadfully wrong. On January 10, I imposed a self-quarantine. The testing—all it amounts to is a litmus test. We took sixteen samples [from different areas of the body] from one animal, and the PBB levels ranged from zero to .7 part per million. Finally in June, we sent one animal's samples in to the Agriculture Department and it was over the level and we were quarantined." But when this animal died, Farm Bureau Services refused to take Zuiderveen's animals to Kalkaska and insisted that his quarantine be lifted. "Ken Jones [the co-op's risk manager] said Farm Bureau Services would pay for all the animals above the tolerance level but not below. But I said all the animals had the poison. Jones told me: 'Either that or nothing.'" Later, Zuiderveen got a call from Red McIntyre, Farm Bureau Services' attorney. "It's your obligation to mitigate your losses," McIntyre told him. Zuiderveen was not familiar with the word "mitigate." Turning to his nephew, Kenneth, Zuiderveen said, "I think we're going to need a lawyer." Jones agreed.

Zuiderveen signed on with Gary P. Schenk, a fast-talking, young lawyer from a conservative establishment firm in Grand Rapids once headed by Philip Buchen, who had become counsel to President Ford. Schenk had teamed up with Paul S. Greer, a more reserved white-haired lawyer in Fremont and the owner of a dairy farm that was among the half dozen hardest-hit in Michigan. Schenk and Greer had pretty much cornered the market on farmers whose animals had been contaminated by PBB but who, because of government and Farm Bureau Services reassurances to the contrary, did not have their cows tested until too late; and by the time they did, the PBB levels had dropped below the quarantine level—meaning they were ineligible for compensation. And now Schenk and Greer were filing property damage law suits against Michigan Chemical and the feed company. The lawyers, as they did with their other clients, told Zuiderveen to either keep his animals as evidence, if that was financially possible, or shoot them. "That's how strongly we felt about it [not selling contaminated animals to the market]," said Schenk. "We advised our clients that if they

158

choose to sell their animals, then we will reevaluate the question of representing them. We truly believe that the animals are a clear danger to everyone."

But even the attorneys were unable to persuade Farm Bureau Services to take Zuiderveen's quarantined herd to the Kalkaska burial site. The day after he ate his Thanksgiving turkey, Garry Zuiderveen shot eighty-seven of his sickest cows. "To depend on the defendants to make restitution is just a pipe dream," he said later. "But there was no glory in shooting the animals. I've been in a war, been shot at; there's no glory in that, either. It was a moral thing. My God, the torture that went into your soul. . . . The government had failed when it forced us to do what we did. It was morally wrong. The system was screwed up. We were searching for answers but all we ran into were dead ends." More than three years later, memories of that day still brought tears to his eyes. Those frustrations also led Zuiderveen to gain a new insight into the emotions that caused the urban riots of the 1960s. "Now," he said, "I know why they burned Detroit."

But that winter his other animals continued to die, and Zuiderveen piled them behind two barns with the intention of properly disposing of them after the spring thaw. Meanwhile the Department of Agriculture lifted the farm's quarantine after the eighty-seven sickest animals were shot and after tests on other cows showed that the PBB levels had dropped to within the acceptable government standards. Finally, in April, just several weeks before the Zuiderveens' suit against Farm Bureau Services was due for trial, the company offered them a settlement, and they accepted. Then the company sent a crew out to pick up all the carcasses but it left the Zuiderveens with all the live animals. "And the Michigan Department of Agriculture encouraged me—although they didn't say I had to—to sell those cows. I had fifty-five thousand dollars' worth of beef that I could have sold. And don't think it wasn't a hard decision to take fifty-five thousand dollars, dig a hole and bury it." But bury it they did, in a 12-foot-deep trench measuring 30 by 150 feet. It took the Zuiderveens three years to rebuild a healthy and productive herd of dairy animals.

The public uproar touched off by the grisly events on the Greens' farm still had not died down when top state officials met nine days later at night in the office of Kenneth G. Frankland, the governor's legal counsel, to review the indomitable controversy. There, the problems were clearly laid out: Many milk and meat processors were refusing to accept animals and other farm products containing PBB even well below the federal standards. Some of these animals were very sick and their owners wanted to get rid of them; but Farm Bureau Services adamantly refused to accept such animals for burial at the Kalkaska pit. The farmers, confused over bureaucratic red tape, were unsure if they could bury their dead cows on their own land with impunity; and so many just let the carcasses be exposed on the ground, including some who had shot their animals. To make matters worse, the settlement fund negotiated by Hettiger and Demlow in February had run out. The two companies and their insurance companies already had shelled out more than $25 million to settle some three hundred and fifty claims. But there were still more than six hundred and fifty additional farms with known PBB contamination but whose animals were testing below the .3 part per million tolerance level. Now these farmers were clamoring louder than ever for a tolerance level reduction so that their animals could be quarantined, making them eligible for compensation and, at the same time, protecting public safety. Almost all the farmers, it seemed, were still mad at Governor Milliken because in September he vetoed a low-interest loan bill for PBB-affected farmers (after it was unanimously approved by both houses of the legislature). And now the Kalkaska burial pit was running out of room. The original estimate that five thousand cows needed to be buried had fallen short by almost twenty-five thousand; and there were still six thousand cows already quarantined, awaiting destruction. Yet the pit had room for only two thousand more cows, at the outside.

The problems were staggering. And few people had any proposed solutions. After the meeting, Kathy Stariha, the governor's special assistant on PBB matters, and another executive staff member, Bill Long, began drafting a detailed memo for Milliken, spelling out the problems and listing several possible courses of action. The four-and-a-half-page memo reached the governor's desk six days later. The first option was to "continue to do what we are doing," which included continuing to tell the public that there's nothing wrong with foods containing less than .3 part per million. Another idea was to develop a second burial pit and then call out the National Guard to help with the work, "thereby reducing the state's cost." But the most innovative idea was a proposal for the state to buy the contaminated but unquarantined food products for use in state institutions such as hospitals, prisons and schools. Or, they further proposed, "the state might attempt to arrange the sale of these animals on the international market." Little wonder that Canada later decided to close off its border to Michigan meat products.

Milliken in essence chose the status quo. By January the settlements resumed, as a result of the out-of-court resolution of Farm Bureau Services' $200 million suit against Michigan Chemical. Also in January, however, the governor sent letters to twenty-five scientists and public health experts across the country, asking them what they knew about PBB and what further government actions, if any, might be needed. In his letter, Milliken admitted the effort was being undertaken now so that he could "obtain full insight into this matter." And then he awaited their replies.

"Most farmers, by this time, were aware there were others with similar problems," recalls Edie Clark, the aide to House Speaker Crim. "But they didn't know who, or where. They weren't organized." Many victims, such as Garry Zuiderveen in Falmouth, had been so successful in isolating themselves from fellow farmers that, incredible as it may seem, they thought they were alone in their problems. But that changed almost overnight in 1976 when state representative Donald J. Albosta formed a special PBB investigating committee and began holding a series of raucous public hearings across the state. For the first time, the farmers had a forum, and they poured out their tales of suffering and neglect and mistreatment. With each session, the hearings gained progressively more media coverage and attendance. And the public began listening. "The eggs apparently have hit the fan and, as many had feared, they're rotten and the smell is fierce," the *Michigan Farmer* magazine reported. "If half of what the farmers said in PBB hearings is true, the state and every resident in it has more trouble than they really want." The trade publication further remarked: "The PBB contamination is blossoming into a horror story of truly monumental proportions. . . . In testimony before a special House committee studying PBB, case histories rolled from the bitter tongues of beaten, damaged, ill farm people, mostly dairymen."

Dr. George L. Whitehead, the Agriculture Department's deputy director, spoke for most state officials with this assessment of the Albosta hearings: "The hearings . . . further

161

stressed the already tense situation. The thrust of the hearings was aimed at lowering the tolerance and trying to direct blame for the problem on state and federal agency officials. The emotional and political aspects of the problem were greatly escalated and this resulted in accusations by some livestock owners of 'payoffs,' incompetence, state laboratory errors, cover-ups, and even threats of bodily harm to state officials."

But more important perhaps than a mere chance to let off steam, the Albosta hearings brought the farmers together, many of them meeting one another for the first time. Together, they commiserated and swapped stories. And with each story, another piece of the puzzle fell into place. No longer were the farmers ashamed to reveal their "poor management" or their families' health problems. Their heart-wrenching stories especially touched one member of the Albosta committee, an unassuming, first-term state representative by the name of Francis R. Spaniola. As the farmers talked of how they had been ignored or mistreated by state agriculture officials or about their own deteriorating health and the medical problems of their families, tears often came to Spaniola's eyes. Quietly he resolved to do all that was within his power to help the farmers. And from the Albosta hearings, the farmers emerged as a force to be reckoned with. "Farmers by this time were well aware that all was not as it should have been," recalls Edie Clark. "Ordinarily quiet, unassuming, self-effacing persons gradually organized and turned into political activists. Many actively lobbied Lansing politicians in an attempt to communicate the extent of the problem."

The actual hearings, particularly at the outset, were fraught with confusion as the lawmakers struggled mightily to comprehend the proportions of the disaster that was unfolding before them and to realize why actions of the state agencies had failed to contain the contamination. At the first hearing in Grand Rapids, Mrs. Jerry Motz, a dairywoman from Athens, told the committee that her husband's PBB level was .35 part per million. And Albosta responded: "Your husband has more than .3 part per million and your herd is not quarantined?"

"My husband," Mrs. Motz replied sternly, "is not a cow, sir; so levels don't apply to him. But if he were a cow, he'd be buried at Kalkaska." Among those invited to testify was Dr. Walter Meester, the Grand Rapids toxicologist whose critique of the state Health Department's short-term study by then had gained widespread attention. But Dr. Meester demurred. "It's a year

162

too late," he said. "Every person in Michigan is now contaminated with PBB."

When Albosta convened his second hearing four days later in Cadillac, a year-round resort city of ten thousand in north central Michigan, more than two hundred persons showed up at McGuire's Restaurant, at one o'clock in the afternoon. Many of them were farmers who, having read about the first hearing, simply wanted to hear the stories in person. Before he called the first witness, Albosta pointed out the presence of Dr. Whitehead of the Agriculture Department and Dr. Isbister of the Health Department, and said that neither of their bosses, B. Dale Ball and Dr. Maurice Reizen, "had the guts" to attend to listen to the people. The audience cheered lustily. And there were shouts that people in Lansing who had anything to do with PBB should be lynched, or at least jailed. The hearing lasted until past 6:30 P.M.

"The reason we put the committee together," Albosta said, "was that we felt the state agencies were not doing enough to help agricultural people, and the Health Department was not doing enough to help the people that claimed to be sick by PBB."

One of the first witnesses to testify was Lou Trombley, an angry dairyman from the community of Hersey, twenty-five miles south of Cadillac. "I had two hundred and eighty head of cattle," he said, after the committee clerk administered the oath, "and one hundred and eight are dead. I sold one hundred and four on the market believing the state's big lies that this stuff wasn't going to hurt anybody. But I was sitting one day eating lunch, reading the paper where a doctor in a Veterans' Hospital [Dr. Corbett] says this is harmful to our health. My cattle has went through the same things that everybody else's has. They've aborted. They wouldn't breed. Lost weight with big appetites. Died for no reason. Our vet's checked them. January fifth of this year I got my first positive test from WARF on one cow: low tolerance. Michigan State [Department of Agriculture] done that cow but they had nothing. . . . This isn't PBB; this is Cattlegate, and we're going to fight if it takes to the end to get this damn thing cleaned up. Our health is going. It isn't only my health, your health; everybody in this state has been poisoned by this."

The audience erupted with applause as Trombley, flushed with indignation, continued: "Governor Milliken can go to hell. We're not going to eat no more of this. I have seventy-two cows left on my farm, and there's other farmers with low—not quarantine level, but low—tolerance herds. Now if the public wants to buy this, and they don't want to label it as PBB and clean it up, we'll feed it to them. . . . What's the Department of Agriculture doing to get this mess cleaned up? What is the Health Department doing? We took blood samples on our children, and they got liver damage last week—to what extent I don't know yet. But my God, I'm not going to sit still for this any longer. We've sat still. It's been going on for three years. This should have never lasted three years. You've got foreign aid for every country if they have a disaster. If you have an earthquake you've got millions of dollars for foreign aid. . . . Has anybody come forward in this room and say they got help from the state for their medical problems? Is there one member?"

"No," nearly two hundred people replied in unison.

"Where is the money that they've had appropriated by the federal government for research to help us people that's sick?" Trombley persisted.

"In their pocket," a voice said in the audience.

"That's right. Somebody's pocket," Trombley answered. Again, applause filled McGuire's Restaurant.

"We have nobody that's being helped. We've got people here that's farmed for over thirty years on welfare. Why are these people on welfare? Their dairy cattle is all dead and buried. They're sick, and they've got to go and apply for relief! Is this the way to treat the American farmer that feeds this world, this nation, the United States, Russia, China and every other country that they can squirm our grain off onto? Where is it right to us? We want this cleaned up. I'll make it short, boys. You tell the governor we got a message for him. He either buckles up and listens to what we're telling him today, and again in Sault Ste. Marie, and if he don't want to listen then, he can call the National Guard because the farmers of Michigan is going to march in Lansing. And we're not going to stop. This is a bicentennial year. Our forefathers were a bunch of dumb farmers like we are maybe. But, by God, they started this country, and we're going to take it back. And we're not going to leave it to the chemical companies and farm bureaus and the rest of these people down here in Michigan. These people from the Department of Agriculture that's telling us that this stuff is not harmful, they're a bunch of liars, and so is the Health Department for getting out here and telling you people this is good to eat—because it's not."

When Trombley finished, the room burst into applause, and Albosta moved quickly to align himself with Trombley's statements, saying that the Agriculture Department had been "lax" in relying on the federal tolerance guideline of .3 part per million instead of lowering that level to .02 part per million. Albosta added, "I think the Department of Health was also involved very deeply . . . in a short-term study that did not prove anything but a big fraud, in my mind. It was invalid. It wasn't carried out properly and, to me, it was an excuse to maintain a level of .3 part per million." The disenfranchised farmers had gained an ally in the state capital.

Not all the testimony was directed at state agencies, however. Some, in fact, was quite personal in nature. Mrs. David Curtis of West Branch gave a harrowing account of her family's health problems.

"Our David, whose birth date is in 1966, had some stomach pains. Stomach X rays were done and were negative. Both children did not gain weight during 1973 and 1975. In fact, my own family doctor, whom I had worked for, looked me in the eye one day and said, 'Are you sure you're not poisoning these children?' And this was before we had any indication at all that we were contaminated. And looking back on other symptoms we remembered that we had: sores on our faces, in our noses and on our legs. We especially remember our scalps being sore and a loss of hair. . . . We each recall aching muscles in joints, extreme fatigue, and a soreness and burning just below the throat in the area of the esophagus. We had sore gums. We noticed a lot of anxiety, which I believe could have been caused partially by psychological reasons. Each of us still has severe joint pains. And my husband was suffering so much from fatigue in the spring of 1975 that he couldn't even get to the fields, and farmers came and helped him put his crops in. We noticed that he had a lot of splitting fingernails. They peeled in layers. My husband was treated in January 1975 for severe rash and abdominal pains. He was treated with cortisone." Mrs. Curtis said her five-year-old girl in 1973 had severe intestinal problems that were not diagnosed, developed blurred vision, including temporary blindness and finally a club foot that

165

required braces. Those symptoms eventually subsided as inexplicably as they had appeared. "We also cut her long hair because it was getting dull and it was falling out," she said.

Several other relatives, including her parents, who also ate foodstuffs from the Curtis farm, experienced assorted health problems as well, Mrs. Curtis said. We supplied milk to our minister's family. Their little girl was born during the time . . . with a club foot and also had to have braces. Their little girl had sores on her face. I have other relatives who have had contaminated chickens who have had physical problems." She dabbed her eyes with a tissue somebody had offered her and returned to her seat.

Next was Ron Creighton, a young farmer who owns forty acres of land just east of Stanwood. Creighton had fourteen head of cattle and an assortment of ducks, geese and chicken—all contaminated by PBB. "We ate our own eggs, made our own butter and milk, rendered our own lard and butchered our own pork," he said. "And we started having our trouble with health about February 1974. My wife Jeannette's legs swelled up to the extent where she had to wear my boots to go into town." He said even a ten-day hospitalization failed to produce a diagnosis. Soon she developed symptoms: no saliva, loss of hair, vision difficulties. In August of 1974, Creighton was visiting with a neighbor when the neighbor was quarantined. "There was a state man there that had the quarantine slip, and Carmen asked him if he thought I ought to have my animals checked. And he asked me if I sold any of the meat or eggs or anything. And I told him no, that we was in the process of raising a dairy herd and was using most of the pork and eggs and milk for our own use at the time. 'Well,' he said, 'don't worry about it, then.'" Shortly after that, Creighton recalled, his own health problems began. "I started having trouble with my feet swelling, as if they were stoned bruised. I had trouble with dizziness. And at that time I was working for the Mecosta County Road Commission, plus doing what chores we had [on the farm]. Then in January 1975 I got so I could hardly stand it anymore." A doctor told Creighton that he had congenital arthritis, which he had to "learn to live with." Despite taking aspirins, he said, "the pain increased, and I kept missing more time at work." Creighton visited other doctors, who examined him for gout and performed liver tests, but nothing turned up. Finally, he heard about, and went to, an osteopathic physician in Big Rapids

166

named David T. Salvati, who had begun seeing many farm families poisoned by PBB. "He told me that I was having a lot of the same symptoms that people with PBB were having, and asked me if I had my animals checked, and I told him, I hadn't at the time." But Creighton took Dr. Salvati's advice. The results showed PBB concentrations as high as 1.7 in some hogs and chickens. The cows also were above the tolerance guideline.

In late February of 1975, Creighton was fired from his job with the road commission. "I got so that I couldn't stand getting in and out of the truck and the vibration from the motor, and the guys that I worked for got so that they was doing my share of the work." Later that year Creighton and his wife had their own fatty tissues analyzed for PBB. He showed 1.46 parts per million, she .54 part per million. "We've been pretty lucky. We haven't had too much trouble with our kids. That winter in 1974 they slept a lot. I'd say twelve, thirteen, fourteen hours at a time. And that's not normal for our kids," Creighton testified. "But they're better now. And we had PBB levels just drew from their blood, and they've all got PBB. My wife still has chest pains, dizziness and her legs still ache. I'm still... I still have trouble with my joints. I've got calcium deposits on my elbows and knees. And it's nothing for me to sleep anywheres from twelve to eighteen hours at a time. I have trouble with dizziness, trouble standing up. And I can be walking along and all of a sudden I feel like I'm going to tip right over. One time my head fell on the coffee table. I've had trouble with headaches. I can't get out of the bathtub by myself. My wife has to help me out. And we had to put extra mattresses on the bed so I could get up in the morning."

By the time Creighton had finished, Albosta was shaking with rage. "Our Health Department has did [sic] a very, very bad job," he said, "and our Agriculture Department the same way. After listening to people like Mrs. Curtis and Mr. Creighton speak, I pretty near had tears in my eyes and I can't help it. I would just like to go over and do some bodily harm to the same people that's did bodily harm to you."

And as each story came pouring forth, the dimensions of the PBB contamination seemed to enlarge. Mrs. Harley Cole, a resort owner in Pickford, located in Michigan's Upper Peninsula, told of the gastrointestinal problems she, her husband and their four children experienced. Her husband, she said, "is having very bad joint problems. He's having back problems. He had a small bowel ulcer. On November 14, 1975, he finally collapsed." Her husband was thirty-three-years-old. "I have a young boy who is six years old; his knees are almost the size of mine. This is very upsetting. The school nurse comes to me and asks me, 'Mrs. Cole, I know you're very responsible to your children. But do you not know that your daughter is ill?' I said, 'Yes, I know it. I have taken her to the doctor. The doctor says he can't find anything wrong—except all the kids do have PBB in their systems.' I think it's time that the state of Michigan realizes that it is not up to us to prove that PBB is harmful. The burden of proof belongs to the federal government and the state of Michigan. We don't have the money that they do and we are the ones who are paying taxes to this state for them to take care of us and to watch over us. And if this is the type of thing that we're receiving, I think we no longer need the government officials we have." Mrs. Cole went on to tell of the mysterious deaths of fourteen household pets within a matter of eight weeks, including one that was "very stout." The veterinarian could find nothing wrong with one dog, but then she simply fell over dead, Mrs. Cole said. The autopsy showed that she had .42 part per million PBB in her fat. Ten of the dead dogs were pups nursed by the stout mother.

"There is another thing I would like to mention," she added. "We are very concerned about the fact that our wildlife is being contaminated. My husband shot a bear this year. We consumed it. He became ill again. He became worse. So we sent a sample in from the bear." Sure enough, the bear somehow had also been poisoned by PBB. "And this is being caused by the state and Farm Bureau not doing anything about dead animals laying around. It's about time that some of these farmers got some help. They've paid enough."

Another nonfarmer who testified was Victor Gleisen, a farm equipment salesman who said he visits hundreds of farms each year. "And I have been instrumental in diagnosing some of these herds as polybrominated biphenyls, in my estimation, before the local vet got to them. I know in Osceola County I told a man he had PBB. His brother was a veterinarian. He didn't believe me. But they found out he has it. I have other people that will verify—some of them are here—that I told them that I thought they had polybrominated biphenyl. You could see about so much of it and you get to know what you're looking at. What I'd like to say is we . . . I have only uncovered the tip of the iceberg. There are a lot more herds out there than you think."

When the meeting finally broke up after 6:30 P.M., the reporters raced for the telephones. The legislative forum had stamped the imprimatur of legitimacy to the harrowing experiences of the farmers. PBB figured prominently in the news the next day, but not merely because of the tumultuous Albosta hearing.

On the same day as the Cadillac meeting, Governor Milliken in Lansing announced a "five-point action plan" to deal with the problem that, he said, "has plagued Michigan for the past two years." The plan's highlight was the appointment of a five-member "Scientific advisory panel" to review all the available scientific data on PBB and then recommend to Milliken any further courses of action it deemed appropriate. "Those recommendations will include an evaluation of whether state guidelines for meat, milk, poultry and eggs are safe or should be lowered, an evaluation of long-term human health implications and whether there are factors other than PBB at low levels impairing the health of Michigan animals." The other aspects of the governor's five-point action plan were the appointment of a three-member oversight committee charged with monitoring and facilitating the progress in the settlement of farmers' claims, a commitment by the state to bury animal carcasses presently remaining on farmers' property, a directive to the Department of Agriculture to complete testing of every animal still under quarantine and, finally, a directive to the Department of Public Health to "intensify its efforts" to help the affected farm families. The action plan, Milliken explained, "is also designed to help end the rumors and half-truths that often surround this issue."

But the five-point action plan did little to diffuse the Albosta road show, which held its third and final hearing on March 12, a week later, in Sault Ste. Marie, a city of fifteen thousand in Michigan's Upper Peninsula and the northern terminus of U.S. Interstate 75, which ends in Tampa, Florida. "It was the worst winter day of the year," recalls Doc Alpha Clark. He left his home well before dawn and arrived by ten. "Hell, I thought nobody'd be there. But when I walked in, three hundred people were there. And they were mad as hell."

The testimony of farmers was similar to the earlier hearings. But at the "Soo" hearing, a young local public health

169

physician showed up to plead for state aid and compassion. He was Dr. James Terrian, director of the Chippewa County Health Department. He said it wasn't until October 1975 that "someone in Chippewa County had raised the question of PBB to me," since state agriculture officials maintained that the Upper Peninsula virtually had been exempt from PBB contamination. "Since that time, the Chippewa County Board of Health has directed me to do all I can within our existing resources to help families who believe that they have health problems which are associated with PBB," Dr. Terrian said. And so with the assistance of the War Memorial Hospital and its staff, fat samples were obtained from surgical patients there for PBB analysis. "These were people in whom we had no reason to expect PBB tissue levels," Dr. Terrian said. But the first thirteen samples all showed PBB, ranging from .05 part per million to as high as 2.94 parts per million. As a result of that startling finding, he told the Albosta committee, the county health department hired a nurse to work twelve hours a day to interview families who needed medical care. "There are people in Chippewa County who are experiencing new, unusual problems. These include such things as weight loss, ulcers in people who have not had them in the past; vague, miserable, uncomfortable gastrointestinal problems; fatigue, sleepiness in people who, in the past, have not been sleeping ten, twelve, fourteen hours a day. Mothers have seen their children stop gaining weight, or lose weight. It'd certainly be troublesome to me as a parent," said Dr. Terrian.

Other disturbing results turned up when he requested the War Memorial Hospital's radiology staff to examine X-ray records for the years 1972, 1974 and 1975 for patients under eighteen. "Between 1972 and 1974, there was doubling of the number of children that had confirmed ulcers. The numbers are small; it was twenty-three in 1972 and forty-seven in 1974." Records for 1973 were omitted deliberately to avoid confusion, since that was the year PBB first contaminated human foods.

Moreover, Dr. Terrian said, the fact that there had been a tripling in the number of persons under age seventeen willing to participate in a series of gastrointestinal tests suggested "there was an increased number of people under age seventeen who had gastrointestinal distress sufficient enough to go through what really is not very pleasant or much fun."

As a result of the assorted information that was collected, Dr. Terrian said efforts were made to obtain further help from the state Health Department in Lansing. "We haven't been successful," he said. "We haven't got [from Lansing] very much in terms of resources; one of those resources is information. The response from some state agencies has not indicated the same level of sensitivity and concern that we have been demonstrating in the Chippewa County Health Department. And I think in this instance the Chippewa County Health Department has assumed the proper stance." He, of course, was right.

"Doctor," Spaniola, the earnest, almost diffident, first-term lawmaker, asked, "are you saying that the department has not responded as they should in the pursuance of the kinds of things you are attempting to pursue?"

"I think that's accurate. The Department of Public Health appears to be expecting a clear scientific relationship which will be dose-related between the presence of PBBs in people and some demonstrable, consistent health impairment," Dr. Terrian replied. "I think that independent of the scientific need to make certain that we maintain absolute objectivity is a human need to make certain that we're responding to people with compassion."

Spaniola asked if Dr. Terrian had felt any repercussions from the state Health Department as a result of his outspokenness and consumer advocacy posture.

"Well, I read in the papers that I'm characterized as an alarmist. And part of that comes because I am young and I don't have a lot of scientific credentials. Maybe by the time I'm sixty I won't be looked at as an alarmist. There's nothing that would delight me more than in fifteen years to say, 'By golly, I should not have gotten so worried about PBB. PBB is a nutrient.'" Interestingly, Dr. Reizen, the state public health director, Dr. Terrian's titular boss, called him two days before the Sault Ste. Marie hearing, inquiring about his planned testimony before the Albosta committee. Dr. Terrian told Dr. Reizen that he, Terrian, could not represent the state Health Department at the hearing because he did not approve of the way Dr. Reizen and others were handling the problem.

Spaniola, whose calm, reasoned approach was a dramatic contrast to Albosta's flailing, give-'em-hell performance, also asked Dr. Terrian why he thought some farm families were

171

being ridiculed and called "outright kooks"—even by state officials—for blaming their animal and personal health problems on PBB.

"It relates to strong attacks on positions that individuals within state government have taken and who, at times, have been attacked personally in terms of their credibility or their integrity," Dr. Terrian replied slowly. "And some of these individuals have responded with some defensiveness, which at times has taken on a form which appears to be an attempt to impugn the motives of the citizens of the state of Michigan who have questions that have not been adequately responded to." One such typical bureaucrat was Dr. Kenneth R. Wilcox, Jr., a tall, dour man who serves as chief of the state Health Department's bureau of disease control and laboratory services. After Hilda Green described her recent gall bladder problems to the Albosta committee in Grand Rapids, Wilcox simply dismissed them as those that "might be expected from an obese woman."

The emotional Albosta hearings greatly exacerbated the mutual feelings of distrust and even hostility between farmers and state bureaucrats, especially agriculture officials. Indeed, the Agriculture Department became so provoked that it deliberately plotted a high-powered campaign in what turned out to be another misguided effort to restore public confidence. Using taxpayer's money, the department publicly singled out Richard Edington, a ruggedly handsome dairyman from the Upper Peninsula, as a typical example of a poor manager who was trying to blame PBB for problems that had nothing to do with the chemical.

The Michigan Department of Public Health reacted with more contrition, however. A week after the Albosta hearings ended, it convened a meeting in Lansing of all local health officers from around the state. It was a soul-searching affair, with Theodore Ervin, the state's deputy public health director, openly lamenting the agency's loss of credibility. And all resolved to do a better job from here on out, including "seeking out and listening to the farmers." Among such farmers would be those with below tolerance PBB levels who are known to be good dairymen, it was pointed out. "There should be some careful looking and listening in order to add what these people are seeing and experiencing to the scientific determinations," Ervin's notes from the meeting said. But when Dr. George L. Whitehead, the irascible deputy agriculture director, later came across Ervin's notes and read that passage, he demanded that the passage be stricken from the official record. But Ervin refused.

As the March 19 meeting came to a close, Ervin cautioned the local health officers (Dr. Terrian among them) to keep in mind that different farmers will have different "perspectives." And then, attesting to the staggering complexities of the PBB controversy, Ervin listed these "perspectives":

A. Families on PBB-quarantined farms who have had sick animals.
B. Families on farms where herds were exposed, but below quarantine level, who have sick animals.
C. Families on farms with no known PBB exposure who have sick animals.
D. Families from "PBB-clean" farms who have no more sick animals than could be normally expected.
E. People who know they ate PBB-contaminated products—and attribute various illnesses to this.
F. People who know they ate PBB-contaminated products—and do not attribute any illness to this.
G. People who do not know if they ate PBB-contaminated products but fear they did, and attribute illness to this.
H. Persons in groups B and C, who see sick animals which they attribute to PBB and fear they may also become sick or cause sickness if the animals are eaten.
I. Persons not concerned (a group growing smaller, rapidly).

But to Ervin's list one must add yet another, and an extremely important, "perspective"—that of whether or not a farmer had been successful in obtaining an out-of-court compensation settlement from Michigan Chemical and Farm Bureau Services Inc. For the most part, farmers who received these settlements had restocked and gone back into business, such as Rick Halbert and Blaine and Adela Johnson of Hesperia. The Johnsons, for instance, had among the most highly contaminated herds in the state. "We think we got sixty pounds of bad feed, and each cow probably got a pound of it," recalls Mrs. Johnson. While they do not doubt the feed was bad, they say it also "could have been a contributing factor—especially if the animals were not well taken care of in the first place." In other words, the Johnsons said, how hard animals were hit by PBB depended on how well they had been cared for by their owners.

173

The implication was clear: It was the "poor managers" (whose farms got very little PBB, were not quarantined and thus ineligible for settlement) who now were doing all the hollering about PBB.

The Johnsons ultimately sent 153 cows to the Kalkaska burial pit. The cows had been appraised at $157,000. But the final settlement the Johnsons got totaled just over $300,000, which included cleanup costs and loss of milk sales. The couple bought a replacement herd, purchased a new tractor and then paid off their farm. "I guess it looked very attractive. But who's to say we wouldn't have felt the same way? The insurance companies paid out too much in the beginning and then later had to pull in their horns. Then they got tighter with their dollars, I guess," Adela Johnson said. She made no bones about why she and her husband vehemently oppose farmers who say all PBB should be prohibited in foods. "We're fighting for our own future, but in doing so it appears we're fighting them."

Her husband, Blaine, put it more bluntly. "Many of us successfully collected our claims several months after the discovery," he said. "There was some publicity on amounts and hoped-for amounts which sometimes included land and punitive damages. In general, the figures sounded better than farming. This had a psychological effect on farmers just below one part per million [the first federal tolerance guideline], and was a strong factor for the lowering to .3 part per million [the second federal tolerance guideline], in my opinion. At that point, I didn't recall any public fright or disapproval. As the .3 group began being paid off, there came a third group of farmers still under the .3 level who began to claim problems in their herds; and later they claimed human health problems. This group was the first to meet resistance from farmers in the high and .3 groups, then from the Michigan Department of Agriculture, Michigan State University, the Food and Drug Administration, some veterinarians, the Michigan Milk Producers Association, and others. This group used the news media heavily to tell their awful story—to the point that it is affecting our markets and our very right to produce and sell our products."

And so many farmers like the Johnsons began publicly denouncing fellow farmers—those who now could only demonstrate low PBB contamination but who demanded a just compensation nevertheless for their poisoned animals. Farmers

174

such as Al Green and Lou Trombley found themselves being openly ridiculed as hypocrites who, grandstanding as protectors of the consumer, shot their cows when all they really wanted to do was bring about a further reduction in PBB standards—thereby qualifying them for quarantines and compensation. These internecine attacks were fueled by agriculture officials who encouraged rumors that such "low-level farmers" were poor managers who did not adhere to good animal husbandry practices—supposedly the true reasons why their animals were sick and dying.

"What we say in public may be inflammatory," Adela Johnson admitted, "but it's the truth as we see it. It's a sad, sad thing to have farmer against farmer. We don't visit with each other anymore like we used to. Things just are not the same as before. And, the sad thing is, we're all Christians on both sides of the fence."

In their counterattack, the low-level farmers, paradoxically, also ascribed the profit motive to the opposition, saying that folks such as the Johnsons, having been justly compensated, now were downplaying the PBB contamination, hoping to go on doing business without further disruption—never mind that they were sending to the market new generations of animals contaminated by PBB residues that cannot be eradicated from the farm environment. Blaine and Adela Johnson purchased eighty new cows in 1974 and 1975. Later, when they tested the fatty tissues of six such cows, all six showed PBB, although at below the quarantine level of one part per million. But if the tolerance level were dropped, they could well be quarantined once more. Selling below quarantine but still contaminated food products did not bother the Johnsons. But they certainly had the courage of their convictions. "Yes," said Mrs. Johnson, "we eat our own meat and drink our own milk. We even had one cow that tested at a hundred and twenty-five parts per million. We just trimmed off the fat and ate it. It was delicious." She said her entire family, including four young children, has quite high PBB levels; yet no one is sick. "If we were cattle, we'd be buried. But do you see anything wrong with us?"

But most others displayed a less cavalier concern toward a chemical about which so little was known, especially in its long-range effects. "My kids, their joints squeak, just like the cows, when walking," said Lou Trombley, the burly dairyman from

Osceola County. "They have skin and respiratory problems. It's nothing else but PBB. And now they're being ridiculed at school. Hell, I've always raised my family with belief in government. Now I tell them government stinks. This is Cattlegate. Nine million people have been poisoned." Trombley had over three hundred cows and sold 103 of them before he even suspected his herd had PBB. "And one of them died right on the scale," he recalls. "But we were never quarantined because the Agriculture Department said our animals were below the tolerance level." Finally, one cool summer evening in 1976, Trombley went out and shot every remaining cow. "They were my cows, and they were sick and dying. What I saw happen to those cattle I didn't want to happen to the public. I didn't think it was safe to eat them, so why should I sell them to others to eat? And now even my neighbors won't speak to me because I openly said I had PBB. To admit PBB is the worst thing a man can do. It's better to have VD." Shortly after he shot his animals, the Trombleys began receiving anonymous telephone threats, prompting Trombley for the first time in his life to sleep with a loaded shotgun within reach.

"If I'm such a 'bad' farmer, why did my bank lend me another $100,000 to buy more cows after I shot 196? I've made a profit every year since we started here in 1969, except the first year and the last year, when we shot the animals. If I'm such a 'bad' farmer, how come I had $17,000 saved, which is what we lived on for over a year?" Trombley's grandparents had been farmers in southern Wayne County, just downriver from Detroit. And as a young man, he worked in a steel mill in Trenton, a suburban Detroit community. At the same time, he bought a farm near there. "But I wasn't happy just farming on the side," Trombley recalls. And so in 1969, after thirteen years, he had saved enough money to buy a farm in the north central Michigan community of Hersey. Since then, he has bought out two other farms to double his original investment. Then the PBB contamination struck his farm in early 1976. Although state Agriculture Department tests showed only traces of PBB in his cows, Trombley said private laboratory tests showed more than negligible PBB contamination. Yet the state never acted to keep his sick animals out of the human food chain. A year after he shot his 196 remaining cows, Trombley put his life's work up for sale "lock, stock and barrel," including nearly a hundred more head of cattle he had purchased after he shot the contaminated animals. "We were both born and raised in Michigan," said Carol Trombley. "Now we never want to see Michigan again. We want to go somewhere and live in peace and quiet. That's what we came here for." Her husband added, "Hell, I can always buy cows again—but not my family and their health. How much more evidence do people need? Do they got to wait until their own family is hit? At least we can die knowing we did what was right."

Farmers such as Trombley soon were being ridiculed in the executive offices of the Department of Agriculture. For instance, one day, shortly after Trombley shot his animals, the Johnsons were in the department's executive offices in Lansing when Trombley's name "just came up," recalls Adela Johnson. Dr. Whitehead said he had something interesting to show the Johnsons. It was test results that showed very little, if any, PBB had been found in some of the Trombleys' cattle. "If you were Farm Bureau," Mrs. Johnson said later, "would you pay $620,000 for his 'damages'?" They have a neighbor who also shot his cattle, she said. "But being a likable sort with an honest face, he has also been able to borrow huge sums of money."

Even before the terrible split in the farm community had occurred, Alan L. Hoeting, the Food and Drug Administration's district director in Detroit, was becoming increasingly puzzled by the persistence of the PBB controversy and what he saw as an unusual turn of events in such a contamination problem. "Ordinarily, we have to defend the 'lowness' of a tolerance level. In this case, it was just the opposite. It was a very different kind of situation. Ordinarily, the FDA tries—has to—prove something is bad. Here it was just the opposite." Here, he marveled, his agency was being excoriated for not being stringent enough. (But there is one important difference he did not mention, however. In matters such as the saccharin controversy, the FDA is governed by the Delaney Amendment, which unequivocally requires the agency to ban any food additive that has been shown to cause cancer in laboratory animals. There the FDA has no choice. But PBB is not a food additive in its intended use, and so the agency in this case enjoys considerable latitude in setting public exposure limits, including economic considerations, in the specious risk-versus-benefit equation.) Referring to Michigan agriculture officials, Hoeting said, "I don't know of any other regulatory officials, in breaking new ground, who have caused so much condemnation of food and animals in carrying out regulatory and consumer protection responsibilities." And so Hoeting, whose office Rick Halbert had called for help in March of 1974, formulated a preposterous theory as to why so many farmers had become so vocal in their complaints. And on April 30, 1976, Hoeting went to Washington to promote his theory in Congress.

"I think, to try to get at the issue of why we are continuing to receive so many reports and complaints and what have you, we would have to go back and look at the total economic environment in agriculture," he told the House subcommittee on conservation and credit, which was chaired by a Minnesota congressman, Bob Bergland, who now is Jimmy Carter's secretary of agriculture. "Dairy farmers throughout the United States have suffered a severe financial squeeze. Their costs exceeded their income. In 1974 and 1975 that was the case. From a tabulation of some data which was prepared by our office from some reports from the Michigan State University department of agricultural economics, it shows that the typical dairy farmer lost an average of $107 per cow in 1974 and had a management loss of $128 per cow in 1975.

"Also, as I sat in my office in Detroit and listened to the complaints and the press reports, I am also very much aware that the bulk of our complaints which we received concerning animal health have taken place during the period January 1, 1975, through May 1, 1976. It just happens in Michigan that the property taxes are due and payable on February 15. I understand farmers' federal income tax payments are due March 1. This is the period of time this year when farmers' stock of hay or grain or what have you, which they have raised themselves, will become depleted. They are then forced into a situation where they have to buy grain from the general market.

"A part of what we are seeing in Michigan at this point is due to complaints of the overall price squeeze that is taking place for dairy farmers."

Representative James M. Jeffords, a Vermont Republican, asked Hoeting, "Thus, you believe, then, that the farmers who have only cattle or dairy herds with .3 part per million or less are complaining primarily because of the economic situation and not because of any loss attributable to the PBB?"

"This," Hoeting replied, "is my judgment. I have reams of data in my files which indicate that most of the individuals who are doing most of the complaining are farmers who have

178

virtually no PBB in their animals. While it is outside of the purview of the Food and Drug Administration, I also read the press clippings and I find that these individuals are in debt in the range of $50,000 to $85,000, or more."

Jeffords apparently was satisfied with Hoeting's outrageous accusations. Neither did Bergland show much interest, saying only that, "I would remind members of the committee that we have six witnesses this morning. Time flies by."

Had it not been for Representative Alvin Baldus, a Democrat from the state of Wisconsin, Hoeting's speculations might have gone unchallenged. "It would seem to me," Baldus said to Hoeting, "that you are suggesting that getting rid of the herds by condemnation would be a remedy for the farmer. But in the dairy business cash flow is better than no cash flow because expenses remain almost the same. Even though you are losing some money, you are not losing as much as if you went out of business entirely. If you get rid of the herd but did not get the money back, the interest on the capital investment continues. So it seems to me that if that was a person's first thought—that is, if he reexamined that—it would not be a very solid foundation for a remedy for a financial problem. It would make it worse. Does that make sense to you?"

"Yes it does," Hoeting answered.

The common sense Congressman Baldus introduced into the debate over low-level farms, however, did not deter Michigan bureaucrats from recirculating Hoeting's speculations at every opportunity. Two weeks after Hoeting made his accusations in Washington, Dr. Whitehead, the deputy agriculture director, wrote a letter to Dr. Kolbye at the FDA, reporting, "The PBB problem in Michigan continues to linger on, and all the controversy is centered around a few low-level herd owners who would like to make a claim for damages. In general, most of them appear to be cases of malnutrition but they are certainly doing their best to get publicity and public sentiment which, unfortunately, is injuring the livestock industry in this state."

Malnutrition, of course, is precisely what Dr. Whitehead and his cohorts told Rick Halbert and many other farmers their cows were suffering from. There were a number of such memos written and circulated by agriculture and public health officials, some of which were sent to Governor Milliken. And at Farm Bureau Services, staff veterinarian Dr. Paul E. Johnson was exhorting the company's top officers to take "strong counteraction and pretty darn quickly." In a three-page vitriolic memo, he wrote, "Regarding belligerent claimants, the more insistent they are on the degree of their problems, the more likely their actual level of contamination is very low. They have used contamination as a garbage can to throw all their problems and losses into without having to show a cause-effect relationship, let alone prove it."

Nearly one and a half years after Hoeting told the Bergland subcommittee he had "reams of data" to back up his allegations against Michigan farmers, another congressional subcommittee demanded to see such information. But Hoeting was unable to substantiate his earlier claims, and the FDA later had to issue a statement retracting Hoeting's 1976 accusations. The panel that demanded to see Hoeting's data was the House subcommittee on oversight and investigations, chaired by California Representative John E. Moss, now retired. After Moss reviewed the documents Hoeting had sent, he wrote Dr. Donald Kennedy, FDA commissioner, "I regret to inform you that of the [four and a half inches of] materials, no more than fifty pages are relevant to the question. Most of the documents supplied carry dates post-dating Mr. Hoeting's remarks before the agriculture subcommittee. A number of documents included are totally irrelevant to the question."

Hoeting's attitude toward the low-level Michigan farmers, one top FDA official conceded later, "was not relevant to our role in the matter." Said John R. Wessel, scientific coordinator of the agency's office of compliance: "Hoeting perhaps got too involved. The farmers are as honest and sincere as any human beings. There's no doubt in my mind," Wessel said. The agency's formal retraction of Hoeting's accusations said that, while Hoeting appeared to have been expressing a personal opinion, "the agency as a whole has not taken a position on or even considered the possible economic motives of Michigan farmers involved in the PBB incident in Michigan."

But in the spring of 1976, the deliberate campaign to discredit low-level farmers seemed to gain momentum. It finally caused *Michigan Farmer* magazine to thunder in an editorial, "We have resented from the beginning of the tragic episode repeated attempts to blame the victims—the farmers— rather than the perpetrators. In our first contacts with farmers whose herds were suffering, we heard repeated complaints that

180

Farm Bureau Services representatives challenged the management, nutrition, and general husbandry practices of farmers in an attempt to shift the blame from the poisoned feed." The editorial continued: "Now an even more insidious campaign is being waged against farmers with low levels of PBB in their herds. And to make it even worse, some of the campaigning is being done by fellow farmers. The basic message we have run into goes: 'There is no proof that PBB at low levels causes any adverse effects in cattle. Farmers with PBB levels in their animals below the .3 part per million level should look to their management and nutritional programs. Some of these farmers just aren't feeding their animals enough. Others are trying to take Farm Bureau and the insurance companies to the cleaners.' We got the same story from representatives of Farm Bureau Services, Michigan Department of Agriculture, Michigan State University, the U.S. Food and Drug Administration, the U.S. Department of Agriculture and in letters and phone calls from farmers around the state.

"And yet," the *Michigan Farmer* said, "we had other information that indicated just the opposite was true."

The magazine had sent one of its reporters, Paul Courter, to tour the dairy farms of Missaukee County to interview low-level farmers and Dr. Alpha Clark. Courter began his report this way:

"Driving through the Missaukee County countryside, you'd think all is well and serene on the farms around the rural community of McBain.

"The fields are bigger, the soil better-looking and the dairy farm buildings and milking parlors more up to date than you might expect in that northwesterly part of the state. The names on the mailboxes and barns of the farms reveal a heavy Dutch influence—Zuiderveen, Kamphouse, Van Haitsma, Molhoek.

"Spend a little time with a few of those dairymen, and you'll quickly learn that all is not well, most assuredly not serene, and hasn't been since PBB contamination was discovered in Missaukee County dairy animals."

Among the many farmers Courter met on that trip was an erect and folksy dairyman with pale blue eyes and a quick smile by the name of Roy Tacoma, whose name was destined to become famous throughout Michigan and make history in the state's judicial history.

What Courter found on farm after farm were sick and

pathetic-looking animals with the now familiar symptoms, lined up in the parlors as farmers tried to coax milk out of their shriveled udders. Before PBB struck, many of these farms were producing 30 to 50 percent above the state average.

Dayton Matlick, editor of *Michigan Farmer*, wrote in the accompanying editorial, "The implications that these struggling, frustrated dairymen have abandoned their hard-won knowledge of husbandry and are starving their animals in order to cash in on the disaster is as asinine as it is heartless. Sure, there may be a few exploiters around—there always are. But the farmers we visited are good dairymen and good people. They developed their herds over generations of breeding and would not sacrifice their animals willingly.

"Regardless of 'professional' testimony to the contrary, we are convinced that many farmers with low-level contamination in their herds are suffering financial loss due to poisoning of their animals beyond their control." Matlick also had generous praise for the red-headed, barrel-chested Dr. Alpha Clark, who, he said "has the perseverance and guts to fight for them [the farmers] against the ponderous bureaucracies—public and private—that grind lesser men to dust."

Bonnie Hughston, who with her husband, Bill, own a trucking operation, later would write about the bitter days of the controversy: "We saw many cases where trusted farm managers were fired when PBB struck because suddenly cattle were dying. In one case, the manager was accused of stealing animals because the owner could not accept the fact that that many animals could die," said Mrs. Hughston. "Every day I read or heard about some farmer saying this PBB is blown up and exaggerated by the press. Invariably I could get out my files and see that this same man who now thinks it is not a problem thought it was very much a problem before we trucked his cattle away and he got his settlement. Others who didn't think it was much of a problem seemed to have a hot line to Farm Bureau," she said. "We have visited farms from every area in Michigan. Many have been in the dairy business for years and years. Suddenly they were being accused of starving their livestock. Some were accused of not having PBB, but iodine poisoning, moldy feed, lice, parasites, you name it—even though they had tests proving they had PBB in their herd."

Two farmers who bore a major brunt of the establishment's public ridicule were Jerry Woltjer and Dick Edington.

Edington, thirty, owned a herd near Pickford in Michigan's

Upper Peninsula. In early 1975, he began noticing unusual health problems among his herd of 256 cows. His veterinarian that spring called the Department of Agriculture for assistance in diagnosing the problem. But Drs. Donald Grover and Frank Carter, the veterinarians who had worked on the Halbert herd in 1974, again were unable to determine the problem. Fat tissues taken from Edington's dead animals were tested for PBB, but the results came back negative. By early summer, Edington decided to stop milking the cows since, in the three previous months, they had consumed $12,000 worth of feed while producing only $9,000 worth of milk. By then only 101 cows out of 256 were still alive; the rest had died, except for 9 which Edington sold for meat. By late fall, Edington had fallen $51,000 in debt to the federal Farmers Home Administration, and so the agency repossessed the remaining animals and sold them for meat. The sale took place less than a week after Al and Hilda Green shot their herd, and when word of the government's role in the sale of a herd suspected of PBB poisoning reached the public, the uproar was instant and came from all parts of the state. "U.S. Sells PBB-laced Herd for Beef," the Grand Rapids *Press* reported. Those who had purchased the Edington cows brought them back to the Michigan Livestock Exchange in St. Louis, demanding refunds. But when the exchange, in turn, requested the Farmers Home Administration to take back the animals, Keith Russell, head of the agency's program in Michigan, refused. Furthermore, he said there were at least forty other herds in the state whose owners were in the same boat as Edington, and that their herds, too, might well be disposed of in the same manner. "As long as the animals are legally salable, we can't see any reason why they shouldn't be sold," Russell said. "We were helping the farmer [Edington] get over a touchy situation. He didn't want the responsibility of putting those animals on the market."

With the Michigan Livestock Exchange left holding the cows nobody wanted, Rick Halbert said, "Somebody dreamed up this idea: 'Hey, once and for all, let's show everybody that this low-level business is nonsense.'" But B. Dale Ball, the state's agriculture director, explained the subsequent events this way, "the Michigan Department of Agriculture and Michigan State University's college of veterinary medicine and college of agricultural and natural resources worked out an arrangement to move the herd to a farm near Mason for study."

Quickly, ninety-four cows from the Edington herd were

hauled to a farm just south of Lansing owned by Frank McCalla, which was equipped for a diary operation but was not being used as one at the time. There the animals began receiving lavish attention from veterinarians and dairy nutritionists from Michigan State University. After eighteen weeks on the farm, state agriculture officials reported that most of the cows had been restored to good health and that their past problems were due to "external and internal parasites, anemia and malnutrition." The department even put out a six-page report, complete with "before" and "after" photographs, which concluded, "The MSU [Michigan State University] scientists have established that the problem with this herd was not PBB poisoning."

The department was so pleased with the results that on April 27, it staged a "show-and-tell" session on the farm for Michigan lawmakers and media representatives. Included on the agenda was a color slide show of the "before" and "after" pictures of the cows. But the Agriculture Department never got to show all the slides, for state representative Don Albosta had shown up with a group of angry farmers, including Hilda Green and Lou Trombley. "It was a three-ring circus," recalls Dr. Thomas H. Corbett. The Ann Arbor anesthesiologist was also there that day. As lawmakers, who were bused from Lansing, and agriculture officials attempted to inspect some of the cows, irate farmers shouted questions at the agriculture personnel, disputing state and Michigan State University test results. Many of the farmers had driven to the Mason farm in cars and trucks that bore a new red-and-white bumper sticker, which read: "Cattlegate—It's Bigger Than Watergate." Trombley approached Ball with a container of milk from one of the cows in the herd, daring Ball to drink it. Ball refused, later explaining, "I wouldn't have drank unpasteurized milk from my own healthy cattle when I was in the dairy business. And I was not about to drink the stuff that he handed me in the middle of the barnyard, not knowing where it had come from. Also, I had had threatening phone calls telling me what was going to happen to me and so forth."

"Albosta was out there working up the farmers, Trombley and that sort of bunch," Ball recalls, "and another guy was asking questions that had nothing to do with the agenda. So we never got to cover the agenda. We never got the thing handled the way it should have been. We had an agenda to discuss it and

184

then see the cattle and so forth. But all the people . . . that sort of switched things around. It was just one of those deals where they just didn't want to hear the facts. They wanted to ask impossible questions."

Among those who had questions was Jane Haradine, the astute reporter for the Grand Rapids *Press* and a former public health nurse who had begun to follow the PBB scandal closely. She wanted to know, for example, why the Agriculture Department in the spring of 1975 could find no PBB in Edington's animals and now admitted three of them had "traces" after a private laboratory, the Wisconsin Alumni Research Foundation, had found PBB in ten out of thirteen samples from the same herd. After further studying the report, she discovered a number of "conflicts" and "discrepancies"—such as why it omitted to mention the presence of PBB in one animal that had died during the "study." Because the amount of PBB found had been considered "insignificant," Haradine was told by Dr. Sam Getty, a veterinarian and clinical professor in the department of large-animal surgery and medicine at the Michigan State University's college of veterinary medicine. "It doesn't mean anything," he said. Another discrepancy Haradine spotted was the absence of records to prove that eleven animals had been tested for PBB. The report also claimed that the herd's milk production now had exceeded the state average; but Haradine discovered that at least two cows—perhaps more—that were poor producers had been excluded from the "average." Haradine wrote, "Even the number of animals with PBB [three] conflicts from the report's conclusion [which shows four] . . . . No mention is made of PBB reported found in the milk tank," a report later confirmed by Dr. John Welser, dean of Michigan State University's veterinary college.

When Haradine pressed Dr. Getty about his record keeping, especially why calving records were glaringly incomplete, he told her it was because some of the cows had aborted, adding, "There was nothing to analyze." Yet, as Haradine pointed out in her story the following day in the Grand Rapids *Press*: "The number of premature births or abortions was not included in the study even though this is a common PBB complaint of farmers."

One person on the McCalla farm that day who was virtually overlooked was Dr. Clinton Grover, Edington's veterinarian. But Haradine walked over and spoke with him.

When he inspected Edington's cows in January and February of 1975, Dr. Grover told Haradine, there was no evidence of parasites. Even stool samples had been negative, he said.

Another reporter who did some snooping around that day was Richard Lehnert, who had replaced Dayton Matlick as editor of *Michigan Farmer.* "I saw abscessed udders in five of the forty cows shown that spring day, heard their joints creak as they moved and wondered at the few that were milking, the few that were bred," he wrote later.

And so, despite all the money and effort to persuade the public that a low-level herd can produce milk and look healthy, "the 'study' didn't prove anything," says Halbert. "Why should public money be spent to slander somebody?!"

At the end of a frustrating day, Ball anounced that, with the study over, the milk-producing cows would be sold to dairymen and the nonproducing ones would be slaughtered for beef, since the cows had below-quarantine PBB levels.

Edington's animals became contaminated because two of the three commercial feed elevators in the Eastern Upper Peninsula had been contaminated by PBB residues in Farm Bureau Services feeds. The concentrations were considered low—traces—by the time testing was finally performed. But one unopened bag of dairy feed #410 found at the Pickford elevator in September of 1974, for instance, had up to 1.2 parts per million PBB.

"I'm sure if Dick Edington had had twenty-five grand to put into that herd, he could have made them look good, too," said Gary P. Schenk, the dairyman's attorney. A year later, *Michigan Farmer*'s editor Dick Lehnert published an editorial headlined, "Sorry, Dick." It called Edington "the most unfairly maligned farmer [ex-farmer] in Michigan today." Edington had gone out of business and now Lehnert was sorry. Then Lehnert revealed the conditions of the cows he had closely examined that day on the McCalla farm in Mason. "But I wrote nothing because there was, and is, no definitive proof of anything. But I'm still sorry for Dick Edington and his wife and kids. His name, among PBB-afflicted farmers and those sympathetic to them, has become part of the language....'To pull an Edington' means to set someone up and destroy his name, reputation, credibility and his future," Lehnert wrote. "I don't know how I might have prevented that, but I'm sorry nonetheless. I don't to this day know what happened to that herd, or what made those animals die. I doubt that it was Dick Edington."

Another dairyman who took it on the chin for no reason was Gerald Woltjer, who bought an eighty-acre farm in Coopersville, a community fifteen miles west of Grand Rapids, in the spring of 1974. The week he moved in, PBB was identified; and he learned that the herd of the previous tenant, Peter Crum, had been poisoned, and at levels among the highest in the state. That, of course, was the first time Crum had heard about PBB as well. Some of Crum's cows had PBB levels up to 1,800 parts per million. Most of them had gone to the market or, as *Michigan Farmer* noted, "We ate 'em." Woltjer diligently followed the cleanup instructions supplied by the Department of Agriculture, but it didn't seem to make much difference, for almost no one that early on had quite appreciated the persistence of the chemical once it escaped into the environment. The only person who did was Dr. George Fries in Beltsville, Maryland, but he didn't tell anyone. "I just assumed everybody knew it. Of course, I should have said something."

That autumn, health problems began appearing in Woltjer's registered Holstein herd of more than two hundred cows. He had a few of the animals checked for PBB, but only traces turned up. Yet deaths and illnesses that did not respond to treatment continued to plague his herd for the next year and a half. On the first day of April 1976, Woltjer took a .22-caliber rifle and shot 235 cows and calves, sparing only some calves that Woltjer thought might survive the poisoning. Then he and his wife, Donna, took the kids and left the farm, and did not return for two days.

"My kids were out of school that week on vacation and we promised we'd go away for a few days. We were under a lot of pressure because of this and we just wanted to get away." When Sergeant Jack Rosema of the Ottawa County sheriff's department arrived at the Woltjer farm at 2:00 A.M. Friday on April 2, he found the 235 animals in two pens behind the barn. Some were still alive. Rosema and several deputies had to locate the wounded animals and finish them off. When they returned after daybreak several hours later, a few still had to be shot. Woltjer said he decided to destroy the cows because "they couldn't go anywhere. I was losing $300 a day trying to milk those cows. We were almost out of feed and out of money. Those animals were miserable. We just couldn't stand it any longer." The estimated herd value was over $140,000. He could have sold the cows legally, but chose not to because, he said, "I don't believe they should have been on the market poisoning the people of Michigan."

Within two weeks after Woltjer shot his cows, eight Coopersville area farmers drove to Lansing to complain about Woltjer to their state senator, Gary Byker. They said they and their families all had been contaminated by PBB but were feeling perfectly fine. They said Woltjer was a person who should not be engaged in dairy farming. Woltjer's dairy, hog and beef barns were "grossly mismanaged." Woltjer was deeply in debt, hounded by creditors. Woltjer had failed in the hog business several years earlier. Woltjer, in short, was "totally incapable" of operating a successful farm. "This group of farmers was universal in condemning Mr. Woltjer as a total failure in animal husbandry, and it was the concensus that PBB played absolutely no part in his difficulties," Dr. Jack Isbister, a disease control officer in the state Health Department, reported to Dr. Reizen afterward.

There was no explanation why he was even present at the meeting in the first place, which had nothing to do with matters of public health. The meeting was held in the Agriculture Department's fifth floor conference room, just down the hall from director Ball's office; it had been arranged by Senator Byker and, told the nature of the farmers' complaint, Ball and Dr. Whitehead made themselves instantly available, on a moment's notice.

A few days later, the rest of the Woltjer herd was quarantined when test results came back showing excessive PBB contamination.

But it was too late to do him any good. More than $800,000 in debt, Woltjer declared bankruptcy. And one day before the U.S. Bicentennial celebration, his farm was sold for $127,000 at a public auction.

Jerry Woltjer was a quiet, brooding man, not given to excessive eloquence. But his emotions and those of many other Michigan farmers are pretty accurately summarized by a letter that arrived at the Detroit *News* in the fall of 1978. It was written by Tom Butler, the Gregory dairyman who because of "bromide ingestion" was unable to obtain additional life insurance.

"Our experience in the PBB episode was contrary to all the great things we have tried to teach and instill in our children— about our country, our government, our political system. But as our children say: 'Can this be the same United States of America that champions human rights for people in other countries when successful farmers are ruined and even ridiculed for the sake of big businesses' almighty dollar and face-saving of the politicians and bureaucrats in Lansing?'" Butler wrote. "When all is considered, we can't blame our children for this skepticism. Then what really shook us most, was when our children started questioning the lack of Christian values involved here. We were at a complete loss for an answer, and could only tell them that apparently we are not dealing with Christian values in the PBB tragedy. One could go on and on about our experiences in this unbelievable nightmare and still conclude that maybe our children are correct in believing that our country is indeed in a sad state of affairs."

If state officials were alarmed when Woltjer shot his animals, they were even more taken aback when he refused to dispose of the carcasses. The press once more jumped on the story. "I don't know who's going to do it. I don't care if it's the township or the state, but I'm not going to touch one of them. They're so full of poison they don't belong buried on any of these farms," Woltjer said.

There were already hundreds of carcasses lying on farms across the state. And even in Michigan's "snowbelt" spring was approaching, and the dead animals soon would begin rotting. Their former owners were demanding action from the government. On Garry Zuiderveen's farm in Falmouth, there were 180 dead cows, and one pile already was starting to bloat and show signs of decay. On John and Eli Argersinger's farm in Leroy to the southwest, another 125 carcasses were strewn behind the barn, covered by ice and snow that was beginning to thaw.

Meanwhile, Dr. Howard Tanner, director of the Department of Natural Resources, was urgently warning Governor Milliken's staff that the Kalkaska burial site "is rapidly nearing capacity" and that plans at once must be made to develop yet another mass grave. Dr. Tanner also was telling the departments of health and agriculture that his agency did not have the manpower or equipment to advise farmers who might be willing to bury the dead animals on their own land.

The health and agriculture departments, however, were unable to decide what to do, still worried that agreeing to help farmers dispose of their animals at Kalkaska would make the state liable for compensation claims later. "Apparently many farmers with sick and dying cows and high feed costs are waiting to see what happens," Harold D. Baar, chief of the Health Department's division of community environmental health, reported to Dr. Reizen. "If the state does remove the cows that have been shot, others will likely start shooting. Some are apparently so angry they may start shooting state officials." Earlier, the idea was advanced that the state accept dead and sick (but below quarantine) animals for burial at Kalkaska. The state would do this, said Harry Iwasko, an assistant attorney general, if the farmers would "give us an absolute warranty that they will not take action against us for the destruction." But when Farm Bureau Services got wind of this proposal, it threatened to "completely abandon" the Kalkaska project, thus shifting full responsibility and liability of all the animals to the state. The idea was dropped. And so now, while the state agencies were still vacillating, farmers once more were left to their own resources to find some solution.

Otto Miller in Lake County, for instance, had thirty-eight dead cows on his farm. He asked the state to take the carcasses to the Kalkaska burial pit, but it refused. When the animals began rotting, neighbors called the Health Department to complain. Local health officers showed up at Miller's farm with a court order giving him twenty-four hours to bury the cows on his farm or face jail and a $100-a-day fine. So Miller buried the carcasses. But a week later, he was charged with violating state pollution laws. Miller had unknowingly buried the cows in a section of land with a high water table at the headwaters of the Pere Marquette River. Miller was digging up the carcasses when county officials appeared again on his farm and threatened him with arrest if he disinterred the animals. But Miller dug them up anyway. He was immediately arrested. The problem finally was resolved the next day when Miller again buried the carcasses. In late summer, the county sent a hauler to the Miller farm, disinterred the cows and trucked them to Kalkaska for burial. Later the county sent the Millers a $635 bill for the trucking costs, instructing them to pay now and then seek reimbursement from Farm Bureau Services. But to this day, the Millers have refused to pay the bill.

Eventually the Agriculture Department—over the vehement objections of Dr. Whitehead, who insisted that farmers themselves bury their animals on their own land—agreed to a Milliken suggestion to pay the cost of trucking to Kalkaska and burying many of the carcasses strewn across the state, including those on Jerry Woltjer's farm in Coopersville.

But in the meantime, a different kind of problem faced Doug and Judy Carroll in Luther, just a few miles north of Otto Miller's place. The couple had twenty-eight cows that died over the winter and they were still lying on the ground. State officials told Mrs. Carroll one day that "we had to bury the cattle in twenty-four hours, or they would give us a $100 fine and put my husband in jail," she recalls. "And we said we didn't have the money at that time to pay for [digging] a hole to be burying our cattle. So I think it was a day or so after, a neighbor of ours got some men with a bulldozer and they came over and dug a hole for us, and we buried the cattle. Ever since we buried the cattle we've been having vandalism at the house." One night, while Doug and Judy were in town four miles away visiting her mother, vandals painted "PBB" and other obscenities all over their house. Since, they have had their yard lights shot out, their tractor tires punctured and even a tractor's steering wheel sawed off. They suspect some of their neighbors might be responsible for these acts, resentful that they buried their cattle on the land, posing a possible health hazard to the community's water supply. The Carrolls were never quarantined, even though they ultimately lost eighty head of cattle. Department of Agriculture laboratory test results on their animals found PBB traces, but not enough to warrant quarantine. Later that year, the young couple went on welfare. In late 1978, they, too, abandoned Michigan.

# 11
# NO MORE
# MR. NICE GUY

"A nice guy who finishes first," they call William G. Milliken. He is a native of Traverse City, born into a political family. His grandfather, J. W. Milliken, had been a state senator at the turn of the century. And so was his father, James Milliken, who served in Lansing from 1939 to 1950. Even Bill Milliken's nice-guy image was handed down; his father was known as "Gentleman Jim."

Milliken graduated from Yale and then flew fifty combat missions as a waist gunner in World War II. After the war ended, he returned to Traverse City and joined the family enterprise, the J.W. Milliken Department Store. But in 1961, Bill Milliken got tired of business. By then already a civic activist as well as the local Republican chairman, he ran for the state senate. He won easily. In 1964 he was elected lieutenant governor. And in 1969, he became Michigan's forty-fourth governor when incumbent George Romney left the state to serve as Richard Nixon's secretary of Housing and Urban Development. In 1970 and 1974, Milliken won election in his own right, capturing many votes in traditionally Democratic strongholds by running on a platform of concern for urban problems and what he calls "pragmatic republicanism."

Along the road to success, he acquired many nicknames. The lollipop governor. Boy Scout Bill. Governor Milquetoast. "Years ago, the kidding bothered me. But not now," says Milliken.

The governor, however, was called many other things—some of them vicious enough to upset anyone—by the angry farmers, who were surprised and then hurt by Milliken's distant attitude and the treatment they got from haughty bureaucrats. The rural farm community, after all, as in other midwestern and plains states, is the backbone of the Republican party; and in Michigan, the farm community is to the Republicans what the influential United Auto Workers union is to the Democrats. "Hell," says Doc Alpha Clark, "we're all Republicans—or at least were."

To many of the PBB-affected farmers, Bill Milliken no longer was "Mr. Nice Guy."

At the outset, he rejected a proposal by his own agriculture director to destroy and bury the affected animals, pay the farmers for them and then sue Michigan Chemical and Farm Bureau Services to recover the costs incurred by the state; this would have encouraged farmers to destroy their contaminated cows instead of dumping them into human food channels.

He signed into law a bill making state forest land available as the burial pit—but barring state funds for the operation; this left the financially devastated farmers at the mercy of the two culprit companies.

His own budget director rejected a Health Department request for money to begin a long-term medical study; this would have provided more quickly a clearer picture of the health problems.

His own staff rejected an offer by perhaps the country's leading environmental medicine scientist to study the effects of the contamination—for free.

He continued relying on his health and agriculture officials, who—having failed to deal effectively with the spreading contamination—now were covertly and overtly ridiculing farmers.

He made little effort to seek genuine federal assistance or disaster aid relief, even after another Michiganian, Jerry Ford, had become president in early August of 1974.

But the worst blow for the farmers came in September of 1975. The Democratic-controlled legislature had passed—unanimously, in both chambers—a bill providing long-term low-interest loans to the affected farmers. But Milliken vetoed it, calling it "a hollow promise to Michigan farmers who are facing economic disaster through no fault of their own." He called the bill "well-intentioned but defective" because of what he considered vague wording.

Milliken's objection was that the Albosta-sponsored bill lacked a specific appropriation for the loan program—even though the legislation indeed had authorized a transfer of funds from the Veterans' Trust Fund. But that provision, the governor said, was "of doubtful validity." The estimated cost of the 3.5 percent loan program was $41.4 million.

Yet, a month after his veto, Milliken, facing a massive budget deficit, borrowed $300 million from the same Veterans' Trust Fund to balance his budget.

As an alternative to the vetoed loan program, Milliken proposed a series of measures that would have levied taxes against feed manufacturers and chemical companies. This revenue, he stated, would finance the loan program, which would be made available even to low-level farmers whose animals were contaminated but seemingly at minute PBB levels. But two top aides later admitted in writing that these proposals were merely "intended to put pressure on Farm Bureau Services and Michigan Chemical," who in August had stopped paying compensation claims after exhausting the settlement pool negotiated by Hettiger in February of 1975.

Many farmers felt Milliken's description of the loan bill he had vetoed—"a hollow promise held out to Michigan farmers" —was a more apt characterization of his own scheme. Garry Zuiderveen said he felt "frustrated, bitter and disappointed," adding, "We've got two cases in federal court now, trying to prevent foreclosures until these farmers get some help. And now this."

In vetoing the loan bill, Milliken again had rejected the advice of his agriculture director, B. Dale Ball, who, ironically, left the job several years later with the public perception that it was he who failed to adequately perceive the needs of affected farmers. In a memorandum urging the governor to sign that legislation, Ball wrote: "While there are certain weaknesses and omissions in the bill, I believe it is better than nothing, and may provide the means for farmers who have suffered great economic losses, through no fault of their own, to remain solvent pending settlement of the claims against the responsible parties. To veto the bill at this time would prevent any assistance to some very deserving farmers and would indicate a lack of sensitivity to the problems of the unfortunate victims of this disaster."

Several weeks after Milliken vetoed the loan program, the shooting of animals began. By mid-January, the governor decided it was time for him to gain a better understanding of the messy PBB problem. Milliken sent letters to twenty-five medical doctors and research scientists from around the country "whose counsel I should seek in my efforts to obtain full insight into this matter." Milliken asked these persons for advice because, he wrote, "my office is besieged by lingering questions which involve three central themes:

1. Is there evidence to indicate that the current action guidelines for meat, milk, poultry and eggs are not safe?
2. Is there evidence which bears on the long-term human health implications of exposure to PBB?
3. Are cattle now contaminated with PBB at low levels suffering health impairment because of exposure to PBB, or is it possible that another causative factor is involved?"

Milliken further told these health experts that he planned to appoint an advisory panel to evaluate all the available information, including their responses.

The governor's letters, seeking a "full insight," went out on January 14—more than nineteen months after he first heard about PBB.

"Nobody saw the magnitude of the thing," William N. Hettiger, the governor's executive secretary and confidant, recalled later. "We were relying on the Department of Public Health and the Department of Agriculture. Nobody thought there was a human health danger, but the terrible impact on the whole agricultural industry. A lot of our attention—perhaps misplaced—was on the economic impact to the farmers," Hettiger said. "But the magnitude kept growing, far beyond what anybody had imagined. It kept going up, up, up, up. Right then [in 1974] I don't know what we could have done differently. We were floundering around right then. The first tests [by the state Health Department] showed no human problems. That's about where we were. Our information was coming from the experts—the health and agriculture departments. But, yes, it's a fair assumption that they didn't stumble over themselves to find the magnitude of the problem we had."

In late January, responses to Milliken's belated search for independent and expert advice began trickling in. One was from Dr. James Terrian, the young director of the Chippewa County Health Department. "No person," he wrote, "can say PBB is safe at any concentration," adding parenthetically, "I do not like the phrasing of this [first] question. The burden of

195

proof rests with those who contend PBB at any level is safe. Let that be proven." Dr. Terrian's five-page letter concluded, "I remain concerned about the continuing exposures of people to PBB in their foods. Serious weaknesses of the MDPH [Michigan Department of Public Health] short-term survey and failure to begin the long-term study are unacceptable facts."

At the other extreme, typically, was the response of John R. Welser, dean of Michigan State University's college of veterinary medicine. The letter, also signed by three other university scientists, stated that there was no evidence that the existing federal PBB standards were unsafe. The letter further claimed that "evidence being accumulated suggests that cattle now contaminated with low levels [.3 part per million or less] of PBB are not suffering health impairment because of exposure to PBB. Other causative factors may be involved." Such factors, the letter suggested, could be malnutrition and diseases brought on by bad management.

The other replies generally fell between the positions taken by Dr. Terrian and Dean Welser. Dr. Benjamin L. Van Duuren, who had worked with Dr. Corbett on anesthetic gases, told Milliken that "it is impossible to provide unequivocal answers" because "the paucity of information is overwhelming." Dr. Irving J. Selikoff, the environmental medicine expert from New York's Mount Sinai School of Medicine, concurred with Dr. Van Duuren, but also warned Milliken that "concern for the current action guidelines is amply justified." Dr. Selikoff offered a number of suggestions, including "an effective environmental sampling program for at least some years to come ... to monitor sources of potential human and animal exposure," he wrote. "Had this been in effect in 1974 and 1975, rendering of contaminated carcasses and use of material in feed to contaminate new animals might have been minimized, for example." Dr. Selikoff also recommended, "The major sources of continued environmental contamination should be eliminated, despite the anticipated cost, e.g., sick animals should be destroyed and discarded [not recycled] whatever the fat levels of PBB." He also warned that the likelihood that PBB will be carcinogenic in test animals "is great."

Other thoughtful advice came from a brilliant University of Michigan scientist named Isadore A. Bernstein. He told the governor, "Hopefully, the advisory panel which you intend to appoint will have sufficient scientific expertise, but no vested interest, so that it can take an unemotional, objective view of existent scientific data and can evaluate the risk to human health against economic pressures."

On March 5, the same day the Albosta hearing was held in Cadillac, Milliken announced his five-point action plan to deal with the persistent PBB crisis. The highlight of the plan was the five-member PBB scientific advisory panel, to be chaired by Dr. Bernstein, who, at the University of Michigan, was a professor of biochemistry in the medical school, a professor of environmental and industrial health in the school of public health and a research scientist in the institute of environmental and industrial health. The other panel members were Dr. Van Duuren, professor of environmental medicine at the New York University Medical School; Dr. Lynn Willett, of the Ohio Agricultural Research and Development Center in Wooster, Ohio; Dr. Walter Meester, the Grand Rapids toxicologist best known for his critique of the state Health Department's flawed short-term study; and Dr. Perry J. Gehring, director of toxicology research at Dow Chemical.

A week after the governor announced the formation of the advisory panel, charged specifically with assessing the safety of the current PBB tolerance levels, a Michigan State University scientist put out a study claiming that many of the problems being seen on Michigan farms were due not to PBB but to iodine. The Great Lakes area has been known to be deficient in iodine, part of a large goiter belt that was erased with the simple addition of trace levels of iodine to table salt. And likewise, iodine also is added to some livestock feed. The study was authored by Dr. Donald Hillman, an extension specialist in cattle nutrition, who had been among the first scientists to visit the Halbert farm back in the fall of 1973. But Dr. Hillman's conclusions came under serious question when it was disclosed that the study had been funded by a $25,000 Farm Bureau Services "research" grant.

Dr. Hillman said he "stumbled" onto the problem in the first place after a perplexed veterinarian sought his help. "There were a lot of sick animals out there. No question about it," he recalls. "Some people tended to jump to conclusions about motives." Dr. Hillman said, "The Department of Agriculture knew of many sick dairy herds that had no PBB. So I proposed to Farm Bureau Services: There's another problem out there besides PBB.... Many farmers were calling to say

197

'Hey, we didn't get any Farm Bureau Services feed, but we have the same problems.'" Dr. Hillman said he found the iodine-caused symptoms were virtually indistinguishable from those caused by PBB.

No one had a more violent reaction to the iodine study than Dr. Donald P. Wallach, a senior research scientist with the Upjohn Company in Kalamazoo. Dr. Wallach was at the farm of his good friends and neighbors, Jim and Alice Fish, in Hickory Corners the day Dr. Hillman arrived at the Lockshore Farms. "He spent about fifteen minutes in one of Jim's barns looking at animals," Dr. Wallach recalls. "He then asserted that the problem was not PBB intoxication but excessive intake of iodine. He had no proof then, nor does he now, that this assertion had any basis in fact." Dr. Wallach was so disturbed by the iodine study that he called Dr. John Cantlon, Michigan State University's vice-president for research and development, at home one night. After a long discussion, Dr. Cantlon agreed to turn the matter over to Dr. John Nellor, associate vice-president for research and development. Dr. Nellor then convened a meeting of top university scientists to review the study. Their conclusion was that there was no problem with iodine toxicity in Michigan cattle.

"Naïvely, I didn't anticipate any problems," recalls Dr. Bernstein, a short balding man with white hair who is extremely popular among his students and research assistants at the university. Indeed the selection of Isadore Bernstein as panel chairman had come as something of a surprise to many people. Because of the steadily widening credibility gap between the public and state and federal institutions, Dr. Reizen, the state health director, had advised the governor not to appoint to the panel any member of Michigan State University or the U.S. Food and Drug Administration. And furthermore, for that very same reason, Dr. Reizen had recommended that the panel's chairman should not even be a resident of Michigan. And so partly for those reasons, the front-runner as panel chairman became Dr. Van Duuren, the tall, erect and reserved South African-born academic. A onetime du Pont scientist, Dr. Van Duuren in 1955 joined the New York University, where he now was director of the laboratory of organic chemistry and carcinogenesis at the NYU Medical Center's Institute of Environmental Medicine. Yet, despite his fame in the world scientific community, the governor's office was unable to locate anyone who had personal knowledge of Dr. Van Duuren in order to confirm that he "possessed the desired personal attributes" to lead such a panel. Dr. Isleib, chief deputy agriculture director, also was unable to contact anyone personally acquainted with Dr. Van Duuren, and so he told Kathy Stariha, Milliken's special assistant for PBB, that Dr. Bernstein would be acceptable as chairman. "I stated to Ms. Stariha," he recalls, "that I prefer any risks attendant with Dr. Bernstein's chairmanship to an unknown leadership quality"—a statement that Dr. Isleib would live to regret.

But right off the bat, the panel became embroiled in controversy. Dr. Meester objected to the presence on the panel of Dr. Willett, who had gotten PBB research grants from both Michigan Chemical and Farm Bureau Services. Dr. Meester said he would not serve unless Dr. Willett was removed. In turn, Dr. Willett pointed out that Dr. Meester, having examined numerous contaminated patients, hardly brought to the panel an unbiased viewpoint. "Right away, we came to an impasse. Willett and Meester each felt the other should leave. Finally the governor appointed a new panel," Dr. Bernstein recalls.

The second panel, still chaired by Dr. Bernstein, was announced on April 5, a month after the five-point action plan was issued. Both Dr. Meester and Dr. Willett were out. And another member of the first panel, Dr. Gehring of Dow, had removed himself because of his involvement with his company's earlier research with PBBs. In their place, four new members were named. They were Dr. Frederick W. Oehme, a Ph.D. and a veterinarian who was director of the comparative toxicology laboratory at Kansas State University; Dr. Nelson S. Irey, an M.D., a clinician and an anatomic pathologist at the Armed Forces Institute of Pathology in Washington, D.C.; Dr. Thomas Tephly, director of the toxicology center of the department of pharmacology at the University of Iowa; and Dr. M. Lloyd Hopwood, of the department of physiology and biophysics at Colorado State University. Dr. Van Duuren, along with Dr. Bernstein, was a holdover from the first panel.

'Our greatest need now," said Governor Milliken, "is to replace the emotionalism surrounding this issue with the best scientific evaluation possible. We must substitute reason and knowledge for fear and rumor. I have asked this panel of distinguished scientists to follow the facts wherever they may lead and to report back to me with their recommendations as

199

soon as is practically possible. I am confident that this panel will conduct its investigation in a true academic spirit—unbiased and unimpeded by the controversy now raging."

Four days later, the Department of Agriculture put out a press release claiming that "less than one-tenth of a pound of PBB is contained in all the 23,500 head of beef and dairy cattle now known to have low-level contamination with the fire retardant chemical PBB." Thus, it said, "the total in all of these animals would be equivalent to less than four tablespoonsful of PBB." The calculations were made by Dr. Isleib, who, less than a year later, would be caught in a blatant attempt to deceive the public. Also on April 9, the federal government finally granted $336,964 to the state of Michigan to begin a long-term study of four thousand state residents exposed to high levels of PBB.

When Dr. Bernstein agreed to serve as chairman of the PBB scientific advisory panel, his awareness about the PBB contamination was "very little—other than cursory knowledge from the newspapers," he recalls. "At the time, it didn't seem so important a problem. There was no body burden data [to indicate 9 million people had been poisoned], and no breast milk information [which suggested that everyone in Michigan had been exposed to the chemical]." But when Dr. Bernstein began studying PBB and the contamination, he quickly became concerned. "I can't escape the feeling that the agency [the Michigan Department of Agriculture] tended to play down the problem and did not actively pursue a determination of the extent of the problem," Dr. Bernstein said later.

The panel scheduled a two-day conference on April 19 and 20 at the Hilton Inn near Detroit's Metropolitan Airport to hear scientists and regulatory officials discuss the panel's main charge: whether or not the present federal tolerance guidelines should be reduced. The press and the general public were barred from the meeting, Dr. Bernstein said, because "we wanted it completely unstressed. And it was." When the somber governor publicly opened the session on Monday morning, he said, "It is time for an end to rumors and half-truths. It is time for hard facts, and it is the job of this panel to get those facts."

The Food and Drug Administration, feeling defensive because its tolerance guidelines were being questioned, held a high-level meeting in Washington the week before the April 19–20 conference. "The PBB problem" was a main topic of discussion at the commissioner's staff meeting. "Mismanagement of herds was discussed," admits Dr. Frank Cordle, a medical epidemiologist at the agency's bureau of foods. "And the commissioner [Dr. Alexander M. Schmidt] felt FDA should publicize this." Among those who presented the Food and Drug Administration's views on PBB at the scientific conference was Al Hoeting, who impugned the motives of farmers and questioned their talents. But apparently he did not impress the Bernstein panel. "Hoeting was so obviously biased, so far out, that it lessened his credibility," Dr. Bernstein said later. Yet, the panel, after hearing mostly from state officials and FDA representatives during its two-day airport conference, came away with the impression that "there was no problem," in Dr. Bernstein's words. But the panel continued reading and reviewing both published and unpublished scientific literature concerning PBB and a related compound, PCB, or polychlorinated biphenyl.

It held a second two-day conference on May 7 and 8 in Chicago, where it heard from still other scientists, including Dr. Selikoff and Dr. Corbett, who described his work with rodents that suggested PBB may cause birth defects.

The panel recognized that "appropriate scientific proof did not exist" to answer the crucial question of whether or not PBB caused acute health problems, Dr. Bernstein said. "On the other hand, the acute administration of relatively low levels of PBB [to laboratory animals] have produced contradictory results, and the results appear to depend on the species and the age and stage of development of the subjects," he continued. "Having agreed that it saw no conclusive proof of short-term effects of PBBs in humans, the panel then turned its attention to long-term effects." But no such information was available. No one had done such work. "The panel then followed the usual toxicological practice of looking at results of exposure to structurally related chemicals, in this case PCB," Dr. Bernstein recalls.

It was at the second meeting that the panel became aware of the work of a toxicology research scientist at the U.S. Center for Disease Control named Renate D. Kimbrough. She had fed PCBs to rats and produced a high incidence of liver cancers. The study, published in the December 1975 issue of the *Journal of the National Cancer Institute*, "clearly related high level feeding of PCBs to rodents with hepatic [liver] cancer," Dr. Bernstein said.

"Once the panel became aware of the animal data on cancer arising from exposure to PCB, it became clear that there was presumptive evidence for risk from long-term exposure to its related compound, PBB, on which no adequate experimental work had been done," he said.

"In fact, the ultimate experiment in human disease—exposure of people—was actually in progress."

At the end of the two-day meeting in Chicago, Dr. Bernstein recalls, "there was a change of attitude." By the time the six panel members met in Ann Arbor to write their report, he said, "We knew what the decision would be. It was unanimous."

The panel recommended that the federal PBB tolerance guidelines be drastically reduced—and swiftly.

The stunning recommendation had the effect of a scab being savagely torn from a healing wound. After being reassured for two years by the government that PBB was not much to get worked up about, the Michigan public was jolted.

The panel's recommendation also enraged most of the state officials. Certainly Governor Milliken was unhappy about it, but he accepted the group's decision graciously. But none was more incensed than the peevish Don Isleib, the chief deputy agriculture director. Like most other key state officials, he had received the Bernstein panel's report on Sunday evening, the night before the panel was to meet with the governor to officially deliver the report and then to meet the press. In the governor's huge conference room on Monday morning, May 24, about twenty persons gathered to await the governor. The six scientific advisory panel members were there. So were Dale Ball and Don Isleib; Dr. Maurice S. Reizen, the state public health director; Kathy Stariha, Milliken's special assistant for PBB; and several of their aides. The atmosphere was tense. Finally the governor entered. "He came in and said he would support our recommendation," Dr. Bernstein recalls. "Milliken may not have seemed to care for the report, but he supported it." During the meeting, Dr. Isleib found himself no longer able to contain his anger. And he snapped, "You always have trouble when you bring in a bunch of academics!"

Dr. Bernstein, caught off guard, retorted, "You wouldn't be in this mess in the first place if academics had been involved earlier." Dr. Bernstein found Dr. Isleib's childish remark so irritating that he almost stalked out of the room. The entire

202

group then went out to meet the throng of reporters who were awaiting the verdict.

The report emphasized that any predictions about the long-term effects of PBB must take into consideration the available information on PCBs, since the organic raw material for the formulation of both compounds is the same, and since the procedures for synthesis also are similar. "Therefore, the carcinogenicity of PCBs cannot be ignored," Dr. Bernstein explained.

While noting it had received no evidence "that significant health effects resulting from PBB ingestion have been documented in man," the panel added, however: "The potential hazard from the continuing presence of low levels of PBB in diet or body tissues of animals has many aspects which must await further study and clarification. The possibility of mutagenic and carcinogenic effects from low body burdens of PBB will only be resolved after long-term exposure." The ultimate experiment.

The report further said, "The panel is concerned that the long-term retention of PBB in human tissues...could increase the PBB levels in those who presently have measurable levels, and could lead to detectable accumulations in those who presently do not. The knowledge that the PCB mixture is carcinogenic and that the PBB mixture—whose effects are similar to PCB—may also be carcinogenic, requires that the potential for increases in body burden of PBB be immediately restricted."

Specifically, the scientific panel urged a prompt reduction of tolerance levels from .3 part per million to .005 part per million in meat; from .3 part per million to .001 part per million in milk, and from .05 part per million to .005 part per million in eggs.

The recommended reductions were drastic. Perhaps they can be more easily understood when expressed in parts per billion, which eliminates the need for decimal points. For meat, from 300 parts per billion to 5 parts per billion; for milk, from 300 parts per billion to 1 part per billion; and for eggs, from 50 parts per billion to 5 parts per billion.

The panel said it specified the new guidelines because those were the lowest levels that science at the time had the analytical ability to detect. But the panel also recommended that these guidelines be constantly reviewed to determine whether they should be lowered further as detection capability improves.

The recommendations caught nearly everyone off guard, including the press. Governor Milliken had opened the press conference with a less-than-ringing endorsement of the panel's principal recommendation. "While I want to emphasize there is no known immediate risk—and it is by no means certain that there are, in fact, long-term hazards—I believe we must, as a precautionary measure, respond to the recommendations of this highly credible scientific panel." Milliken explained that a 1913 state law requires a public hearing by the state Agriculture Department before the department can adopt lower tolerance guidelines than the federal ones. "Therefore," he said, "I am today directing that the Michigan Department of Agriculture promptly schedule the necessary public hearing with the objective of following the panel's recommendations."

Dr. Oehme, the veterinarian and director of the comparative toxicology laboratory at Kansas State University, was asked about Dr. Hillman's study. "In my opinion, the dosages of iodine that have been reported for the herds in this area and the other potential interactions have not played a role in contributing to the PBB problem as it is currently existing. Based upon the evidence that we have right now, yes, I would [rule out iodine]," he replied.

The atmosphere of distrust had become such in the spring of 1976 that Dr. Bernstein felt obliged to state publicly that the panel "particularly wishes to indicate that it did not experience any undue pressure to arrive at one or another specific position."

(But it wasn't only the actions of the health and the agriculture departments and Michigan State University's iodine study—all downplaying PBB—that fueled deep public mistrust. Indeed the governor's own office had by this time come under fire as well. While the Bernstein panel was meeting in Chicago on May 8, the Detroit *News*, in a page-one story, revealed that Dr. Selikoff had offered to conduct a broad human health study in Michigan in 1974—but was snubbed by both the Agriculture Department and Milliken's office. As a result, wrote reporters Stephen Cain and James Cnockaert, "virtually nothing is known about the possible harmful effects of PBB to thousands of Michigan residents....")

204

At the press conference, Dr. Bernstein elaborated on why the panel had recommended such a severe reduction of the federal guidelines that the state had followed for more than two years. "Once one decides that carcinogenicity or long-term effects are involved, it would seem that the level of nondetection be the standard, especially since, in this particular case, it appears reasonable and probable that the PBB level—the PBB contamination—can be circumscribed and eliminated," Dr. Bernstein said. "What we are concerned about is the continual exposure and build-up over a long period of time of very low levels in the environment being retained and accumulated as body burden for the citizens of the state."

A reporter in the audience looked up from his notepad and commented, "If I ate PBB-contaminated meat and I read this report saying that you lowered it to 5 parts per billion, I would not feel very confident that I was going to be healthy."

"Yes, of course," replied Dr. M. Lloyd Hopwood of Colorado. "The thing is that you're looking at this as eating a single steak or something with a little PBB in it. The thing that is of concern, when we're talking about trace amounts, is to continually eat PBB every day in your meat. And this is what we would like to have no one doing. I wouldn't want to subject myself to eating it every day."

Because the Agriculture Commission, the policy-making body of the Agriculture Department, once already—in the spring of 1975—had refused to lower the PBB guidelines, reporters pressed Milliken about what he expected now of the commission, whose members he appoints. "I would expect them to be lowered," the governor said of the guidelines.

But Milliken hedged when asked if he would "insist" that the commission lower the guidelines in order to minimize further public exposure to the chemical. "I think this panel's recommendations should be very carefully pursued because I think that the word, the recommendations of this panel—not only with me but with the legislature and with the public—will carry a good deal of weight.... But the fact that this panel, assembling all of the information, has come up with these recommendations causes me to believe at this point that we should reduce tolerance levels lower even than the FDA had recommended."

The panel's recommendations produced instant reactions. Gary P. Schenk, the Grand Rapids lawyer who was representing eighty-odd claimants, lavishly praised the report. "The panel performed a monumental task and service," he said. "What they said is what farmers have said for two and a half years: This stuff is dangerous. It has vindicated our faith and pride in our clients, who would rather keep or kill these animals than sell them for consumption by the public." But at Farm Bureau Services and Michigan Chemical, the processing of claims came to an abrupt halt as the companies reassessed the situation.

Elton Smith, Farm Bureau Services president, saw the report as causing "economic havoc." *Michigan Farmer* magazine quoted him as saying, "It will be consumers who will pay the tremendous costs of testing and enforcement through higher taxes and food prices. It will be consumers who will suffer if Michigan's number-two income producer—agriculture—goes out of business because they [the producers] have no markets for their products." The battle of the guidelines once more was under way.

Two days after the Bernstein panel delivered its report to Governor Milliken, B. Dale Ball decided to schedule the mandatory public hearing for June 10—fully knowing that Dr. Bernstein would be out of the country then.

On May 24, with members of his panel and top state officials seated around the large conference table in his well-appointed meeting room, Milliken had made clear that state law required the Agriculture Department to hold such a hearing before adopting tolerance guidelines more stringent than federal standards. "At that point," Dr. Bernstein recalls, "I indicated to the governor that I had a commitment which would take me out of the country, to Japan, very shortly—I think the next week—and that I would be gone for three weeks. I indicated to the people around the table that the members of the panel—and the the panel was present—would be happy to be present [at the public hearing] if called. We did not know, at that time, on what date the hearing would be held. I did go away. Prior to my departure there was no indication of the date of the hearing. On my return, on my desk there was indeed an official invitation to the hearing."

The Agriculture Department had held its hearing during Dr. Bernstein's absence, and the Agriculture Commission then unanimously voted not to follow the Bernstein panel's recommendations, thus defying the governor as well. None of the other members of the advisory panel—all from out of state—showed up to testify at the June 10 hearing.

Ball has claimed that all the panel members were notified of the June 10 hearing. But when Dr. Bernstein checked back with each member of the panel, he found that two of them—Dr. Van Duuren and Dr. Irey—never received such notices. Dr. Oehme was notified by telephone, but was unable to attend, as were Drs. Tephly and Hopwood, who were notified by mail. "Nobody told the others that they were not going to attend," said Dr. Bernstein. "But nobody [in the Milliken administration] went out of their way to get someone there, either. Not Ball. Not Reizen. Not the governor's office," he added. Ball said he was "very disappointed" that no panel member showed up.

Even so, no state official made any effort after the June 10 hearing to contact the panel members to see if any of them wished to submit a written statement before June 22, the date the Agriculture Commission was to vote on the panel's recommendations. Indeed, Ball closed the hearing record immediately after the public hearing ended. "We had a complete hearing and we had asked them to be there. We were so busy summarizing [the hearing testimony] and so forth," Ball said, "I don't think anybody else took the initiative to try and contact them." Ball said the staff recommendation to the members of the policy-making Agriculture Commission was unanimous. "We based it on the hearing record, and no one asked to leave the hearing record open, and everyone wanted something done in a hurry," said the agriculture director.

Dr. Thomas H. Corbett accused Ball of "rigging" the June 10 hearing. "The program was loaded," he recalls. The day-long hearing was held in the Michigan National Guard Armory in Lansing, as was the 1975 hearing, which had been delayed by the Agriculture Department to accomodate Dr. Kolbye of the Food and Drug Administration.

About six hundred people showed up, a crowd beyond most people's expectation, and they were mostly against the Bernstein panel's recommendations. The huge turnout perhaps had been due largely to the efforts of Franklin Schmidt, an Ottawa County dairyman who sent out 14,500 letters under the banner "Concerned Michigan Farmers" to rally opposition to the Bernstein panel's report. The campaign was financed by the Michigan Farm Bureau.

Ball opened the hearing by noting the absence of members of the governor's advisory panel, and then called on Dr. Kolbye. Dr. Kolbye gave two reasons why it was now "inappropriate" to lower the PBB standards. "First, such a policy is not necessary for the protection of the public health," he said. "Second, the source of PBB residues in the Michigan food supply has changed."

He explained that the continuing contamination of foodstuffs was no longer due to the original mix-up—which could have been avoided—but to the unavoidable contamination of new animals exposed to areas contaminated in the first place.

"PBBs are extremely stable and persistent," he said, "and they have been occurring in waste products from livestock and feeding areas affected by the original contamination incident. The environment of Michigan farms so contaminated will probably remain that way for some time in the future. New livestock introduced on these farms would also be exposed to this indirect source of PBBs, and food derived from these animals could contain low levels of PBBs despite farmers' attempts to prevent contamination. In other words, the complete elimination of PBBs in the Michigan farm environment is presently not possible."

And so even though the analytical capabilities had improved to detect much lower PBB concentrations, Dr. Kolbye said, any further reduction of the PBB standards was not now in order because of the "unavoidable" nature of the continuing contamination. When such "inevitable contamination of food occurs as a result of environmental pollution," he said, the FDA cannot simply "ban the unavoidable substance as a means of eliminating its presence in food." Dr. Kolbye added, "While I wish it were that simple, the cost factor of the matter is that we are talking about banning food itself, with the end result being the elimination of a major portion of the nation's food supply, particularly fish, meat, milk, eggs, corn, peanuts, cotton seed meal, etc., because all these products, no matter where produced in the United States, or elsewhere in the world, could contain some environmental contaminant."

John Wessel, scientific coordinator of the FDA's office of the associate commissioner for compliance, later tried to explain the concept this way: "It is our mandate to prevent food from entering the consumer channels whenever the contamination could have been avoided; and that's the key: 'could have been avoided.' It is our judgment that the mix-up could have been avoided; therefore, we could not allow any amount of PBBs to enter the food supply. And the only way we could enforce this or translate it to an everyday, enforceable practice is to define a level by our available analytical methodology." At the time the PBB mix-up was discovered, that level was 1 part per million, Wessel said. The tolerance guidelines were lowered in November 1974 when the detection capability improved.

"Subsequently, when our analytical methodology improved again, the situation in Michigan also changed," Wessel explained. "The source of contamination, this recycling of PBBs back into the animal, is such that there is no way that anyone can avoid this from happening. A farmer cannot clean up his farm to the extent to totally rid the farm environment in Michigan of PBBs. Any live animal introduced into this environment could pick up these contaminants. So this is the case: We consider it an unavoidable contamination and a separate section of the law applies."

He added, "The setting of tolerance guidelines is one of the most difficult things in the world to explain. It's a balancing act, really; but a lot of work goes into it. It's not like a bunch of people sitting in a room and a magic number emerges." Dr. Kolbye explained later, "The transition point between the avoidable presence and the unavoidable presence is like drawing a bright line in a gray zone." And he told the June 10 hearing, "Human ingenuity cannot currently prevent low levels of PBBs from occurring in food produced by some Michigan farmers."

Another scientist who testified that day against the Bernstein panel's recommendations was Dr. M. L. Keplinger, a pharmacologist with Industrial BIO-TEST Laboratories, Inc., of Northbrook, Illinois. He said the panel had "considerably overstated the total picture of PCBs and certainly the situation with PBBs." Dr. Keplinger added, "Well, many materials accumulate in the body." He said BIO-TEST's studies with rats and dairy cows and calves show that "rather high body burdens" of PBB may be sustained without bodily injury, even though the laboratory found low levels of PBB had induced liver changes. But Dr. Keplinger dismissed the liver function changes as "normal responses to a chemical which is foreign to the body." BIO-TEST also had been retained by the legal counsel to Michigan Chemical.

Another consultant to Farm Bureau Services and Michigan Chemical who testified was Dr. Thomas E. Spike, a dairy farmer who also holds a Ph.D. in biochemistry. He, too, was against any further reduction of the tolerance guidelines. "There have been several hundred people with PBB in their bodies for two years now at much higher levels than anyone who had no PBB in their system would get from eating meat and milk under the present guideline levels. Many of these people have had greater than 1 part per million in their systems for two years. If there were going to be deleterious effects at these levels, I would expect we would have seen some by now," he said. The Bernstein panel's recommendations, Dr. Spike said, "are, in my mind, entirely unwarranted and would be absolutely devastating to Michigan agriculture."

Even state agriculture and public health officials testified against the Bernstein panel's recommendations, including, Dr. Donald Muentener, chief of the Agriculture Department's laboratory division, and Dr. Kenneth R. Wilcox, Jr., chief of the Health Department's bureau of disease control and laboratory services. They disputed the panel's statements about the analytical capabilities in the detection of PBB—despite Dr. Kolbye's earlier statements.

Among the few who favored a reduction in tolerance guidelines were two veterinarians who daily saw the ravages of PBB, Louis Blesch of Sturgis, a town of ten thousand in southern Michigan just a few miles north of the Indiana border; and Susan Jacoby of Constantine a village of seventeen hundred about fifteen miles west of Sturgis. "A lot of it [PBB] has been cleaned up because a good many of the high level herds have been buried. But still, our problems exist," Dr. Blesch said. "Most of our herds today are the low levels that aren't under quarantine. They are still selling milk—some of them selling milk and meat, and their animals are still dying." He said that he practices in both Michigan and in Indiana, but that the problems stopped in Michigan, at the Indiana border. "I have not had a single case of this type of toxicity or poisoning in any farmer that feeds anything but Farm Bureau feeds." Dr. Blesch added, "They've been solely confined to my clients who use Farm Bureau Services feeds. For this reason, I seem to discount other factors such as iodine and so forth that's been mentioned."

Dr. Jacoby said at least ten of her clients had so-called low-level PBB contamination. "I have known them thoroughly and I am personally acquainted with the herds, so I think I can tell if there suddenly was a definite difference in the incidence of diseases and problems that had never occurred in that amount and in that seriousness previously," she said. "I have found some definite differences in diseases and reaction to diseases in these cows after they have been exposed to PBB. There were differences in the time lapse." Whereas in the past, cows in stress could be saved, she said, "now they just die on us.... Now they just wither away and die." Dr. Jacoby concluded, "We should eliminate PBB off the farms as soon and as thoroughly as possible."

A number of farmers both opposing and supporting the Bernstein panel's recommendations testified, as the hearing soon became a rerun of the 1975 hearing. Larry Crandall, a Battle Creek dairyman and neighbor of Halbert's, noted, "Here we are again! Same place, barely a year after the last attempt to reduce PBB guideline levels. I ask: Has anything changed in the past year?"

What has changed, of course, is that more PBB had been allowed to get into the human food channels, a fact Crandall did not seem to acknowledge.

If the Bernstein panel's recommendations are followed, Crandall said, "The farmer's livelihood will cease, employees will be released and everyone will suffer. Many farms will become uninhabitable for livestock, and certainly unsalable for livestock purposes. Is the state willing to buy these farms?"

But another farmer, Tom Glass, noted, "The level has to be lowered to get the situation cleaned up because if people say it's not a disaster now, all they have to do is go to Kalamazoo and walk in a restaurant—and I don't know how many of them there are—but you walk in and you see a sign that says: We Do Not Feed Any Michigan Meat or Milk on These Premises. Or you have school systems that don't want to buy any Michigan meat or milk. Now if that's not an agriculture disaster, then I don't know what is!"

Farmer Harley Hinkley also urged the adoption of lower tolerance guidelines. "All we've had on our farm is low toler-ance. We've had veterinarians come to our farm, cut the animals open, lay them there, look at them, study them and say, 'We don't know what they died from.' It is just something terrible. There's no justification nowhere. When our cattle started dying, I said, 'Son, by George, you don't know nothing about cattle and I forgot all I ever did know.' And that's all I ever done in this world was take care of cattle.... Now I don't know where you want the tolerance; I think it ought to be lowered. But I do know we ought to come up with something to stop these cattle from dying. There is nothing sickeninger than to doctor and doctor and doctor, and can't get no results.... I told them [Farm Bureau Services] I had PBB and they laughed at me. Had I been a young man, I probably would have went to prison because that manager—I would have rolled him. But I was older and I controlled my temper. They don't care whether we make it or whether we don't. Nobody else does. They just start the farmers a-bucking against each other. By George, Abraham Lincoln said, by George, let's see: 'Unite together, divided you die'—or something, some such statement as that Abraham Lincoln said. And that's the way it is with us farmers. If we don't unite together, we're all going to hang separately. Now I'll tell you, I've got PBB in my blood. I got an enlarged liver. I don't know whether there's anything the matter with me or not. Last spring in April, they put me on total disability. What in the devil is a young man like me doing—as strong and healthy as I am and as hard working as I've done in my life—on total disability? Who in the dickens can answer them foolish questions? There ain't a dag-burn man in this building, nor there's been in here today, that, five years ago, could have kept up with me or went ahead of me. Today, I'm worthless. Just as worthless as teats on a boar hog."

The testimonies continued all day and into the evening. Toward the end of the hearing, Yvonne Yarnell, a Missaukee County dairywoman, offered a trenchant observation. "I've been standing and sitting, and listening to people who have been quarantined and are on their second herd and hearing them say they had no health effects. At first I just couldn't believe it. And then I got to thinking; maybe it's the fact that they found out they had PBB, were quarantined, and got rid of it right away. Maybe the fact that we got so sick and had so many complications was the fact that we had been eating it for three years, and drinking the milk. So we ate it at least probably two to two and a half years longer than they did before we found out."

212

Interestingly, independent medical scientists later would offer the same postulation after examining more than a thousand poisoned Michigan farm dwellers.

A week after the June 10 hearing, Ball got a letter from Ken Jones, Farm Bureau Services' risk manager, containing a thinly veiled threat. "We wish to inform you on another aspect that may not have already been brought to your attention, that is the reaction of both United States and Lloyds of London insurance representatives concerning products liability," Jones wrote. He said the insurance carriers "are already very apprehensive about products liability exposures and will severely restrict, if not withdraw entirely from, the writing of products liability coverage on food products in Michigan if the effective tolerance is lowered to zero." But Jones need not have worried, for midway through the June 10 public hearing, Ball remarked privately, "There is no scientific evidence to support it [lowering the tolerance guideline]."

On June 22, the Agriculture Commission, appointed by the governor, defied Milliken by rejecting the Bernstein panel's recommendations, thereby retaining the existing tolerance guidelines. "A review of the scientific testimony reveals it to be predominantly in favor of retaining the current guidelines, but personal testimony was conflicting and inconclusive," concluded Ball, who recommended to the commission that they reject the Bernstein panel's advice. "State law requires that a public hearing must 'clearly establish a necessity' for any change from the federal guidelines. This the hearing did not do," he explained later. Ball said his recommendation "was based on advice and testimony from highly qualified national and worldwide scientists, including cancer specialists, whose business it is to protect the public health—just not adequately but with substantial safety factors." He failed to mention, of course, the unequivocal recommendations of the only group of scientists who had ever reviewed all the available literature on PBB and its close relative, PCB. Ball said further that his department received 386 letters opposing the Bernstein panel's recommendations and only 38 favoring them. In his recommendation to the Agriculture Commission, Ball once more relied on the state Health Department's discredited study: "The department is impressed by absence of medical testimony associating human health problems with PBB exposure, even in the group of farm families with highest exposures." At no time did the

Food and Drug Administration mention its own human health survey in which precisely such health problems had been reported—and at high incidences.

The refusal of B. Dale Ball and the Agriculture Commission to go along with the Bernstein panel's recommendations not only stunned the general public but took Milliken by surprise as well.

That same afternoon, the governor held a press conference to discuss the Agriculture Commission's decision. "I do not agree with the position the commission has taken," he said. Milliken that morning had met with the commission in East Lansing "to be sure that they understood the point of view which I have felt and the attitudes that I have expressed so that they would have what I consider to be the broader view of this problem.... I do not approve of the decision the commission has made." Milliken said the commission may have acted in a manner consistent with what it thought, "but what they thought is not what I think."

A week later, he sent a detailed memorandum to the legislature proposing that the lawmaking body now exercise its authority to lower the PBB tolerance guidelines. "Now we have before us the need to take strong, decisive, unilateral action on a problem that is almost uniquely Michigan's—the problem of PBBs," Milliken declared. As a "precautionary measure," he proposed a "partial lowering" of the federal standards from 300 parts per billion to 100 parts per billion (compared to the 5 parts per billion recommendation by the Bernstein panel) for meat; from 300 parts per billion to 150 parts per billion (compared to the Bernstein panel recommendation of 1 part per billion) for milk; and from 50 parts per billion to 10 parts per billion (compared to the panel's recommended level of 5 parts per billion) for eggs. Reductions also were recommended for poultry, rendered animals and animal feeds.

Milliken estimated that if his recommended meat tolerance level was adopted, about four thousand head of cattle would exceed 100 parts per billion, thus requiring their slaughter and burial.

This time, however, Milliken further recommended that animals violating any new tolerance level be disposed of by the state and that the owners of these animals be reimbursed. "I believe that the public interest requires that owners of contaminated animals have a clear source of reimbursement. It is

214

my judgment that the state has a responsibility to compensate a farmer for an animal that has become, in a sense, a public nuisance," he said. The irony, of course, is that such a policy is precisely what B. Dale Ball had advocated two years earlier, which both Milliken and the legislature rejected. Had that policy been adopted in 1974, much of the PBB mess would have been over by the spring of 1976—and without all the hardship so many farmers were still enduring.

In his June 29 memorandum, Milliken also asked for a $117,500 appropriation for the state Public Health Department to establish a control group for the long-term study being sponsored by the U.S. Center for Disease Control, the Food and Drug Administration and the National Cancer Institute. And, finally, in a forward-looking proposal, he requested an additional $300,000 to set up at Michigan State University an animal diagnostic clinic.

"For a variety of reasons," Milliken recalls, "the legislature approved only three of the bills I supported in my memorandum: the bills to reduce the tolerance in animal feed, to fund a control study group and to establish a diagnostic animal health clinic. My proposal to reduce tolerances in human food was among several proposals not acted upon."

One of those reasons, recalls Edie Clark, was that Milliken's proposals were made only several weeks before the legislative session adjourned for the summer. "We just didn't have enough time," she said. The proposals that did pass were uncomplicated and noncontroversial and thus sailed easily through both chambers.

In any case, with the Bernstein panel's report and the Agriculture Commission's refusal to heed its recommendations, intense public attention now was focused on the question of human health and the risk of further public exposure to the chemical. What has PBB done? What will it do?

Within six months, the public would find out, for Dr. Selikoff at last had been officially invited to Michigan to conduct his broad health survey, scheduled to be held right after the autumn harvests. But the urgency of such a study was once more underlined even before the New York scientists arrived.

In 1976, the state Department of Public Health was involved in a nationwide survey to analyze human breast milk for the presence of pesticides. And so the department's laboratory in Lansing had available milk samples from women living in a number of different states. In August, the laboratory decided to look for PBB as well in those samples, including some from Michigan.

The results stunned the health officials. Twenty-two out of twenty-six Michigan samples contained PBB. But ten other samples—from Connecticut, Massachusetts, New York and Ohio—were all negative. All the Michigan samples contained PBB at levels higher than what the Bernstein panel thought should be allowed in cow's milk (which was expected to be diluted with clean milk before reaching humans). Moreover, all six Michigan samples from Wayne County had turned up positive; Wayne County is the state's largest, and includes the city of Detroit. PBB no longer seemed to be only a rural-farm problem. Urban dwellers had not been exempt after all.

"I believe we have a very serious situation on our hands," Dr. Isbister told his boss, Dr. Maurice S. Reizen, the state's public health director. "The results to date have been alarming," he told Reizen.

"That was the first time we got struck with the idea that the general population may have PBB," Dr. Reizen recalls. "It was a credit to people in our lab to get going on breast milk. Nobody stimulated us to do the breast milk tests."

Shortly before the breast milk findings emerged, Milliken signed the bill lowering the amount of PBB allowed in animal feeds from 50 parts per billion to 10 parts per billion. Representative Don Albosta noticed the irony: Animals were now better protected against PBB than people—whose foods were allowed to contain up to 300 parts per billion.

The potential significance of breast milk findings can be seen in context by considering the fact that a nursing infant consumes about one-tenth of its entire body weight in maternal milk each day.

Since the PBB contamination was discovered in May 1974, blood tests have revealed high PBB concentrations in women from quarantined farms; and that led to warnings by state and federal health officials that these women should not breast-feed. But the discovery now that the breast milk of women in the general population also contained PBB clearly was not something that any health officials had expected. And there was special cause for concern because, unlike polluted cow's milk that is diluted with uncontaminated milk before reaching

216

humans, "in [human] breast milk there is a single source/single recipient relationship without influence by dilution," as Dr. Isbister put it.

From these milk sampling results, another important piece of information about PBB emerged: The chemical in the human body can be up to two hundred times more concentrated in milk than in blood. And so now a negative blood test no longer was sufficient reassurance for a woman who wished to breast-feed.

But the Health Department did not immediately make any of such information or findings available to the public, particularly to the estimated thirty thousand nursing mothers in Michigan.

First Dr. Reizen called a meeting to discuss the finding of PBB in breast milk. Among those at the August 19 meeting were Lieutenant Governor James J. Dammon, Pat Babcock and Kathy Stariha of the governor's staff, Dale Ball and Don Isleib from the Agriculture Department; Frank Cordle and Alan Hoeting of the U.S. Food and Drug Administration; and Dr. Renate D. Kimbrough, the U.S. Center for Disease toxicologist whose PCB findings had alarmed the Bernstein panel. At the end of the meeting, a poll was taken to determine whether or not the department should release the latest findings. The majority said no. But Dr. Isbister pointed out that not releasing the breast milk results would invite more charges of official cover-up. Hoeting concurred. And so the Health Department later that day issued a press release about the breast milk findings.

"Although we are dealing with chemicals which may have some potential for harm in the long run, we have insufficient evidence at this time to recommend discontinuing breast-feeding," it said. The department then set out to gather additional milk samples for further study.

The second effort involved gathering for PBB analyses the breast milk of ninety-two women who gave birth in Michigan hospitals during August. Fifth-three of the women were from the state's Lower Peninsula and thirty-nine from the Upper Peninsula.

The results confirmed earlier suspicions: More than 96 percent of the Lower Peninsula women had contaminated breast milk, as did 41 percent of the women from the more sparsely populated Upper Peninsula. All the contaminated

217

women had higher PBB levels in their milk than what the Bernstein panel had recommended as the safe standard for cow's milk. Eight women in the study had higher PBB levels in their milk than even the existing Food and Drug Administration tolerance guideline level for cow's milk. The highest individual sample contained 1,220 parts per billion.

Even though Dr. Reizen privately called the milk findings "a chilling revelation," his department told the public: "The levels of PBB are not sufficient to discourage Michigan mothers from breast-feeding if they so desire."

But from Ann Arbor, two dissenting opinions were heard. One came from Dr. Isadore Bernstein at the University of Michigan, who said the findings had "grave, ominous overtones," adding, "I hope this information will stimulate the governor and the Department of Agriculture to reconsider the panel's recommendation that the tolerance levels be dropped." He said, "Infants and children are more highly susceptible to carcinogens than adults. So mothers should stop breast-feeding. Period. I'm not against breast-feeding. It's good—but not in this state." Dr. Thomas Corbett added, "Reizen says there is no proof that PBB in breast milk is harmful. But my position is that there is no proof that it is safe. I take a more conservative approach." He said he also would advise women not to breast-feed. "You are subjecting children to a possible cancer risk. You're taking a chance on jeopardizing their health and welfare for the rest of their lives just to be breast-fed."

In early 1977, the Health Department arranged for new Michigan mothers to have their milk analyzed for PBB if they wished. The cost, about $25 each, was picked up by the state if a woman's regular medical insurance did not pay for the test. The legislature, in one of its final actions before adjourning for the 1976 Christmas holidays, appropriated $112,000 for the reimbursement program. Over the next few years, several thousand women from all over Michigan availed themselves of this service, reflecting a genuine concern despite state assurances of the continued benefits of breast-feeding.

"I want to emphasize," Dr. Reizen had declared in October of 1976, "that available evidence makes it clear that no toxic effects have been demonstrated from the amounts of PBB found in milk of Michigan mothers."

Yet even today it would be premature and unrealistic to conclude that babies of Michigan women are necessarily free of untoward effects of PBB which had contaminated their mothers. Experience with halogenated aromatic hydrocarbons and other similar chemicals have taught us that the effects of contamination are generally delayed and appear over long periods of time. Furthermore, they are hard to predict or to measure accurately. For instance, who could pinpoint a cause-and-effect relationship if the child of a PBB-contaminated Michigan woman should turn out to be just a little bit less alert than than average, or a little more prone to memory lapses, or a little more susceptible to illnesses? (Indeed nearly two years later, one study among Michigan children would demonstrate the serious consequences of the state Health Department's indifferent attitude.)

But in the autumn of 1976, only uncertainty prevailed. And into this atmosphere of anxiety came Dr. Irving J. Selikoff, the urbane, white-haired environmental health pioneer, bringing with him his renowned team of scientists to begin the nation's long-awaited first mass human health survey to learn the effects of an environmental contaminant.

# 12

# THE WHITE-HAIRED FIREMAN

Dr. Irving J. Selikoff had offered to conduct a human health study assessing the effects of PBB in the fall of 1974. But both he and Dr. Thomas H. Corbett, who relayed the offer to Milliken's office and the Agriculture Department, were surprised that state officials did not follow up on the gesture. "But we didn't think there was any more we could do about it," recalls Dr. Corbett.

Among those who had never heard of Dr. Selikoff then was Edith Clark, who in January of 1975 had become a member of the House Democratic staff. Earlier, the twenty-nine-year-old woman, a Michigan State University graduate, had done public relations work at Oldsmobile in Lansing. Because she had grown up on a farm and was a known animal lover, she was assigned to pay special attention to agricultural issues. By the autumn of 1975, she was practically working full time on PBB. "I was amazed nobody else [in the legislature] was working on the issue. So I began working on weekends, making contacts, taking reading material home," Clark recalls. Even by that fall, few scientists—with the exception of Dr. Corbett—had raised questions about the potential dangers of PBB and about the way the state agencies were mishandling the problem.

In early 1976, Edie met Dr. Alpha Clark, the McBain veterinarian who also had become a vociferous critic of the Milliken administration. The two Clarks began comparing notes and sharing information. "My God," recalls Doc, "you wouldn't believe what we went through to find out what the [state agencies] already knew! We were like kids in a cave, trying to deal with those bureaucrats." The two Clarks became friends, and soon Doc had Edie out visiting farms that the Agriculture Department said had only low levels of PBB which did not affect the animals. She was shaken by what she saw, and later reported to her boss, House Speaker Bobby D. Crim: "Cows were aborting. Of the calves which lived, abnormally high percentages were born blind, or with twisted limbs, bald patches, enlarged heads and otherwise hideously misshapen bodies. Of these, many did not live long. Some adult cows were afflicted with deteriorating limbs which would gradually become disconnected from the rest of the body, and disintegrating ears and tails that would wear down to stubs."

That spring, as the Albosta hearings were being held, and the farmers had begun to organize, Edie Clark finally went to Speaker Crim to request formally that she be assigned full time to the PBB investigation. Crim agreed instantly and instructed her to report to him daily.

By then Clark already had become a one-person clearinghouse for PBB information. Maps of Michigan with circles showing the areas hit by PBB were interspersed among the beautiful animal pictures and posters on the walls of her tiny office. One April day, she got a call from Republican state representative E. Dan Stevens. He said he was interested in learning more about the toxicity of PBB, and asked where he might go for such information. Clark suggested that Stevens call Dr. Corbett in Ann Arbor. Stevens did, and he made a date with Dr. Corbett for Friday, April 16.

Clark decided to tag along. During the course of their discussion over lunch in the University of Michigan Hospital's cafeteria, Clark recalls, "Corbett told us that about a year or a year and a half ago, he had been in touch with Dr. Selikoff, who expressed an interest in sending a team of specialist to Michigan to conduct research on the possible human health effects of PBB. He told Dr. Corbett there would be no charge involved, and all he needed was an invitation from the state." Dr. Corbett also told the two how the offer had been spurned brusquely by Dr. Whitehead at the Agriculture Department and not acted upon by the governor's office. When he finished, Dr. Corbett remarked, "Wasn't that nasty?!" Clark thought his information was "huge, colossal." Dr. Corbett recalls her reaction: "She lit up like a Christmas tree," which he found disappointing. "It then became a political thing, not something done with public health in mind." (At the time, Clark's boss, Bobby Crim, a Democrat, was frequently mentioned as the likely opponent of Republican Bill Milliken in the 1978 gubernatorial race.) When Clark and Stevens finished lunch with Dr. Corbett, Stevens asked the

221

doctor to send him a memorandum recounting the events surrounding Dr. Selikoff's overture.

Clark could barely contain her excitement. After all this time when the Milliken administration was telling the public no evidence existed that PBB caused human health problems now she had learned that it rejected an offer by the nation's top environmental health scientist to provide precisely such information—and for free. But she "sat on the information" for ten days, partly because she felt it was "Stevens' information." Too, Crim at the time was vacationing in Florida. Finally she called Dr. Selikoff on April 26, asking him if he had heard from Stevens. He said no. "He said he was still interested in sending a team to Michigan but thought that perhaps Michigan had enough qualified personnel that were interested in the subject to perform the study themselves," Clark recalls. "I replied that this may be the case, but that the issue had become so emotional that many qualified personnel had become allied with either one side or the other, and that we were in the need of an objective source."

When Speaker Crim returned, she told him of the events that had transpired, including a trip she later made to New York City to meet personally with Dr. Selikoff. "All that is needed now," she told him, "is a formal invitation from you to Dr. Selikoff."

To Clark's relief, the Speaker approved of her actions. She had been especially worried about the unauthorized trip to New York. Crim then called Dr. Reizen, asking about the spurned offer. Dr. Reizen denied any knowledge of it even though his own department's records later showed the contrary. "We never heard of it," Dr. Reizen said of Dr. Selikoff's offer. "When Crim brought it up, we thought, 'What was wrong with that?!'" Clark, who was present during the Crim-Reizen meeting, said, "Reizen swore up and down—did everything but cross his heart—that he absolutely had no idea."

The belated invitation was issued jointly by Crim and Dr. Reizen. And Dr. Selikoff quickly accepted. The actual clinics, however, were postponed until after the Bernstein panel's work was done.

Epidemiology is the basic science of public health, involving the study of disease patterns in various populations. An epidemiologist, thus, is different from a doctor who treats individual patients, which is what Dr. Selikoff did many years ago as a young physician in the working-class neighborhoods of New York and New Jersey. There he first began seeing cases of occupational diseases. "Right away, he was smitten with the fact that these poeple had these conditions. He was immediately disenchanted with all these people [employers] because he saw how all the workers suffered working for them," recalls Celia Selikoff, the doctor's wife of more than thirty years.

The United States Public Health Service began a formal epidemiologic training program in 1951 at its Center for Disease Control in Atlanta, Georgia. "It began at a time when there was great fear in this country of biological warfare and a perceived need to be on guard," said Dr. Michael Gregg, deputy director of the epidemiology division at the Center for Disease Control.

There are perhaps two hundred full-time practicing epidemiologists in the entire country, but far fewer who specialize in cancer, as Dr. Selikoff does. "Epidemiology is not a highly populated profession because the emphasis is still on cure rather than prevention and, generally, it is not as remunerative financially as being in private practice," explains Dr. Gregg.

An epidemiologic investigation is complicated business because it involves many scientific specialties, each analyzing different specimens, different pieces of the puzzle. A bacteriologist, for instance, looks for bacteria; a virologist looks for viruses; an immunologist looks for damages to the body's immune system; another looks for fungi. In such an investigation, the chief clinical epidemiologist (such as Dr. Selikoff) gathers all the available information and then postulates theories as to the cause of some widespread illness. In a sense, such a scientist often has to play detective, trying to unravel a mystery by reconstructing how a criminal operates. Is the bad actor lethal? Does it spread from person to person? If so, how quickly? How long does it take to strike down its victims? And in what manner? Does it cause cancer of the lung or the stomach or some other site?

Such investigations often result in massive and confusing data and numbers. But that's what epidemiology is all about: the manipulation of figures, comparing one thing to another, looking for a statistical variance that might help solve unanswered questions. The scientific process called epidemiology, then, is not nearly as precise or straightforward as some laymen might presume. Epidemiologists don't always move steadily

223

from one point to another, methodically peeling away the layers of mystery; they proceed in much more random fashions.

Epidemiologists don't like to waste time when starting an investigation because important evidence can disappear quickly—and undetected. And the human body is incredibly efficient in breaking down or excreting a disease-causing agent that may pose a threat. Even in routine cases, often by the time an epidemiologist arrives to collect samples for laboratory analyses, the agent may have disappeared or been broken down by the body's marvelous metabolic process into a new form that cannot be so easily recognized and its damages so easily detected.

This is why Dr. Selikoff, upon hearing about a chemical contamination in Michigan, proposed immediately to begin an epidemiologic investigation. When the invitation at last arrived, Dr. Selikoff recalls, "we did not hesitate to agree to this research. At first blush, this may have seemed overly ambitious. Such a survey had not been accomplished before, we would be far from our home base, there were numerous uncertainties. Yet we were confident in our immediate assent."

The PBB disaster in Michigan, he says, makes "a natural experiment—a paradigm of environmental contamination. Since PBB was made for a limited time in only one place, and the contamination is still essentially limited to Michigan, we had the opportunity to properly research the effects of a pollutant, comparing what happened to exposed people to those who were not exposed." In Dr. Selikoff, Michigan probably could not have invited a more qualified person to conduct the PBB epidemiologic survey.

Over the years, he has built the Environmental Sciences Laboratory into one of the largest and the most active in the country, flying from disaster to disaster looking for causes and effects of health hazards—at the invitation of labor, business, government or other scientists. "Selikoff has built a group of colleagues who work with him; but he also has started what is really the first program of its kind in the country: essentially a residency in environmental medicine. He's got teams of people who, as a part of their training, are experts in doing PBB-like investigations, says Dr. Sidney Wolfe, head of the Ralph Nader-financed Public Interest Health Research Group.

The Environmental Sciences Laboratory is a part of the Mount Sinai Medical School in New York City. It has a full-time

224

professional staff of some forty-five persons, including neurologists, chemists, physicists, behavioral psychologists, internists and even two mineralogists, who have played major roles in the laboratory's work on asbestos—for which Dr. Selikoff is most known, all over the world.

Asbestos, about 4 million pounds of which are produced each year, is an inexpensive and ubiquitous mineral well known for its fire-retardant properties and resistance to wear. It is used in countless items, such as brake linings, potholders, water pipes, curtains, spackle, ironing-board covers and textiles. Once asbestos was thought to be biologically inert—without any effect on the body's tissues, that is—but Dr. Selikoff's yeomanlike work has proved otherwise. As his studies showed, asbestos years—decades—later would wreak havoc in the bodies of workers who mined and fashioned it into the endless products society so casually took for granted.

The microscopic asbestos fibers enter the body easily (mostly through inhalation) and then they stay put. Dr. Selikoff eventually followed more than seventeen thousand asbestos workers and showed that their death rate from lung cancer was five to seven times greater than what would be expected in a normal population. Deaths from cancer of the gastrointestinal tract were about three times greater. Even more interestingly, he found that lung cancer in asbestos workers seemed to develop at a rate beyond normal especially when they were cigarette smokers. The interaction of tobacco and asbestos multiplied the effects of each individual substance. A synergistic effect of this kind is what worried many people in Michigan such as Dr. Corbett, knowing that Michigan's residents now had one more chemical burdening their bodies. Would PBB be the one that might trigger such an event?

Dr. Selikoff's findings on asbestos were immensely important because the air in all urban areas is filled with asbestos fibers, expecially at street corners where vehicles must come to a stop, thereby releasing tiny fibers from brake linings into the air. These studies ultimately prompted the Johns-Manville Corporation, the country's largest asbestos maker with more than twenty-five thousand employees in 110 plants all over the country, and the international asbestos union to each donate a quarter million dollars to find possible cures for asbestos related cancers. All asbestos workers, whether they smoke or not, are further prone to an otherwise nonexistent cancer

225

called mesothelioma, a disease affecting the lining of the chest or abdominal cavity, which thus far has proven invariably fatal. Years after these studies, Dr. Selikoff's continued interest in asbestos revealed further that not only workers but their families as well were more likely to develop asbestos-related cancers. Mesothelioma, for example, also began showing up among the millions of Americans who worked in shipyards during World War II, where asbestos was used in ships as insulation. Dr. Selikoff reported that as little as one week of working in a shipyard may have been sufficient to plant the seeds of cancer that would not become known until decades later.

In May of 1978, Joseph A. Califano, Jr., secretary of the U.S. Department of Health, Education and Welfare, issued a public warning that 8 to 11 million Americans have been exposed to asbestos and thus are now at risk of developing a wide range of cancers and other diseases.

"Dr. Selikoff has become the archbishop of environmental medicine," says Dr. Maurice S. Reizen, Michigan's public health director, himself a preventive medicine specialist. Ironically, Dr. Selikoff's stature today as an environmental health researcher has all but obscured a vital contribution he made as a young Staten Island, New York, physician who played a major role in the discovery of a drug that has revolutionized the treatment of tuberculosis throughout the world. The main reason for that is Dr. Selikoff's own reluctance to talk about himself, his personal life or the past. "Time is the one thing he cannot buy," says Celia Selikoff, herself an accomplished sculptress and musician. As a result, even his closest friends and colleagues know very little about Dr. Selikoff's background—for instance, the childhood polio he overcame to become a talented tennis player and later a catcher for a semiprofessional baseball team.

The rotund native New Yorker is a self-effacing man with snow-white hair, rock-steady blue eyes and a toothy grin that drops instantly at the mention of his favorite subject: cancer. While he is not without a sense of humor, most of his jokes reflect his obsession with environmental epidemiology. At the end of a conference on saccharin, for instance, he was in a hurry to catch an airplane. Twice, he paused to ask, "What is the calculated risk time to get to the airport?"

He begins his workday at 4:00 A.M.—seven times a week— but still he doesn't find enough time to do all he would like. So

226

he often compensates by reading while walking, and eating while behind the wheel of his Lincoln Continental, dictating into a recording machine in between bites.

"He comes home and continues to work. Every day. I mean Saturdays. Sundays. Holidays. Even our most important holidays are spent in work. There is no weekend. There is no change in Selikoff's life," says Celia Selikoff, who, like most people, calls him Selikoff.

At the countless scientific conferences the scientist, in his mid-sixties, attends, Dr. Selikoff often is the center of attention. When he enters a room—usually late and lugging a bulging briefcase he is likely to forget upon departure—heads turn; people try to catch his eye to be acknowledged. When such meetings break up, Dr. Selikoff invariably attracts a crowd. Usually several colleagues would vie for his attention, often speaking at once, while still another scientist would be shaking his hand. Throughout the commotion, Dr. Selikoff remains unflappable, systematically tucking away notes and business cards into his pockets, which serve as filing cabinets when he's away from home.

When Dr. Selikoff talks about the subject he knows best, environmental diseases, his statements, never made from prepared notes, are forceful and convey a sense of purpose and meaning. His undeviating message is that the proliferation of cancer-causing chemicals in our environment leaves little time to waste.

"We now have entered an extraordinary new phase in the battle against cancer. For the first time in human history, we are learning the causes of diseases. This brings two new opportunities—and responsibilities. First, the chance to control exposures, to prevent problems in the future. And, second, to help those already exposed and now, as a result, are at high risk of developing neoplasms [cancers].

Not surprisingly, Dr. Selikoff has many critics, particularly among the chemical industry. Yet even scientists such as Dr. Perry J. Gehring, the Dow toxicologist named to Milliken's first PBB scientific advisory panel, holds begrudging admiration for him. "If you're talking about people who have made a real impact in environmental medicine, I'd have to say he's one of the best." Others accuse Dr. Selikoff of being an alarmist. But among many colleagues who come to Dr. Selikoff's defense is Dr. David P. Rall, director of the National Institute of Environmental Health Sciences. "Sure he raises the red flag. But you either do that or do nothing, which alarms nobody. But if there is a problem, that helps no one at all." Another admirer is Dr. Corbett of Ann Arbor. "His motives are totally unselfish. He doesn't do things for personal aggrandizement. He doesn't need to at this stage of the game. I can't think of another man who has done more to protect the health of common man than he has. Dr. Selikoff is a unique national resource. He's a true patriot. And I've never seen a man who works harder than Dr. Selikoff. He has a workload that would fatigue a man half his age. I don't know how he does it." But another Dow Chemical scientist, Dr. Etcyl Blair, now vice-president and director of health and environmental sciences, complained, "The thing about Irv," he said, "is that he constantly talks about 'the tip of the iceberg' of carcinogens. He fans the problem. He tends to incite. And he knows what he's doing—it adds to more people talking about Selikoff; as a result, he's a big name."

When suspicions arose in 1973 about the safety of the drinking water in Duluth, Minnesota, a city of a hundred thousand, which draws its water from Lake Superior, it was the Environmental Sciences Laboratory the federal government turned to for help. The Environmental Protection Agency flew several gallons of the lake water to the lab, where Dr. Selikoff's team stood by waiting. They worked all night, and by morning the answer was known. The laboratory had found large amounts of asbestos-laden rocky wastes in the clear blue water, water thought so pure that Duluth didn't even bother to filter it. It is such work that Dr. Selikoff's name and his team has become known for all over the country, synonymous with the occurrence of environmental disasters, places like Vernon, California; Toledo, Ohio; Monaca, Pennsylvania; Indianapolis, Indiana, St. Louis, Missouri; Hudson Falls, New York; Michigan; South Africa. The list is almost endless.

"We also do long-term research, of course. But we're like firemen. When the gong sounds, we can drop it for a number of weeks to respond to the emergency," Dr. Selikoff says. Michigan, he says, was one such emergency.

"Once on the scene, Dr. Selikoff began making waves," wrote John R. Emshwiller, a Detroit-based *Wall Street Journal* reporter. In various newspaper interviews, Dr. Selikoff questioned the assurances of state and federal health officials that food with low levels of PBB was safe. "I just don't think meat with PBB is good to eat," he said. Dr. Selikoff also challenged the recommendations that mothers may continue breast-feeding, pointing out that PBB concentrates in milk.

Dr. Selikoff's comments drew hundreds of calls from worried parents—and a state Health Department release reiterating that it "continues to recommend that mothers not living on farms that had been contaminated who choose to breast-feed should continue to do so, even though their breast milk contains trace amounts of PBB."

Dr. Selikoff's remarks had not been made without due consideration, however. He had begun planning and laying the groundwork for the PBB study for months; and as result, the accumulating information about PBB had made him duly cautious about the chemical.

The first trip a member of his staff made to Michigan to learn about PBB, of course, was in October of 1974, when Dr. Henry Anderson visited with Dr. Corbett in Ann Arbor. After the official invitation from Michigan was issued on May 11, Dr. Selikoff went into action. On Thursday before the long bicentennial weekend, he called a meeting in his pasture-sized office at the Environmental Sciences Laboratory, located in Upper Manhattan at 101st Street and Fifth Avenue across from Central Park. About twenty people attended, including Edie Clark, whom Dr. Selikoff asked to begin arranging for a centrally located testing site for the health survey. No state public health official attended, although they had been invited. Dr. John L. Isbister, the disease control officer, was unable to get out of Detroit's Metropolitan Airport because of bad weather in New York City. He waited all Wednesday afternoon at the airport, but at 6:00 P.M. learned that he could have a standby ticket for a 9:00 A.M. flight Thursday morning. "I said to hell with it and came home." Among the other topics discussed at the meeting was Dr. Selikoff's intention to visit Michigan in late July to collect firsthand information and see a few farms.

The basis of discussion at the July 1 meeting was information provided by the laboratory's toxicologist, Dr. Kingsley Kay, who had conducted a review of all the data then available on PBBs. "It was concluded," recalls Dr. Anderson, "that the Michigan PBB accident was of great public health and scientific interest and that the Envirnomental Sciences Laboratory could best make a contribution to the understanding of possible human health effects of PBB ingestion by conducting a broad, comprehensive clinical and laboratory evaluation of presumably exposed individuals."

On July 20 and 21, Drs. Selikoff, Anderson, Kay and E. Cuyler Hammond, director of epidemiology of the American Cancer Society, went to Michigan. They wanted to check out the Kent Community Hospital in Grand Rapids, the site of the planned clinic, and to further visit with Michigan doctors and scientists. "In order to appreciate the actual farm conditions, we visited two dairy farms to inspect the animals and ask questions of the farmers," Dr. Anderson recalls. "These visits provided valuable experience to enable us to better understand the farmer's terminology and experiences as they would later be told to us during the survey." As an additional step, Dr. Selikoff had asked Edie Clark to set up a "farmers' advisory council" because, Dr. Anderson explained, "We felt it was essential to develop direct contact with various groups of the farm community. It was hoped that such communication would minimize misinterpretation, misunderstanding and distortion of our goals and, later, our findings." He added, "We specifically asked that all types of experience be represented. She [Edie Clark] did an admirable job in bringing together a workable council of thirteen men and women.... The council did not and was not intended to have any role in the design of the study. They were to pretest the clarity of our letters of invitation and questionnaires. They were able to advise on such matters as what time of year was best for the examination, the most convenient location, how far we could expect individuals to drive, what percentage of participation we could expect, and to provide information we needed about dairy farms and their operation." The council members, Dr. Anderson said, also were asked to serve as volunteers during the clinical examinations.

Among the members of the farmers advisory council was Lou Trombley of Hersey. He advised Dr. Selikoff to pay special attention to low-level farmers because, Trombley said, the highly contaminated farmers knew much earlier to stop consuming their own milk and to stop butchering their meat. But the low-level farmers did not, since they were told their farms had not been contaminated. Dr. Selikoff was impressed with Trombley's acuity. "You'd make a good epidemiologist," he told Trombley, whose chest swelled with pride.

The group from New York had a hectic schedule during

its two-day visit in Michigan, touring farms, meeting with the advisory council, attending meetings with agriculture officials, sitting down with health officials to explain the purpose of the epidemiologic study, discussing matters with Governor Milliken, holding press conferences. Dr. Hammond, the American Cancer Society epidemiologist, suggested to state health officers that an urgent area to research was how to eliminate PBB from the body "in order to lower the likelihood of development of cancer, assuming that PBB is carcinogenic."

During these two days, state officials already had preliminary information from the breast milk studies, and indeed they were discussing the ramifications of the findings. But at no time did they mention the information to Dr. Selikoff, who had been open and cooperative with state officials. The Michigan bureaucrats clearly felt threatened now by the emergence on the scene of a famous environmental scientist who attracted national attention.

Dr. Isbister, the Health Department's disease control officer, for instance, complained that Dr. Selikoff's closest contact in Michigan was Edie Clark, the aide to Democratic House Speaker Crim. "I am still concerned," Dr. Isbister said after the July 20–21 visit, "as to a number of problems which may arise in the next few months in spite of the expressed willingness of Dr. Selikoff to cooperate with us at virtually all levels." Among other things, he continued, the state's recently funded long-term study "is in significant jeopardy because of the attractiveness the Selikoff approach will have to the farm families.... It seems entirely possible to me that those individuals participating in the Selikoff study will not be available to us." Dr. Isbister also objected to the farmers' advisory council which, he said, "appears to have a majority made up of those who have been highly critical of our efforts in the past and cannot be counted upon to be objective in supporting our long-term study as compared to that of Dr. Selikoff." Dr. Isbister, however, did find "one or two" council members who "past experience suggests are reasonable and well-founded people." One was Franklin Schmidt, the Ottawa County dairyman who implemented the Farm Bureau Services–financed letter campaign rallying opposition in 1976 against the Bernstein panel's recommendation to drop the federal PBB tolerance guideline levels. "It appears highly probable that Dr. Selikoff was 'snowed' by the farmers with whom he talked. I very strongly question that he has any kind of an accurate picture of the emotion, self-interest and lack of objectivity on the part of many of the farmers involved in the PBB episode," Dr. Isbister concluded in a report of the Selikoff visit.

At the end of July, the Environmental Science Laboratory also invited Rick Halbert to New York to share his personal experiences and observations with members of the laboratory who would be conducting the field survey in Michigan. Afterward, Halbert didn't even bother to turn in his travel expenses; instead he sent the laboratory $100 as a contribution. "I felt it was my obligation," Halbert said. In early August, Dr. Anderson and another young physician from the laboratory, Kenneth D. Rosenman, visited Michigan to meet with the farmers advisory council to hear the farmers' comments and suggestions about the upcoming study. The clinical examination dates and location also were set: November 4 through 10, after the harvest, at the Kent Community Hospital in Grand Rapids. In mid-September, the New York research team opened a field station at that hospital to schedule examinations and to obtain from each farm family that was contacted names of other families who had regularly purchased foods from their farms.

On September 22, a week after the field station was set up, Drs. Selikoff and Rosenman met in Washington with federal officials representing the National Institute of Environmental Health Sciences, the Center for Disease Control and the Department of Health, Education and Welfare to review the objectives and protocol of the upcoming study, which had begun to attract national attention because of its unprecedented scope. The design of the study is noteworthy because later it would be criticized by people such as Alan L. Hoeting of the Food and Drug Administration and others in Michigan who did not like what Dr. Selikoff found.

"The principal objective was to investigate possible human health effects of PBB exposure. Therefore," Dr. Selikoff recalls, "it was considered advantageous to evaluate the status of those presumed to be at greatest risk: farmers and members of their families residing on farms quarantined by the Michigan Department of Agriculture." He later added, "We realized that not all could be invited to participate; we therefore selected farms in a statistically random fashion to receive invitations from this list [supplied by state agriculture officials].... There was criticism that our study was 'not representative' and participants 'not randomly' selected. We never intended them to be either of these and the criticism is misdirected and uninformed.... because no attempt was made to select survey participants to be representative of the general population or any other specific population."

From the list of quarantined farms, Dr. Selikoff's staff selected 125 farms in a statistically random fashion and sent each an invitation to be examined in the November examinations; this effort resulted in 30 individuals who later were examined. "Recognizing, however, that it took only one action-level cow to result in quarantine of a farm," Dr. Selikoff said, "we listed the farmers by the number of animals they had destroyed, and by the time at which quarantine had been initiated." Invitations then were sent to 50 farmers, beginning at the top of the list. In a similarly methodical approach, 99 "consumers" also agreed to be examined; this group comprised people who do not live on farms but had purchased food products directly from quarantined farms. Another group to be examined was made up of 129 dwellers of contaminated farms—but at below the quarantine levels, the so-called low-level farms. In addition 25 invitations then were sent to farms which had been tested for PBB but had no detectable levels; of this group, 2 families agreed to participate in the examinations. A second group of 71 "consumers" also was invited—comprising those who purchase foods from low-level farms. The total examination group was to be 604—404 persons associated with quarantined farms and 200 nonquarantined farms.

But as Dr. Selikoff and his team were finalizing their study design, they began to fully appreciate the atmosphere of anxiety and uncertainty that prevailed in Michigan. Dozens of doctors from all across the state called, reporting patients with inexplicable health problems. The team also received numerous letters farm families had sent to their lawyers, requesting the attorneys to somehow get them enrolled in the Selikoff study. The public interest was enormous.

And even after the November examinations were under way, Dr. Selikoff recalls, "We received many calls, and had people arrive at the examination site without prior appointments, some having driven several hundreds of miles. ... simply walked in and said, 'Here we are, please examine us.'"

In all, 1,029 persons were examined, including farm

233

families from as far away as the states of Washington and Maine who had lived in Michigan. They returned—at their own expense—to be examined. The overall response rate to the Selikoff invitations was extraordinary. Dr. Selikoff had never seen anything like it in his career: 50 percent of those invited showed up.

Yet, Dr. Selikoff later admitted, "Very frankly, we did not expect to find very much. We had been sensitized with the PCB issue, vinyl chloride, dioxin, that, generally, with these chemical diseases, it is pretty difficult to detect gross clinical changes even though the metabolism of the body is being affected in a serious way."

The Selikoff team also had enrolled fifty-five employees of the Michigan Chemical plant in St. Louis, Michigan. "Since our experience in evaluating toxic environmental agents has taught us that if toxicity is not seen among those with the greatest likelihood of excessive exposure, it would be unlikely that a serious problem would be found in those only lightly or casually exposed," Dr. Selikoff explained. Realizing he could not identify a Michigan farm population that had not been contaminated by PBB to use as a control group, Dr. Selikoff selected Wisconsin, a neighboring dairy state, as the site to obtain a control group. The Wisconsin studies would be held in March of 1977.

Finally, on November 3, 1976, Dr. Selikoff, in his Hush Puppies, a black bow tie and lugging his ever-present leather briefcase, arrived at the Kent County Airport in Grand Rapids. It was the morning after election day, and the city was virtually in mourning because its native son, Jerry Ford, had been defeated by Jimmy Carter. At the airport, where a huge mural depicting Ford's life had been unveiled a day earlier by the president himself, Dr. Selikoff held a press conference, questioning the wisdom of the existing PBB standards and of breast-feeding.

The next morning, the examinations at Kent Community Hospital began promptly at eight. Soon the entire hospital wing, which had been set aside for the mass health screening survey and had stood eerily silent for several days, came alive with activity as farmers and their families checked in at the second-floor nursing station. Among them were Chris and Donald Rehkopf and their two-year-old son, Thorin, who had flown to Grand Rapids from Brewster, Washington, their home

234

since the spring.

One by one, each person filed through the examining procedure, at a rate of nearly two hundred per day, starting with a seemingly endless questionnaire exploring their medical, family, work and dietary histories. Then they moved to other rooms to give blood and urine samples for laboratory analysis, undergo examination of their eyes and skin, complete physicals, behavioral tests, neurological examinations, pulmonary function tests; and some were asked to submit to a fat biopsy for PBB analysis. The medical team wanted to know how every organ system was working: liver, kidneys, lungs, heart, brain.

After two years of heated medical and political controversy, during which little was done by state officials to check out farmers' complaints of health problems, participants in the examination were grateful to see Dr. Selikoff and his team. "They are the first people that are really helping us," said Mrs. Donna Woltjer, wife of Gerald Woltjer, of Coopersville. And Edith Clark remarked, "This is the first time the farmers' complaints were written down instead of written off."

The study was funded by the National Institute of Environmental Health Sciences, an arm of the Department of Health, Education and Welfare, as a part of the government's long-range effort to develop better ways to deal with environmental emergencies. The Michigan survey was unprecedented in the history of epidemiology because it was the first to assess the effects of a chemical among a broad population (as opposed to, say, a group of industrial workers), and the first to include entire families.

The examinations kept the Selikoff team working late into the night, and by the end of the clinic, more than six thousand tubes of blood and urine samples and more than forty thousand pages of data had been collected and were awaiting analysis.

But even after the first day of the clinic, a pattern had begun to emerge. Dr. Alf S. Fischbein recalled: "Joint problems, fatigue, dizziness, memory problems, excessive sweating, sores that won't heal, darkening of the skin, sensitivity to sunlight— many people seem to have these problems."

Other complaints heard by Dr. Fischbein and the other physicians on Dr. Selikoff's team included lack of energy, muscular weakness, diarrhea, visual disturbances, sores and skin rashes. Some of the children had lost weight despite

235

balanced diets; others had lost patches of hair and developed a kind of acne typically associated with chemical contaminations.

The symptoms were not unlike those seen in the PBB-poisoned farm animals. The examination team earlier in the year had been shown films of such PBB-sickened animals by Gary P. Schenk, the Grand Rapids attorney representing numerous farmers seeking compensation for the farms and livelihood they lost due to PBB pollution.

By the end of the six-day clinic, the New York team was disturbed by what it had found. Said Dr. Sidney Diamond, a neurologist, "How much of the problems are organic and how much is emotional overlay may be a valid scientific question [to be studied]. But in terms of the lives of these people, it's really not a relevant issue. These people's lives are destroyed, and that is as important as pain in their joints. You can't take fluid out of the soul and show PBB."

On the morning of November 7, a Sunday and the fourth day of the clinic, the Detroit *Free Press* reported in a banner headline: "PBB Probe Finds Farmers in Bad Shape." The story, by Bob Calverly, said, "What Dr. Diamond is finding frequently are avid card players who no longer can keep track of their cards, seasoned farmers who now can't plow their fields straight, and drivers with previously good records who get five tickets in a month or who accidentally drive through barn doors. These symptoms point to neurological damage, Dr. Diamond says. 'A lot of accidents. They seem to have a lot of accidents.'"

Dr. Diamond also said most of the patients typically attempted to blame themselves, perhaps their personal shortcomings, rather than embellishing their symptoms. One woman with memory lapses told him, "I must be getting old." She was thirty-five.

But Dr. Diamond and the other scientists cautioned that such problems could not be linked with PBB until much more laboratory analyses were done.

During the course of the six-day clinic, Dr. Selikoff allowed the media open access to most areas of the examination site. He also agreed to allow the Michigan Health Department to set up a recruiting station in the hospital wing in order to solicit participation in the state's long-term study.

"We made no effort to silence anyone or exclude any press or federal agency representative from observing the examinations. We assumed that all such guests would exhibit proper respect of the rights and wishes of the participants and the staff," Dr. Anderson recalls. "We regret that some regulatory agency representatives abused our generosity and hospitality to the extent of eavesdropping on personal telephone conversations and taking notes of their contents."

On Monday, November 8, Raymond K. Hedblad, a supervisory investigator with the Food and Drug Administration stationed in Grand Rapids, was instructed by the Detroit office to ask Dr. Selikoff about the accuracy of quotes attributed to him, especially certain statements about FDA's tolerance guideline levels and about the dangers of breast-feeding. But Hedblad learned when he called Kent Community Hospital that the entire Selikoff team had taken the day off to visit the farm of Edie Clark's family south of Holland, Michigan, on the shores of Lake Michigan. When Hedblad went to the hospital the following day, a receptionist told him Dr. Selikoff would be out of town for several days. He was directed to Dr. Anderson. But Dr. Anderson, the gregarious young assistant to Dr. Selikoff, had a number of reporters lined up waiting for interviews. So Hedblad went to a reception area to wait. While he was sitting there, Dr. Corbett, who was participating in the examinations, came into the room and began a telephone conversation with someone he addressed as "Jane." Hedblad furtively listened, and then later wrote a memorandum reporting: "The conversation was with a 'Jane,' believed to be Jane Haradine*, a reporter with the Grand Rapids *Press*. Dr. Corbett asked the other party to take into consideration that he had been tired on the previous day when he was interviewed. He also asked that he not be directly identified with certain statements when the results of the interview were published. He stated that she should understand that he was not part of Dr. Selikoff's group. He therefore did not want his 'inflammatory statements' to reflect badly on the study. He stated that the study group was being conservative in statements which they provided to the press."

Dr. Corbett's conversation ended shortly afterward, and he left the room. Hedblad continued waiting for Dr. Anderson, but he eventually left without seeing the physician.

The eavesdropping incident and Hedblad's memorandum came to light during public hearings in March of 1977 held by

*Actually Jane Brody of *The New York Times*.

237

the U.S. Senate subcommittee on science, technology and space, chaired by newly elected Michigan senator Donald W. Riegle, Jr. The disclosure prompted Riegle to remark, "Even if [Dr. Corbett] were speaking loud enough for you to have overheard the conversation, I personally don't think it's very good practice for people in the federal government to be reporting private conversations of that sort in that manner."

"It's the practice," Hedblad explained, "that when you do an assignment like this, we always reduce it to written form." Dr. Kolbye of the FDA's bureau of foods, explained, "Certainly there is no intent to be a big-brother-type federal investigatory agency here. I think, on the other hand, when there are bits and pieces of information that sometimes shed some light or perspective on the matters that we deal with that are important to the public health that, on the other hand, we cannot tell them to disregard information. It may be of some use to us." Later, Dr. Kolbye claimed that, "For all practical purposes, our investigators are like FBI agents. We even investigated people who said PBB was safe. It's our obligation as a law enforcement agency to investigate. Anybody who took a strong stand we would ask a few questions about. Is the witness credible? Why is this guy saying that?"

Al Hoeting, Hedblad's superior, told Riegle, "I'm very pleased that [Hedblad] reported that information to me. And I think it's a pertinent bit of information." The issue was dropped with Riegle commenting, "Well, I don't know. You are not the FBI and you are not a surveillance organization insofar as I know it. If you have the suspicion of a criminal law violation, that's another matter. But I don't want everybody to feel that if somebody is around from the FDA that they have to go into another room to talk to somebody else."

Dr. Selikoff had been scheduled to announce the preliminary findings of the Grand Rapids survey in December, but personal illness caused a delay until January. In the meantime, however, Harold Humphrey, the state Health Department epidemiologist, came up with a bright idea to take advantage of Dr. Selikoff's illness.

The department had collected about two hundred blood samples at Kent Community Hospital in November, thanks to Dr. Selikoff, who allowed the department to set up a recruiting station during his week-long clinic. Now Humphrey proposed that these samples be quickly analyzed for PBB. "This gives us some time to perhaps get a jump ahead of him [Selikoff]," Humphrey wrote to Dr. Kenneth Wilcox, who is in charge of the laboratories. "If we could have test values available for his review when he comes to Michigan, we might steal some of his thunder, enhance the department's image and set a benchmark against which his group would have to compare," Humphrey wrote. For some reason, the suggestion was not followed. And so, despite Dr. Selikoff's open cooperation with the state Health Department, the department would continue to try to interfere with Dr. Selikoff's work—now that efforts to keep him out of Michigan in the first place had failed.

On January 3, Dr. Selikoff flew to Michigan from New York City to meet with Governor Milliken, Speaker Crim and the largest gathering of media representatives in the state capital in recent memory to deliver his report. "The preliminary report," recalls Edie Clark, "changed the tenor of the PBB issue almost overnight. Although Selikoff's report did not contain good news, it provided a measure of vindication for contaminated Michigan farmers, many of whom had for years complained to deaf ears.... It appeared, then, that the farmers had been right all along. There were health problems, and despite the severity of their problems, they had gone unnoticed by, and without attention from, the state agencies."

After his private meeting with Milliken, Crim and state public health officials, Dr. Selikoff and the entire entourage emerged grim-faced to confront the press.

The Selikoff findings were in direct contrast to the 1974 state study, which could find no human health problems due to PBB exposure. Dr. Selikoff found that PBB indeed had caused widespread and significant human health problems.

"We found health problems that we did not anticipate and would not anticipate among people in general," Dr. Selikoff said gravely. The study revealed that nearly one-third of the 1,029 persons examined had suffered adverse health effects.

"We also found that perhaps where individuals live may not be the whole story," he continued. "For example, one of the highest blood levels we've so far seen of PBB was in a man who did not live on a quarantine farm but ate twenty-one eggs a week." Dr. Selikoff cautioned, however, that his results could not be extrapolated to include the state's general population. "Most people in Michigan don't live on farms."

Although noting that two-thirds of those examined "told

239

us that they felt no deterioration of their health over the past three years," Dr. Selikoff said, "at this time no class or group of people of those examined by us can be said to be free of risk."

He said he had no explanation as to why "there was clearly much individual variability in response to PBB"—that is, why one person might suffer ill health but not another, even though both had been poisoned by PBB. "Why this is so we just don't know. You might add, 'Well, what about the future?' We don't know about the future."

Dr. Selikoff said he was surprised by the high percentage of those with neurological problems. ("In retrospect," he said later, "perhaps we should not have been surprised; because we knew that PBB was lipid soluble, and that the brain tissue and nerve tissue have a high lipid content. It was reasonable to understand that we would find PBB in brain tissue, and that it might have an effect.") Neurological problems, Dr. Selikoff added, were the most general expression of toxicity apparently caused by PBB poisoning. Marked fatigue, a striking decrement in physical and intellectual endeavors were among the most prevalent symptoms. "It wasn't unusual," he said, "for men to need fourteen, sixteen, eighteen hours of sleep per day. This is particularly striking in the population studied since most of the individuals were accustomed to a long working day with an average of six to seven hours of sleep. Men in their thirties sometimes reported that, although they had usually eaten at home, they would take their lunch into the fields so that they could 'sneak' a noon nap and their wives would not know about it and become concerned."

Dr. Selikoff also spoke of young men who suddenly found themselves unable to perform the chores they were used to— "men reporting being unable to comfortably lift one-hundred-to one-hundred-fifty-pound sacks and switching to fifty-pound lots in order to be able to manage their chores. Equipment that previously could be maneuvered in and out of storage by one person now required the aid of an assistant or power equipment," Dr. Selikoff's report said.

Dr. Anderson, his top aide, added, "Memory and judgment deficits were sometimes quite striking. Farmers who had plowed a field in the same way for many years found themselves sitting on a tractor being unable to recall how to begin. Women who had been active in organizations found themselves unable to keep bookkeeping records or meeting minutes adequately,

240

and had to resign from these jobs. In order to remember simple telephone messages or whether jobs had been done or not, some farmers found they needed to carry notebooks."

Dr. Diamond commented, "Many of the people looked neurologically like an aged population but were, in fact, in their thirties."

Another of the striking findings was the prevalence of arthritislike changes, such as joint pains and swellings, and deformities especially among young men in their early thirties. "The knees and ankles seemed to be most often affected," Dr. Selikoff reported. "But the small joints of the fingers and hands were also frequently involved.... It is very unusual to find this arthritislike syndrome as an effect of a toxic substance, and PBBs may be quite unique in this respect."

Many others complained of gastrointestinal problems such as stomach pains and diarrhea; still other complained of a variety of skin problems, including lesions, dryness of the hands, sudden increased sweating, loss of hair, deformities and sharp changes in the growth rate of nails. Some of the children as young as eight and nine years old had a form of acne typically associated with chemical poisoning, according to Dr. Joseph Chanda, chief resident in dermatology at the University of Michigan, who had participated with the Selikoff group in its study. Many patients, Dr. Chanda said, reported more problems than he was able to find. But that seeming discrepancy could be explained by the fact that the questionnaire addressed itself to the problems over a three-and-a-half year period—whereas any objective findings consisted only of those abnormalities that were still present during the examination, at the end of the three-and-a-half-year period, he said.

"It is common knowledge that many dermatological conditions are acute both in their onset and their resolution, and that once they are developed and subsequently resolved, there is no evidence of their persistence other than by historical information provided by the patient," Dr. Chanda explained. (Elaborating later, Dr. Chanda said his Michigan patients consistently reported more symptoms than the Wisconsin control group.) "Probably the most interesting complaint which was related to me during the examination was a complaint of sudden, unexplained increased fingernail or toenail growth," he said. In the Michigan group, sixty-five persons said they had in the past three years begun cutting their nails at a frequency of once or twice a week, whereas normally they cut their nails once a month or once every six weeks. This was particularly interesting, Dr. Chanda said, because one of the symptoms noted in contaminated cattle was abnormal growth of the hooves. (No one in the Wisconsin control group would complain of such abnormal nail growths.)

Out of the 1,029 persons in the Michigan study group, Dr. Chanda found 21 cases of halogen acne, which is associated with chemical exposure and is noted for its sudden occurrence, in unusual places, such as the arms, and involving persons normally not expected to have such acne problems. (Again, Dr. Chanda would see no cases of halogen acne in the Wisconsin group.) Twenty-three in the Michigan group had hair loss that could not be explained by age, medication, stress or illness, Dr. Chanda said. (There would be no such cases of unexplained hair loss in the Wisconsin farm group.)

Dr. Chanda said what he saw were signs of acute human toxicity caused by PBB.

Another University of Michigan physician who took part in Dr. Selikoff's health survey was Dr. Mason Barr, Jr., a pediatrician. He reported he found nothing unusual during the November clinic among children under ten, who made up 17.5 percent of the total 1,029 study group. However, Dr. Barr added, their medical histories revealed an unusual number of symptoms such as nervousness, irritability, headache, muscle pains, frequent colds, joint aches and upset stomachs.

"Personally," he said, "I think there are some PBB effects on the children. So many had such similar symptoms, and it's hard to imagine that muscle and joint pains were caused by the emotional turmoil that disrupted some of the families whose farms were devastated by PBB." He said most of the symptoms apparently had disappeared or abated by the spring of 1976. "We should have looked one or two years ago," Dr. Barr said.

In all, he examined 343 Michigan children under the age of sixteen. Thirty-five percent of them reported multiple adverse health symptoms (compared later to only 2 percent of the children in the Wisconsin study group). Charted by years, Dr. Barr said, the rise in symptoms began in 1973 and rose dramatically in 1974, began to level off in 1975 and finally dropped in the first half of 1976. (Again, this was confirmed after Dr. Barr compared the Michigan and Wisconsin results.)

At first, Dr. Barr was surprised that the Michigan children from quarantined farms were "significantly less likely" to have had multiple health problems than Michigan children from nonquarantined farms. "We had gone in, I guess, presuming that those from quarantined farms would have higher exposure," he recalls.

But Dr. Barr soon realized the possible explanation. "The fact that the farm was quarantined may have served as a warning not to continue eating the meat and drinking the milk. On the other hand, a nonquarantine status could have been taken as assurance that the meat and milk were fit to eat. Thus people on nonquarantined farms continued to eat PBB-containing food and, even though the PBB levels were perhaps below the action level, continued consumption could have resulted in appreciable body burdens of PBB and symptoms of ill health," the tall, bearded physician surmised.

What was the basis for this postulation? While tests showed that PBB levels in fat were similar between the children from quarantined and nonquarantined farms, the blood PBB levels were a great deal higher in children from quarantined farms than in children from nonquarantined farms. "This is an indirect support of my hypothesis—that those from quarantined farms may have suffered an acute high level ingestion, which resulted in high blood levels; whereas those from nonquarantined farms ate less contaminated food over a longer period of time, never achieving a very high blood level but continually storing the stuff in the fat so that those levels built up over a period of time," Dr. Barr said.

"We have come across one or two unusual observations and we don't know what to make of them so far," Dr. Selikoff added at the packed January 3 press conference in Lansing. "So we are continuing, as an offshoot of our November 4 to 10 survey. We are proceeding with some additional studies."

"What are those observations?" a reporter asked.

"Well, we are not prepared to say that there are significant effects on the immunological status of people who have been exposed to PBBs. This is a possibility which was placed before us by our colleagues in the laboratory," he replied.

The human immune system's work is performed largely by living cells that constantly circulate through the blood and lymph vessels—sort of like sentries or security forces patrolling the farthest reaches of the body. The immune system's mastermind is a white blood cell called a lymphocyte. Each person has millions of lymphocytes. It wasn't until the mid-1960s that scientists realized that lymphocytes control the immune defense mechanism, and that there are two basic types of lymphocytes, each controlling different parts of the immune system. One is called the T-lymphocyte, which originates in the thymus; the other the B-lymphocyte, which originates in the bone marrow. The thymus-derived lymphocytes, when normal, combat against bacteria and viruses and are involved in organ transplantation as a rejection process. The B-cells are involved in the formation of antibodies, which fight against infectious organisms.

The red flag concerning PBB's effect on the immune system was raised nearly by accident. Just before the Selikoff team left New York City for Michigan in early November several members of his staff passed Dr. J. George Bekesi, a Mount Sinai immunologist, in the hallway.

"They asked me if I would like to have some blood samples. I asked what this was about. Since Mount Sinai has on any given day about three thousand patients, we were not exactly in short supply of blood samples," recalls Dr. Bekesi. They briefly described the PBB contamination problem to him. But still Dr. Bekesi was not interested. "However," he recalls, "the final word was when the gentlemen made reference to the fact that some of the livestock in Michigan died from wasting disease. That caught my curiosity. This was a clue. People in immunology—either human or animal—know that, whenever you see wasting disease, you usually suspect some problem of an immunological nature."

(Indeed that possibility had been raised as early as March of 1975 by Dr. Paul E. Johnson, the Farm Bureau Services veterinarian, after visiting some thirty quarantined farms. While losses attributable to direct toxicity are minimal, he reported, breeding problems and milk production losses could not be attributed to other causes. "The possible interference effect of PBB on the normal immune response to infection— less than normal resistance to the common variety of diseases— may account in part for many reported losses in young calves and health problems in cows.")

Hearing about wasting disease, Dr. Bekesi agreed to test five human blood samples from the Grand Rapids survey. "We examined five of the farmers for their immunological status, as reflected in B-cell and T-cell changes. The results provided some surprises," Dr. Selikoff added. "In our experience dealing with people suffering from a variety of illnesses at Mount Sinai," Dr. Bekesi continued, "we found these five samples were extraordinarily different from what we see among the normal population." The changes sufficiently alarmed Dr. Selikoff that in the middle of the Northern Michigan winter he dispatched a team headed by Dr. Anderson to Reed City to collect another forty-five blood samples from farm residents.

"We invited forty-five farmers whom we had previously examined, some with symptoms, some without," recalls Dr. Selikoff. "Because of winter driving conditions, participation was limited to dairy farm families living within fifty miles of Reed City, where a field station was established." As a control group, blood samples were taken from New York City residents for comparison.

"Dr. Bekesi soon told us that the New York people were all normal and that there were problems with the Michigan farmers," Dr. Selikoff said. "At that point, we still did not know that this was necessarily PBB. After all, we examined dairy farmers; how did we know that this wasn't something on dairy farms? There are many chemicals used on dairy farms." Next, the Selikoff team went to Marshfield, Wisconsin, in late March.

In the course of examining 235 Wisconsin dairy farm dwellers who served as the control group to the Michigan survey conducted the previous November in Grand Rapids, the Selikoff team drew blood samples from 46 Wisconsin residents specifically for immunological studies. The Wisconsin group was studied precisely in the same manner as was the Michigan group.

"We found that—whatever the reason—Michigan dairy farmers are very different compared with Wisconsin dairy farmers. For example, almost three times as many Michigan farmers complained of fatigue as did Wisconsin farmers. Headaches were almost three times as common," Dr. Selikoff reported later. "Joint symptoms were twice as common. Neurological symptoms—sleep disturbances, memory defects—were almost absent in Wisconsin; in Michigan, they were common. About 20 percent of liver function tests were abnormal in Michigan; only about 5 percent were abnormal in Wisconsin."

245

But the most alarming results came with the comparison of immunological competence between the New York, Wisconsin and Michigan groups.

Blood from eighteen of the forty-five farm Michiganians showed serious deficiencies of immunological function on a variety of standard tests. The abnormalities found resembled the immunological defects that occur in some cancer victims and in patients deliberately treated with drugs to suppress the immunological response. Only one of the forty-six Wisconsin farm residents showed such an immunological deficit, and that person had cancer. All seventy-nine New York City blood samples behaved normally when tested for immunological competence.

The findings suggested the possibility that some persons exposed to PBBs are likely to experience increased susceptibility to infections and perhaps, in the future, cancer.

Dr. Bekesi added that, while the twenty-seven other Michigan samples showed no gross abnormalities, they, too, were not entirely normal. "None of the [Michigan] individuals can you characterize as A-okay," he said. "We truly do not see this among normal or on diseased patients we are studying at Mount Sinai." Dr. Bekesi's findings later were duplicated by Dr. John A. Moore of the National Institute of Environmental Health Sciences in laboratory rats and mice. Dr. Moore found similar immunological (as well as behavioral and neuromuscular) defects in a large portion of several hundred such test animals fed PBB through a stomach tube for four weeks.

Dr. Bekesi said he could not say with any assurance what the long-term health picture might be for the Michigan study group. "But, certainly, I would not like to walk around with this suppressed immunological defense in my body," he said.

At the time of the January 3 press conference, of course, the Wisconsin field survey had not yet been done; too, the full immunological studies had not yet been carried out. All Dr. Selikoff had at the time were his Michigan preliminary findings. But even so, the reaction to his preliminary findings were swift and strong.

The first response came during the press conference itself when Speaker Crim, noting that he wished the Selikoff study had been done "much sooner," said, "I think there's reason enough now for us to begin a look at lowering the [PBB tolerance guideline] levels somewhat."

Dr. Selikoff, asked if he had "any fears about the state food supply," replied, "Nobody wants to eat toxic chemicals." Would he eat bacon and eggs from Michigan each morning? The usually imperturbable, distinguished doctor hesitated, drew a finger across his upper lip, and finally replied, "Well, the answer is yes, I would—because I'm only going to be here a short time."

A nervous laughter rippled through the crowd, but two people who nearly blanched were Governor Milliken and Dr. Reizen.

"Based on what you found," reporter Tom Greene asked Dr. Selikoff, "what would you advise the people of the state?"

Again, Dr. Selikoff paused dramatically. "Based on what I have found," he said slowly, "I would urge the people of the state to prod Governor Milliken as much as you can to get the levels of PBB in food to as low a level as he possibly can."

There it was. A flat, unequivocal exhortation to severely drop the PBB standards, and coming from one of the country's top environmental scientists and the only one who had studied the human health effects of PBB. Coupled with the Bernstein panel's unanimous recommendation from May, the stage was set for the legislature to, for the first time, take the lead in dealing with the unending debacle.

Milliken, who had appointed the Bernstein panel and who had appointed members of the Agriculture Commission, which rejected the Bernstein panel's advice, found himself on the defensive.

"But," he told the press conference, "I don't know that, looking back on this whole unfolding of events from the time the PBB first found its way into the state's environment, that you could say the state would have or could have done many things differently.... It's the nature of the complex problem that we're dealing with. There are no simple yes and no, black-and-white answers to this question. And I suspect that as we look ahead into the future, five or ten years from now, we're going to still be living with this problem or related problems.

"I would say," Milliken concluded, "that there will be no final definitive answer, probably, in our lifetime to the problem of chemicals. We just have to deal with them and cope with them as we go along."

The governor said he wanted his Health Department's "experts" to conduct "an immediate internal review" of Dr.

247

Selikoff's report "with the thought that it may then serve as a guide for any further actions that those of us in the public arena may be called upon to undertake."

Even at this point Milliken would not take a leadership position to reduce the PBB standards and get the chemical once and for all out of the human food supply of 9 million people.

But no matter. Powerful forces had been unleashed finally that soon would bring about the recommended changes without needing the support of the governor and his administration.

The powerful United Auto Workers called for the resignation of B. Dale Ball as agriculture director, a demand also supported by the Detroit *News*. The PBB Action Committee launched a signature-gathering campaign to recall Milliken. Once more, signs all over Michigan were seen in supermarkets and restaurants saying, Free of PBB—Buy Iowa Beef Here, and No PBB—Shipped Directly from the Old West.

But most significant of all was the introduction in the house of a bill to reduce the PBB standards. Its sponsor was a young wiry Democratic representative from a heavily Republican district who was known for his integrity and sincerity. His name was Francis R. Spaniola, the shy young man who, as a member of the Albosta hearings in March of 1976, had vowed to do the best he could to help resolve the PBB controversy. He had introduced the bill in 1976, but it got nowhere because there was little popular support for the reduction of PBB levels at the time. But there was no doubt now that the bill would be enacted, and perhaps finally put an end to Michigan's PBB nightmare.

# 13
# THE ENDURING LEGACY

The Spaniola bill was introduced in February. Its chief feature was a reduction of the federal PBB tolerance level from 300 parts per billion to 20 parts per billion. All the animals above 20 parts per billion would be slaughtered and buried by the state, and their owners would be reimbursed for their losses. The reimbursement policy is precisely what B. Dale Ball, the agriculture director, had recommended immediately after the contamination was discovered, an idea rejected by both Governor Milliken and the legislature.

Now, three years later, the governor and most lawmakers were in favor of the bill. Even more surprisingly, the Agriculture Commission did not openly oppose the bill. In fact, the commission said it supported the proposal. The reason soon became evident.

The Spaniola bill, as with previous PBB proposals, was expected to land in the House Agriculture Committee, which was not known to be predisposed to the measure. But House Speaker Crim referred the bill, instead, to the Public Health Committee. Chaired by a young liberal from Detroit, Representative Raymond W. Hood, the panel was known to favor the adoption of more severe PBB standards. Instantly, the Agriculture Commission withdrew its support of the Spaniola bill. The commission finally readopted its posture of token support after each member received an angry letter from Governor Milliken, who had appointed them to their seats.

Subsequent hearings on the bill in both the House and the Senate followed the predictable patterns set in earlier public forums. But there were two surprises.

One was testimony of Dr. Maurice S. Reizen, Michigan's public health director. Finally he admitted, "I am convinced there are some adverse health effects in humans from these farm families and others who consumed the higher levels of PBB in 1973 and 1974. This did not come to me as a blinding revelation from above, but stems from bits and pieces of information accumulated over these many months." Then Dr. Reizen, a man with sharp features, threw his lukewarm support behind the Spaniola bill. "If one couples the question of potential adverse health effects stemming from the current 300 parts per billion FDA level with that of restoring public confidence in the food products they consume, then I believe there is ample justification for lowering the limit," he said, adding, however, that "I feel the public health would be protected at 50 parts per billion."

The other surprise witness was none other than the governor. He told one standing-room-only audience packed with farm families at a Public Health Committee hearing that passage of the Spaniola bill "will be a major step toward restoring consumer confidence in Michigan-produced meat and dairy products." It was only the second time in Milliken's nine years as the state's chief executive that he has personally testified on behalf of a particular bill; the other occasion involved a budget bill.

At the same hearing, Gregory dairyman Ron Thomas also testified, talking about his family's health problems, especially that of his four-year-old son, who has an enlarged liver. "I don't know what's going to happen to him. But if anything does, there's going to be all kinds of hell to pay in this state," Thomas said. Then he wept.

Touched by such suffering and angered by the way state agencies had mishandled the contamination problem from the very beginning, the Hood committee surprised everyone by amending the Spaniola bill, adopting an absolute zero as the PBB guideline. Such an amendment, however, had no chance of legislative approval. It would have created total chaos if it became law. The panel rescinded the amendment only after Spaniola pleaded and pleaded with its members. By this time most major industry organizations in the state had gotten in line behind the Spaniola bill, including the Michigan Cattlemen's Association, the Michigan Milk Producers Association and the Michigan Livestock Exchange.

The Spaniola bill ultimately was approved by the legislature without great difficulty, surviving several sabotage attempts, including one by Representative Paul Porter, chairman

250

of the House Agriculture Committee. While the Spaniola bill was being debated in the Public Health Committee, Porter rammed through his committee a bill that would have retained the existing PBB standard but allowed any farmers with contaminated animals, no matter what the level, to have their animals destroyed and paid for by the state. The Porter bill did not take into consideration human health. And it never got to the House floor.

Interestingly, although the Michigan Agriculture Department has said the bill would cost the state as much as $41 million, the eventual Spaniola bill contained only $27.6 million. Why the discrepancy? "I don't believe what they are telling me," said one member of the House Appropriations Committee.

"Does the MDA [Michigan Department of Agriculture] suffer from a credibility gap?" asked *Michigan Farmer* magazine. "You bet it does. Statements from the MDA are being routinely discounted by legislators, the news media, consumers groups and even farmers. The intriguing question is how MDA acquired its credibility gap. MDA is a nonpolitical agency, staffed by reputable scientists and public servants, with a previous reputation for demanding superior standards in the state's food supply."

That credibility gap became a canyon in 1977. In February, the agency released a report claiming that only 2 out of 409 samples of food products tested in the previous six months contained even a trace of PBB. And these two samples, it said, were well within the federal standards. What the department did not report, however, were the results of two other surveillance programs conducted during the same period.

These programs found that 75 our of 734 food samples had PBB, two of which were above the federal standards. Both meat samples ended up being sold because of the delay in getting the test results from the laboratories.

Confronted with the deception, Dr. Donald R. Isleib, the chief deputy agriculture director, asserted, "We do hundreds and hundreds of regulatory tests, and that information was not considered appropriate for release in that news release."

The Spaniola bill was signed into law by Milliken on August 2, 1977. "I believe that the procedure and the safeguards built into this law will assure consumers that Michigan has 'gone the extra mile' in attempting to prevent exposure to PBB," the governor said.

251

The law requires that every dairy animal be tested before it is sent to the slaughterhouse. If tests reveal PBB in excess of 20 parts per billion, the animal will be destroyed and the farmer will be reimbursed for the fair market value of the animal. Exempt were dairy animals born after January 1, 1976, because they were born well after the major contamination was over, and thus presumed to be PBB-free. The law further requires that every dairy farm's bulk milk tank be tested. If that milk exceeds 5 parts per billion, the milk will be quarantined; and each individual cow's milk then will be tested to isolate the sources of the PBB contamination.

For the state's nine thousand dairy farmers, Public Act 77 meant a severe disruption of their normal marketing routines. And as Dick Lehnert, editor of *Michigan Farmer*, pointed out, "Farmers will not make a nickel on this law. Rather, they will have new headaches. The law makes the marketing of cull animals subject to a whole series of actions the farmer is responsible, under penalty of law, to instigate every time he wants to sell one. Further, his premises will be routinely invaded by new hosts of inspectors probing his cattle and his milk tank. For his trouble, he will get a ten-dollar bill [later raised to thirty dollars] for holding and maintaining cattle during the testing period." But for the bureaucrats, Lehnert noted bitterly, "the new PBB law means jobs and wages." He added:

"The major problem with PBB is that it is costing millions of dollars to verify, document, elaborate on, legislate against, etc., effects that were clearly visible and had their greatest effects on farm people and their livelihoods. And the millions are not going to the farmers, but to scientists and bureaucrats who have been mostly obstructionists and now are the beneficiaries."

As he signed Public Act 77, Governor Milliken commented, "This law represents a major step in restoring consumer confidence in Michigan's agriculture business," adding that the measure now also should help "secure reentry for Michigan beef into the Canadian market."

In early 1977, Canada, appalled by Michigan's handling of the PBB disaster, imposed a rigid testing program that amounted to an embargo on Michigan meat products.

Shortly after Dr. Selikoff's preliminary report, delivered in Lansing on January 3, a Canadian Broadcasting Company crew from Toronto came to Michigan to film a one-hour documentary about the PBB disaster. "Overnight, the Canadian film had a measurable impact on Michigan," recalls Edie Clark, whose statements to that network state agriculture officials blamed for Ottawa's action. "The Canadian government imposed a testing requirement on all shipments of Michigan beef entering their country. No cattle with any detectable levels of PBB were permitted to cross the border," she said. "Canadian slaughterhouse managers were understandably unwilling to house and maintain shipments of Michigan beef on their premises while fat biopsies on the animals were collected and analyzed—a process involving upwards of two weeks. For all practical purposes, the border was closed to shipments of Michigan beef." And it remained closed despite the new Michigan testing program that took effect on October 3. Canada was Michigan's largest single out-of-state beef market. Milliken appealed to the heads of the Food and Drug Administration, the U.S. Department of Agriculture and even the State Department for help. But Ottawa remained adamant. It did not want its citizens to be exposed to any PBB whatsoever. And soon, results of Michigan's testing program reinforced the Canadians' conviction.

Many Michigan farmers, such as Rick Halbert, whose herds were wiped out in the original round of PBB contamination, had begun anew with new animals—purchased from out of state. But prior to restocking, most of them went through elaborate cleanup procedures to get rid of PBB residues from the farm environment. But even those who, like Halbert, had spent tens of thousands of dollars to clean up found that nothing seemed to get rid of the chemical. It was everywhere. It clung to barn wood. It clung to the feed troughs. It clung to the silos. It was in the soil. And the new cows were picking up PBB from all these sources. The chemical even penetrated three inches of cement.

The state's new testing program also revealed the inadequacies of earlier programs. Almost right off the bat five farms, which never used any Farm Bureau Services feed, were found to have highly contaminated animals. The five farms were from diverse regions of the state, and agriculture officials had no idea how their animals had become contaminated. "Some of this we just can't explain. I'll have to admit that," said Dr. Duaine Deming, an agriculture veterinarian.

One dairyman from Lake Linden in the Upper Peninsula, for instance, grows all his own feed and buys his additives from a feed store in Dollar Bay. The feed store got all its products from Minnesota. Two other farmers said they had bought their feed from Farm Bureau Services' principal feed competitor in Michigan.

The new testing program also showed that a greater percentage of animals tested at Michigan slaughterhouses had detectable PBB levels than in 1976. About 2 percent of the animals tested were found to have PBB exceeding the new 20 parts per billion level, requiring their destruction.

"We've got the whole business of soil contamination," remarked Dr. Reizen, the state health director. No one knew how long it might take for PBB residues to disappear from the environment. "The overriding question is whether many Michigan farms will ever be able to support PBB-free animals again," said one grim agriculture official.

Among the farms quarantined as a result of the new testing program was Rick Halbert's. Ironically, two cows exceeding the PBB standards were found on the farm of Elton Smith, president of Farm Bureau Services. Like the others, Smith, a Caledonia farmer, was reimbursed for his above-tolerance-level contaminated cows. He received $705.65.

The evidence of PBB's persistence in the Michigan environment resulted in new legislation in July of 1978 which expanded the testing program to allow the Agriculture Department to test all bovine animals, sheep, swine, goats, chickens, turkeys, geese and ducks on any suspected farm.

Although Public Act 77 had exempted dairy animals born after January 1, 1976, it had become apparent that some of these young animals also were being contaminated, especially on farms, such as Halbert's, that were the most heavily contaminated. Halbert's calves, for instance, aren't even tested; the state simply comes to pick them up, pays him for them and then destroys them. "We tested about forty at first," said Van Patten, "and all but two or three were violative. So it's just cheaper to buy them than test them. It's a residue problem now—just like pesticides. It'll be around for a long time." Adds Dr. Reizen: "It's down to a dilution process. Just like DDT, it will dilute itself out."

Yet nearly half the offspring of cows that exceeded the first federal guideline (1,000 parts per billion) now were in violation of the new state standard.

In all, "violative" cows were found on more than five hundred farms.

"They [the state officials] drew up a list of procedures which one was to follow and, presumably doing that, one would take the necessary precautions to prevent recontamination of the animals entering the farm. But bear in mind once a persistent chemical is released from the environment, you cannot pluck away every molecule that has been released," said Rick Halbert. "You cannot do that."

Eventually, Canada became convinced that Michigan now was sincerely trying to keep PBB off the market, and lifted its embargo in the spring of 1978.

In a normal year, Michigan exports more than $30 million worth of beef products to Canada. The full economic toll taken by the PBB contamination may be virtually impossible to estimate. For instance, even with the slaughter and burial of tens of thousands of contaminated dairy cows, Michigan breeders did not report extra business; indeed their business suffered because owners of destroyed herds as well as other potential buyers purchased animals from other states.

The contamination, of course, ended up affecting every type of animal farm in the state. Between one-fifth and one-sixth of Michigan's poultry flocks were destroyed because of PBB. Figuring conservatively at $2 a bird and rounding off the number of chickens destroyed at 1.2 million, that means $2.4 million were lost in adult laying hens—plus more than $10 million lost in 1974 alone in egg production. And these dollar estimates do not include contaminated feed that had to be destroyed or the cost of cleaning up premises.

"Concerning the hog marketing situation," one industry official said in March of 1977, shortly after the Canadian embargo began, "presently one of Michigan's largest pork packers is not purchasing Michigan hogs because of refusals by a major chain to purchase the product. This is costing the pork producers $5,000 per marketing day."

William Byrum, executive vice-president of the Michigan Cattlemen's Association, estimates that the eventual loss of cattle and hog sales due to PBB disaster would total "tens of millions of dollars." Larry Martin, president of the Michigan Meat Provisioners Association, said among the hardest hit were processors and wholesalers. For instance, Dahl DeBoer, a wholesaler in St. Johns, normally slaughters a hundred head of cattle a week. But in early 1977 he was down to seventy animals a week, and his sale of boneless beef for ground meat was off about 50 percent. In Owosso, William Mallory, owner of the West Side Market, reduced his purchases from DeBoer after he, Mallory, lost a $20,000 ground beef account with the Memorial Hospital in Owosso because he refused to sign an affidavit stating he used only out-of-state beef.

The Michigan Dairy Foods Association figures it lost 13 million pounds in sales of dairy products just in 1976. "We might have expected a two- to three-million pound drop," said one official.

The economic impact, then, rippled through Michigan's farm community, since rural towns are so heavily dependent upon agriculture as a source of revenue for local business.

Not yet taken into account is the cost of public administration over the years, or the farmland that may have to be taken out of production, or the years of business progress lost. "Losses in Michigan will exceed $1 billion before this is over," predicts Senator Riegle. "And we still don't know what the full social implications will be in terms of health effects."

And such consequences may have impact well beyond Michigan. At the National Institute of Environmental Health Sciences, for instance, Dr. David P. Rall, the director, has had to reprogram hundreds of thousands of dollars for PBB research. "We took it from other projects," he said. "We took it from Peter to pay Paul. We'll make it stretch. It may be difficult at times. I think that certainly we won't be able to move as fast as we would like. But, also importantly, it limits our ability to respond to a new PBB problem from another source. If something comes up next year, it will be much more difficult for us to try to respond to that issue, because we have used funds for the ongoing investigation in the PBB problem."

About the same time Canada lifted its embargo, the Michigan Department of Agriculture launched a $250,000 promotional campaign to restore public confidence in Michigan food products. The department's international marketing division had received concerned inquiries from all over Europe, Asia and the Middle East about the effects of PBB on Michigan fruits, vegetables, grains, as well as meats and dairy products. Margaret McCall, an Agriculture Department information specialist, said Michigan apparently had developed a "wasteland image" all over the world.

Among the few Michigan farmers who came out ahead are brothers Mick and Dick Kokx, two taciturn young Newaygo County farmers. They were the low bidders when the state was searching for a farm to hold all the contaminated animals being identified in the new PBB testing program. Such a holding site became necessary primarily because, as in the case with the Kalkaska burial site earlier, the second pit was running into legal challenges from local residents. As a result, what had been seen as a short-term holding plan became an indefinite and lucrative baby-sitting operation for the Kokx brothers. And the state was under contract to pay them $2 each day per animal. Eventually, they made about $500,000.

The second burial site turned out to be 2.2 acres in a corner of the Au Sable State Forest, about nine miles north of Mio in Oscoda County and fifty miles east of Kalkaska. After the predictable and protracted legal challenges by local residents, the issue finally was settled by the state supreme court and the Mio pit went into operation in early August of 1978.

Effigies of Milliken, Ball and Dr. Howard Tanner, director of the Department of Natural Resources, were hanged. Even a personal visit from the governor failed to quell the boisterous protesters. Standing in a blue parka in the steady rain, Milliken tried to tell about a hundred of them that the pit, lined with twenty feet of clay, presented no danger to their wells or other drinking water sources. "You're either a fool or a very good liar," someone shouted. "I understand your concerns," Milliken said. "But I honestly believe the precautions that have been taken fully protect the health and welfare of the people. We've got to find a place to bury the PBB, and this has been proven the safest way to do it." As he left, an angry woman jabbed her umbrella at the window of Milliken's car. The protesters even sent a telegram to the Kremlin appealing to chairman Leonid Brezhnev for help.

Instead of meek acquiescence from nonpolitical Amish and Mennonite families, state officials encountered outrage and determined opposition in Oscoda County, population 6,300. The county, one of Michigan's poorest and least populated, draws its livelihood and joy from its timber-rich woods and the celebrated Au Sable River, one of the country's finest brown trout streams.

"This is God's country," said Connie Dallas, owner of the Au Sable-Manistee Realty Company. "People come up here for the clean air and water; you know, when they leave they fill up jugs of our well water to take home with them. Now they want to put the poison in our ground. They want to take it all away from us."

Such fears, however, were displayed not only by local residents. Even tourists passing through Oscoda County avoided the drinking water. When his waitresses told him customers were leaving their water glasses untouched, Paul Pasternak, owner of a hotel and restaurant, was incredulous. "At first I didn't believe it. But then I started checking myself. And they were right." Few people disturbed their glasses. "PBB has put Mio on the map," said Nelson Yoder, a member of the Oscoda County PBB Action Committee. "But for the wrong reasons."

By 1978, public concern had become widespread over the potential dangers of burying animals ravaged by PBB. The findings by Dr. Selikoff and other independent research scientists had awakened most of the state's 9 million people to the risks associated with PBB exposure. Soon that public anxiety rose another notch with a stream of disclosures that hundreds of thousands of tons of PBB wastes and contaminated feeds and food products had been buried almost haphazardly in landfills across the state, some without the knowledge of state environmental officials.

Michigan Chemical had buried 269,000 pounds of PBB wastes in a twenty-acre landfill in Gratiot County from 1971 to mid-1973. The landfill, owned by the county, was operated by a private contractor. The chemical company later switched to a landfill in New York, sending 251,000 pounds of PBB wastes to Chemtrol Pollution Services near Lewiston, New York. At both of these landfills, the U.S. Environmental Protection Agency later discoverd leaching. The burial of wastes at the Gratiot landfill was not known by Michigan officials until January of 1977, when Michigan Chemical, after a prolonged delay, revealed the information to the U.S. Environmental Protection Agency, which then relayed the information to Lansing. Subsequent tests by the Department of Natural Resources found ground water near the site but in areas within the landfill had become contaminated.

Besides the Gratiot landfill, seven others scattered around Michigan were used to dump contaminated feed and food products. And because the existence of some of these landfills was not known for years, monitoring for leaching was not begun until much later. Not surprisingly, PBB also began showing up in the state's wildlife—once officials thought to check. Rabbits, coyotes, ravens, gulls, starlings, Norwegian rats, pheasants, raccoons, bear, deer—they all had PBB.

"The state had not been sufficiently careful where materials like PBB and others like it have been buried," admitted Dr. Tanner who was not director of the Department of Natural Resources in 1973 and 1974. But one who was with the department then, William Turney, director of the department's environmental health division, explained, "The scenario is this: Back in 1974 and 1975, the state Agriculture Department and Farm Bureau had a serious problem after they discovered there was PBB-contaminated feed. They started checking grain elevators and found some incidental concentrations of PBB, and came to our agency and asked how to get rid of it. We gave them the names of five landfills where grain could be safely disposed of. We did it with the full knowledge of the landfill operators and, in most cases, the local health department supervised it." The only problem was that more than just those landfills approved by the Department of Natural Resources were used, as the department found out later. The agency did not learn until October of 1978 that at least two other landfills— in Washtenaw County near Ann Arbor and in Lenawee County in southern Michigan near the Indiana border—were used to bury PBB contaminated wastes. "It was an honest oversight," Dr. Tanner said. His department did not learn of the existence of the two landfills until it came across two Agriculture Department memos alluding to them after new public concern arose during Governor Milliken's reelection bid in the fall. One of the landfills, the one in Lenawee County, had been specifically prohibited by the Department of Natural Resources from accepting any PBB-contaminated feed because it was too close to the Raisin River. After its existence was known, testing at the Lenawee site found PBB in the Raisin River—a source of water supply for several communities in that region. The landfill was lined with clay, but the leak developed because rainwater collected inside the clay-lined areas until the water welled up over the top, carrying the contaminated liquids into the river.

The "oversight" leading to burial of contaminated feed in the landfill occurred as a result of lack of interagency communication. The Department of Natural Resources on June 20, 1974, sent a letter to the owner of the landfill, telling him no

PBB feed could be buried there. But the letter arrived after the Agriculture Department authorized the landfill to accept some thirty tons of contaminated feed. Agriculture officials said later they released the feed for burial there after the landfill owner had told them he obtained authorization from the Department of Natural Resources. The Agriculture Department never bothered to check with the Department of Natural Resources.

In all, several hundred pounds of contaminated feed and food products were buried in eight landfills around the state. In addition, another 4,525 gallons of chemical waste containing an unknown amount of hexabromobiphenyl, the major ingredient of Firemaster, were buried in Kawhawlin, near the Saginaw Bay north of Bay City in Michigan's Thumb region from 1971 to 1974.

But even as the existence of such landfills were still being discovered, the state's PBB animal testing program began to phase out. After costing $16 million in the first year, the state legislature on April 15, 1978, adopted a resolution exempting the entire Upper Peninsula from further testing because few contaminated animals were being identified, except on a small number of farms. Soon entire counties also were being exempted. By fall, more than four thousand farms were exempted from any testing.

The exemptions were based on an elaborate set of criteria. They were granted if at least 15 percent of the cows in a herd were tested and found to have no PBB. Farms also were exempted if their animals had PBB, but only at 5 to 10 parts per billion (that is, below the state standard of 20), and did not constitute more than 25 percent of all animals tested. Even a herd with a single violative animal, up to 40 parts per billion, might be exempted when a "representative" sample of the herd was tested and those results were nondetectable. A "representative sample" was defined as "the square root of the herd size but never more than eighteen or less than six animals."

The testing program, in requiring fat biopsies of every cow before marketing, meant that veterinarians all over the state had to learn the procedure, as Alpha Clark did earlier. Some, however, apparently did not learn very well because several dozen cows across Michigan died shortly after such biopsies, prompting new lawsuits. The deaths resulted from infections at the site of the incision, which traveled to the cow's stomach, inflaming the lining. "A lot of farmers are complaining because

260

they didn't want the biopsies in the first place," said Dr. Deming, the state veterinarian. "We try to pacify them and tell them it's the law. This is a consumer protection law. But it imposes quite a burden on the farmer. It wasn't designed to aid the farmer. We've interrupted the normal marketing of their culled cows."

Besides the reduction in PBB standards and a statewide testing program, Dr. Selikoff's January 1977 report also had an impact in Washington, including a set of U.S. Senate hearings that ultimately resulted in a law to create a team of scientific experts with the capability to respond quickly when another PBB-like contamination occurs in the future.

The Senate hearing was the effort of Donald W. Riegle, Jr., a Michigan congressman who had been elected in the fall of 1976 to the seat of the late Philip A. Hart. Riegle requested and obtained permission to hold such hearings almost the minute he was appointed to the subcommittee on science, technology and space, on which Michigan's other senator, Robert P. Griffen, also sat. Riegle wanted to examine particularly the role of the federal agencies in the handling of the PBB disaster. "This is something that's going to happen over and over again. That's why the senator thought it was important to hold the hearing," recalls Dan Jaffe, a subcommittee staff member.

Four successive days of hearings were held at the end of March in different parts of the state, and later two more days of hearings took place in Washington in late April and early May. "It was extraordinary, unconscionable, how long it took to get things together in Michigan," commented Mike Brownlee, another key member of the subcommittee and one who had played a major role in the five-year struggle that led to the passage of the landmark 1976 Toxic Substances Control Act. Brownlee had been particularly struck while in Michigan as he was interviewing farm families in an anteroom while the hearings were going on. "Some came up in crutches, others shaking. They were in very bad shape. Yet there was very little we could do—we couldn't even tell them where to go for help. No place. It was frustrating."

Riegle, long after the hearings were over, told a joint session of the Michigan legislature, "It is clear that all agencies of government failed to respond adequately in the early stages of this problem and, as a result, public confidence in federal and state agencies has been severely damaged." The senator even proposed the creation of an independent administrative body "completely separated and apart from any existing state government agency that has previously been involved with the PBB issue and which can monitor the activities of the various state agencies actually charged with carrying out the work." Riegle's and Brownlee's assessments of the performance of public agencies echoed those made by *Michigan Farmer* magazine several years earlier: that the agencies have "creaked and groaned slowly along in their attempts to help the stricken farmers, slowed by legislative restrictions, shortages of funds and manpower, and bureaucratic red tape."

On top of the Selikoff report and the Riegle hearings, yet another measure of vindication came in the spring of 1977 when a small group of Michigan farmers were invited to the White House to attend a meeting to which a number of federal officials had been summoned to account for their agencies' actions.

In the fall of 1976, Chip Carter, campaigning in Michigan for his father, had met several of the PBB-affected farmers. And one of them, Theron Carter of Grand Rapids, began calling Chip Carter at the White House incessantly after Jimmy Carter was inaugurated. "Chip had only one woman handling all his calls; so she called me and gave me Theron Carter's name and number," recalls Jane Wales, associate director of the office of public liaison. "So I called him back and after he told me the story, I immediately wanted to get more background information. I knew nothing about PBB; this was in February or March."

Wales soon called Lester O. Brown, the mustachioed investigator who was looking into the PBB disaster in preparation for hearings to be held by Congressman John Moss's subcommittee on investigations and oversight. "I was in Cincinnati for a hearing when I got this message to call the White House immediately," recalls Brown, chuckling. "I thought, 'What the—?' It was Jane Wales. She wanted me at the White House the next morning for a briefing. So I went."

After the briefing, Wales drafted a memorandum for her boss, Midge Costanza. "It was clear that public officials were sitting on their hands," Wales told Costanza, adding that White House intervention was in order. "The thought was for Midge to go to Michigan," Wales said. "I knew if she saw the cattle, she'd never let go of this issue." But senior staff members

262

opposed the idea, saying it would not be good form for a Democratic White House to swoop into Michigan to publicize a problem that was plaguing the administration of a Republican governor who was the subject of a recall attempt (which later fell far short of the mark). And so a White House meeting was decided upon.

"I was flabbergasted when they called," recalls Pat Miller, a diminutive but energetic Lake County woman who had begun taking an active leadership role in the PBB Action Committee. The White House meeting was set for May 10. It was a beautiful time of the year to be in Washington, The Michigan delegation consisted of Miller, Garry Zuiderveen, Theron and Pam Carter, and Dave Curtis and his wife. Doc Clark had been invited; Wales wanted very much to meet him. But he declined. "I wanted them to hear directly from the farmers, the people who were affected," Dr. Clark said. He did, however, sell a calf to finance Miller's trip. Among a room full of government officials at the meeting, held in the Roosevelt Room, were Lester Brown and Dr. Kolbye of the Food and Drug Administration.

Miller spoke of the financial needs of the farmers, the need for more research money, more medical assistance for the contaminated people and a lowering of the PBB guidelines. The meeting was chaired by Wales, although Costanza was also present during much of the discussion. She chewed out several of the officials around the table, especially representatives of the FDA. "A number of matters were brought up and then we passed on everything to Mike McGinnis [of the Department of Health, Education and Welfare]. That's the role of the office of public liaison," Wales said. "Our job was to get people with problems together with people who supposedly could solve the problems. And so our role—the White House role—ended very quickly."

When the two-hour meeting ended, Costanza took the Michigan farmers down the hall into the Oval Office. The President was in London attending a NATO ministerial meeting. Costanza then led the group into the Cabinet Room, took them through the Rose Garden and peeked into the President's private study before ushering them out on to Pennsylvania Avenue. From Washington, Miller sent Edie Clark a postcard of the White House and wrote, "There is hope!"

"When they left that meeting, they thought things'd change overnight. But nothing happened, at least not right

263

away. Eventually, the federal government doubled its allocation for PBB research," said Edie Clark.

Another outcome of the White House meeting was that Lansing officials, particularly at the Michigan Department of Public Health, began taking more seriously Pat Miller and members of the PBB Action Committee. Shortly afterward, they conferred in Big Rapids with committee members to explain the department's plans for providing medical attention to PBB-poisoned farm families. One such effort was a pilot program to enroll people into major medical centers for exhaustive studies "to see if we can find some common denominator among the individuals," the state health officials said. The program would start with six people.

Miller and the other committee members were mildly pleased. It was better than nothing, and seemed to signify a change of bureaucratic attitude. "So now the Health Department finally realized it had to deal with us, too," said Miller. "But what can they do? They made a mistake and now won't admit it."

The hearings by the House subcommittee on investigations and oversight were held in Washington in early August. It, too, focused on the role of the federal agencies, and particularly the Food and Drug Administration, in the PBB disaster. It was during this two-day hearing that Mt. Sinai's Dr. Bekesi reported his immunological findings on the Michigan farm residents. Also revealed at the hearings, as a result of Lester Brown's digging, was the FDA's disregard of its own information that nearly 40 percent of farm residents its inspectors visited had suffered serious medical problems. Such disclosures prompted one member of the subcommittee, Congressman Thomas A. Luken, an Ohio Democrat, to remark, "Since I have been a member of this subcommittee, I cannot remember receiving testimony which more clearly illustrated the government's failure to prevent injury and assist the sick and needy. Federal action has been too slow, uncoordinated and ineffective."

On August 2—ironically, the day Dr. Bekesi's findings were made known in Washington—Governor Milliken in Lansing signed into law the Spaniola bill to begin the massive testing program of all dairy cows in the state. The Bekesi findings also touched off new public concern—and demands that, once and for all, medical studies be done to find out the effect of PBB on the state's general population of 9 million. The anxiety elevated even further in late October when still more disturbing information about PBB emerged. By this time, not only did Dr. Selikoff have updated results from his November 1976 survey but also many scientists who had begun animal research with PBB now were ready to give their reports. The forum, sponsored by Michigan State University, was a "Workshop on Scientific Aspects of PBB," held at the university's Kellogg Center.

Out of his original study group of 1,029 persons, Dr. Selikoff said, a subgroup of 102 nonfarm residents turned out to have just as many health problems as those who lived on farms. And many of these nonfarm dwellers weren't even aware their health had deteriorated. "This brings the level of concern one step closer to Michigan's general population," Dr. Selikoff said, because the 102 nonfarm familes were different from the general population only because they bought their foods directly from farms, some of which later were quarantined but some of which were not. So, many such farms also supplied the state's supermarkets as well.

Breaking down the group of 102 nonfarm residents further, Dr. Selikoff found that food purchased by thirty-five out of the group had come from farms that were not quarantined. And, surprisingly, the prevalence of illnesses among these thirty-five were greater than the other sixty-seven persons in the group who had eaten foods purchased from quarantined farms.

This seemingly curious finding, however, supported the earlier postulation of Dr. Mason Barr and several farmers themselves. Their theory held that families whose farms were quarantined and their direct customers took the quarantine as sufficient warning to stop consuming the farm's produce; and so while they may have had an intense exposure to PBB, it lasted only for a short time. On the other hand, the theory goes, families whose farms were contaminated but never quarantined and their direct customers took the nonquarantine status as official government certification that such farm produce was safe to consume; and so these people ended up getting more PBB in the long run. Is the human body more efficient at absorbing low concentrations of PBB over a long period of time than at absorbing massive doses in a brief span? "It's a cumulative affair," said Dr. Selikoff. "The intensity and the duration can subtly intermingle." That certainly did not bode well for the state's general population, since only about five hundred dairy farms (out of nearly nine thousand) were ever quarantined, even though many, many more were contaminated but never quarantined.

Among Dr. Selikoff's other findings included abnormal elevations of liver enzymes, which are associated with liver damage; abnormally high levels of carcinoembryonic antigens, a general indicator that the body may not be well; widespread skin, neurological and joint problems. In all, the variety of health problems among Michigan residents were "significantly" more prevalent than in a comparison group of Wisconsin residents. Both groups had been remarkably similar in the absence of such health problems until 1973, the year PBB entered Michigan's food supply. Then, starting in 1974, Dr. Selikoff said, adverse health symptoms among the Michigan group began climbing sharply while the Wisconsin group remained the same.

At the Michigan State University conference, Dr. Selikoff was the only scientist among dozens who had human health data to report. All the others were laboratory research scientists. But they also had interesting—and often contradictory—results to share. And their conclusions generally were easy to predict. With few exceptions, independent and federal scientists found problems with PBB. On the other hand, some who could find nothing or very little wrong with PBB either had financial ties to Farm Bureau Services or to Michigan Chemical, or both; or else were affiliated with Michigan State University, which had come under the suspicion of some farmers.

Dr. Renate D. Kimbrough, the U.S. Center for Disease Control toxicologist who first implicated PCB with cancer, found tumors in livers of rats given a single dose of PBB. She said these tumors almost certainly would have become malignant had the animal not been sacrificed prematurely to get a quick reading on PBB.

Dr. James R. Allen, a well-known University of Wisconsin pathologist, fed seven pregnant monkeys a diet containing PBB at the same level—.03 part per million (or 300 parts per billion)—that the Food and Drug Administration said (and still says) is safe for people. Five monkeys gave birth to offspring that showed growth retardation. A sixth monkey aborted a mummified fetus. The seventh gave birth to a stillborn.

266

"This suggests that even at extremely low levels, there are subtle effects on reproductive changes and fetal development," Dr. Allen said, adding prophetically, "One may not observe these changes in an average human population in that they would not be looked at. A mother may have a small baby but not concerned about it. What I'm saying is that we'd better start looking for these effects because they occur in nonhuman primates"—the animal closest to man.

All seven of the mothers themselves had suffered weight loss, and four had prolonged menstrual cycles, indicating possible abnormalities in the hormones. Past research has shown that such nonhuman primates respond to chemicals like PBB in a manner very similar to man. Interestingly, too, Dr. Allen said, the five offspring with growth retardation had been breast-fed only. Other researchers, at the National Institute of Environmental Health Sciences, said rat experiments showed that the transfer of PBB through breast-feeding "appears much more important to the appearance of PBBs in newborns than does placental transfer [before birth]."

Dr. Corbett and a colleague, Dr. Allan R. Beaudoin, of the University of Michigan's department of anatomy, reported on their work showing that a single high dose of PBB is lethal to a rat embryo and sufficient to produce birth defects as well.

Dr. Allen's growth retardation findings were confirmed by scientists at the U.S. Department of Agriculture's agricultural research service of the animal physiology and genetics institute. Among the researchers was Dr. Joel Bitman, who has a laboratory next to Dr. George Fries and who had become interested in PBB research in the early 1970s. They found that young rats who nursed mothers exposed to PBB "do not grow as well." They also found PBB induces liver injury to delay reproductive maturity and interferes with fat metabolism.

Dr. John A. Moore, associate director of the National Institute of Environmental Health Sciences, and his colleagues confirmed in rats and mice PBB's damage to the immune system that Dr. Bekesi of Mt. Sinai had found in humans. Other scientists at the federal research institute, Drs. H. A. Tilson and P. A. Cabe, found PBB significantly decreased the motor activity of rats, including grip strength. They said their studies indicate that "oral administration of PBBs results in signs of skeleto-neuromuscular dysfunctions, a finding similar to that reported for humans chronically exposed to PBBs."

267

And then there were the reports given by scientists who were hired by Farm Bureau Services or Michigan Chemical, or who were affiliated with Michigan State University. Reported Dr. Lynn B. Willett of the Ohio Agricultural Research and Development Center in Wooster, "Surprisingly high concentrations of PBB can be accumulated in tissues of cows without apparent signs of toxicity." Dr. Willett, who had been named to Governor Milliken's first and ill-fated PBB Scientific Advisory Panel, added, "Claims that PBB causes toxic responses and death among dairy animals environmentally contaminated with trace levels of the compound must be seriously questioned." His work, it turned out, was sponsored by the FDA—the same agency that employs Alan L. Hoeting, who first began the campaign to impugn the motives of the so-called low-level farmers.

Dr. Willett said heifers, both pregnant and nonpregnant, showed no evidence indicative of adverse effects from PBB exposure. Calf mortality was zero and milk production was the same as a group of control animals not given PBB. What's more, Dr. Willett said, birth weights of calves whose mothers had been highly exposed were "significantly greater" than the birth weights of calves whose mothers had only low exposure.

Dr. Willett said he had given some calves such massive doses of PBB that their tissues resulted in PBB concentrations 100 times greater than the FDA's standard of 300 parts per billion. Yet, he said, "This dose produced no clinical signs of toxicity."

Another study, reported by scientists at Industrial BIO-TEST Laboratories, Inc., of Northbrook, Illinois, found signs of toxicity only in animals given an extremely high dosage. In all other lower doses, they said, no overt signs of sickness appeared, even in the calves. In a second study, involving adult cows, they also found no health problems. And two of the cows gave birth to healthy calves. Furthermore, they said PBB had no effect on milk production, body weights or amount of food consumption. The laboratory had been retained by counsel to Michigan Chemical. It also was under investigation in 1977 by four federal agencies because of its sloppy procedures and questionable findings.

Dr. John R. Kateley, an immunologist in the department of pathology at Lansing's Edward W. Sparrow Hospital, said he found no immunological abnormalities in cows given PBB. His work was funded in part by both Farm Bureau Services and Michigan Chemical.

Dr. Marvin E. Wastell of Farm Bureau Services also did some experiments but found "no abnormal observations."

Michigan State University scientists reported on a variety of studies. One, by the department of crop and soil sciences, said there was no evidence that above-ground plant life picks up PBB from the soil. The only exception was carrot, which had only "minor quantities" of contamination. This settled a concern harbored by those who had purchased fertilizers to grow their own produce. Another study found that PBB apparently did no harm to growing pigs. The department of pharmacology said PBB does not alter liver function, although "this compound may sensitize the kidney to toxicity produced by agents administered secondarily." That conclusion seemed to dovetail with another study which said excessive iodine given to PBB-contaminated rats seemed to cause toxicity. Iodine, of course, was the explanation offered by the university's Dr. Hillman as being the cause of the widespread illness among farm animals.

Interestingly, by the time of the Michigan State University seminar, Dr. Hillman had come up with a new theory. It was not PBB—or even iodine—after all, he said. It was excessive fluorine, Dr. Hillman had discovered. Fluorine is an inevitable contaminant of rock phosphate, a soft mineral and a nutrient that is mixed with feed to nourish bones. But too much fluorine, Dr. Hillman said, produced the "classical signs" of PBB contamination: weight loss, reproductive problems, susceptibility to many infections, lameness. Four of the herds he said earlier had iodine poisoning actually had fluorosis, Dr. Hillman claimed. "We just didn't recognize it until a few years later that it was fluorosis, and it was a more serious problem." He reported seeing one cow so weak it had to walk on its knees, another with such rotten teeth that it could not drink cold water.

Yet, even the Michigan Department of Agriculture's John C. Dreves, assistant chief of the plant industry division, later said the state had tested dairy cattle feed and was unable to find excessive fluorine. "We're aware of Mr. Hillman's allegations. We also have checked feeds, and we can't support what he is finding as factual."

But Dr. Hillman was undaunted. He went on to call for "a thorough investigation by the U.S. Department of Justice" of farmers who claimed PBB problems and their lawyers, who, he said, "have more to gain than any of the plaintiffs." Dr. Hillman also began questioning Dr. Selikoff's 1976 health survey, saying that its sampling method may have been biased because the study included people like Al and Hilda Green. "I think there was definitely a conspiracy to perpetrate a hoax by convincing the public of a PBB problem," he said later. For example, Dr. Hillman continued, look at the Greens' animals. They were "in a state of gross malnutrition," which clearly demonstrated that Al and Hilda Green "obviously were not very knowledgeable about the feeding and management of dairy cattle." As he had done at Jim Fish's farm in Hickory Corners earlier, Dr. Hillman reached his conclusions after simply looking over the animals. "He [Green] didn't have to tell me; I could tell just by looking," Dr. Hillman later explained. "I believe it is time that some of us who have observed such nonsense let the public know our side of the story," he said. "My conclusion is that if any of the cattle on farms with traces of PBB are sick, it is due to something other than PBB."

Dr. Hillman's outspokenness soon made him one of the most controversial figures in the PBB disaster. And a hush of anticipation fell over the audience of several hundred persons in the Big Ten Room at the Kellogg Center as he approached a floor microphone to question Dr. Selikoff, who sat at a head table on a raised platform with several other scientists.

"Four years after exposure and perhaps a million dollars spent on research in this state, is there any direct link between PBB and any human health problem that has been documented with laboratory data that is statistically significant?" Dr. Hillman asked.

"The answer is yes," Dr. Selikoff answered sharply. "There is no way to explain our information other than there was something peculiar that happened to these farmers we examined. Now if they never lived on a farm and PBB had never been there, then it was due to something else. Otherwise it doesn't make sense."

Standing in the middle of the room, Dr. Hillman assumed an exaggerated look of skepticism.

"And they didn't have fluorisis," Dr. Selikoff snapped, slamming down a hand microphone he held.

But Dr. Hillman would not give up so easily. "Did you show any relationship between levels of PBB in serum [blood] and any symptoms?" he asked, his voice, too, rising.

"Of course we have. You didn't look at the slides," Dr. Selikoff retorted.

"They went by pretty fast," Dr. Hillman answered.

"They went by pretty fast, but the posters are stable," said Dr. Selikoff, whose findings also had been on display for two days on wall posters.

Now sullen, Dr. Hillman concluded, "I take exception with it and you have not considered any other possible toxins."

Confusion, more than anything else, emerged from the Michigan State University-sponsored workshop. But one thing became clear: If scientists by this time still were unable to reach agreement on PBB's effects even in laboratory animal research, the answers likely may never be known. The reason? There was no more left of the original Firemaster FF-1 involved in the 1973 mix-up. From then on, scientists doing PBB research would have to use other mixtures; and each PBB mixture can vary greatly in content from batch to batch. In other words, scientists in their research would have to use something different from what made Michigan's farm animals and people sick.

Not surprisingly, then, enough conflicting evidence emerged from the Michigan State University conference to back up almost any argument a person wanted to make about PBB, ranging from its absolute deadliness to its absolute safety. And this was clearly demonstrated almost exactly a year later when a court decision was handed down at the end of the longest trial in Michigan history in which a judge was asked to decide if low levels of PBB had damaged a herd of dairy cows.

# 14

# DISSENT FROM COURTHOUSE HILL

In the autumn of 1978, PBB seemed to be in the news nearly everyday. Previously unknown landfills were being discovered; leaching at others was coming to light. And most of all, concern about human health—and the Milliken administration's handling of the PBB crisis—once more became a matter of public debate. The election campaign of 1978 was under way. Governor Milliken was seeking reelection, and his Democratic opponent, state senator William B. Fitzgerald, had grabbed the PBB issue as his campaign keystone. That choice seemed wise, for many powerful interests in the state had become critics of Milliken on the PBB issue, including the influential United Auto Workers union. The consumers of Michigan, Douglas Fraser, then international UAW vice-president, had said in 1977, "have not been protected by our government from the errors and greed of private interests. We have not been protected by Governor William Milliken, the agriculture commission he appoints, or the Agriculture Department it controls. We have not been protected by the FDA or the USDA." He testified at the 1977 Riegle hearing, "Governor Milliken must personally bear his share of blame for the PBB disaster." Fraser, now head of UAW ticked off a list of specific complaints against the Milliken administration, and then singled out the "sorry record" of the Department of Agriculture for special attention. "It has not acted in the best interests of Michigan consumers," said Fraser. "It has not acted in the best interests of Michigan farmers. All too often it has acted to protect the short-term economic interests of the Michigan Farm Bureau." He said that, on hindsight, the UAW "should have moved a lot faster than it did to criticize the whole PBB affair."

Another strong critic of Milliken's handling of PBB was the Detroit *Free Press*. Like Fraser, it also said it wished it had spoken out sooner. "We have had to confess than in the earliest phases of that tragedy we along with many others did not fully grasp the implications," the paper commented in an editorial a month before the election. "Nor," it added, "is there any indication that Senator Fitzgerald did, although in fairness it should be said that responsibility for strong early action rested more with the administration than with the legislature."

Fitzgerald, a combative six-feet-four, former college basketball player, seized the PBB issue with vengeance, calling the handling of the disaster "symptomatic of indecision, drift and mismanagement of the Milliken administration."

If elected, he said he would fire the bureaucrats involved, including members of the Agriculture Commission. "The mechanism of our government that is there to serve people in times of crisis broke down. That's the failure of the Milliken administration," Fitzgerald said. He had the backing of the UAW, the Michigan Education Association, another powerful group in the state, the AFL-CIO and the right-to-lifers. As the campaign reached a climax, both President Carter and Vice President Mondale campaigned in Michigan for Fitzgerald, an Irish Catholic with a popular name in state politics.

His campaign clearly put Milliken on the defensive, who was asked about PBB everywhere he went. "Contrary to some suggestions," the governor said to a group of college newspaper editors, "I did not slip out in the dead of night and mix that feed myself."

But two events in October deflated Fitzgerald's campaign. One was the candidate's own doing. He simply overplayed his hand. Radio and television spots prepared by media consultant Charles Guggenheim talked of PBB's grotesque effects without clearly noting that some of the symptoms were found in laboratory animals only—and were produced by much higher doses than people ever got. One such thirty-second radio spot featured this dialogue:

> *Announcer:* "Want to know the truth about PBB in Michigan? Then listen to the people who know."
>
> *Voice:* "Loss of hair, memory loss, blindness, liver cancer..."
>
> *Voice:* "Birth defects ... the brain developing on the outside of the head."
>
> *Voice:* "Yes, genetic mutations..."

> *Voice:* "They figure 95 percent of the people of Michigan have been contaminated with PBB."

> *Voice:* "Everybody is going to get a taste of this stuff before it's all over with. Right today, you may still be ingesting PBB...."

At this point, the announcer breaks in to say that a governor is supposed to protect the health and safety of the people. Then another unidentified voice said: "I became concerned just as a physician and a scientist. And I called the governor's office, and nothing happened. It's a disaster and it's a disgrace to the state of Michigan." The speaker, of course, was Dr. Tom Corbett, who was referring to Dr. Selikoff's rejected offer to conduct human health surveys in Michigan for free.

The ad concludes with Fitzgerald saying, "The buck has to stop with the governor."

Reaction to Fitzgerald's ads was swift and emotional. Milliken called them "a cruel hoax" and "reckless advertising." The incumbent wrote to his challenger, "You simply cannot rewrite medical science and scientific research," adding:

"There is no research to justify your exceeding the bounds of decency and good taste and resorting to such disgraceful scare tactics. You have gone too far. Your campaign for governor has achieved a new low in Michigan politics. A campaign for Michigan's highest office requires higher standards than you have demonstrated. Your advertising offends good taste, insults the intelligence of the voters and should be taken off the air."

Most editorial writers in Michigan agreed with Milliken that the ads revealed Fitzgerald's own lack of judgment.

But when Fitzgerald returned to Michigan from Rome after attending the funeral of Pope John Paul I, he rejected Milliken's demand that the ads be yanked. "This is a scary issue that people have to face," Fitzgerald said upon his arrival at Detroit's Metropolitan Airport. "He [Milliken] doesn't really seem to understand that this is a human problem." Fitzgerald then composed a written reply to Milliken's letter, saying, "... you've consistently downplayed the magnitude of this tragedy, even when your obligation to inform the public should have dictated otherwise. Now you're doing it again." Fitzgerald did, however, say he would review the ads, perhaps with modifications in mind.

Fitzgerald's position further eroded with a page-one story in the Detroit *News* in which Dr. Corbett himself called the ads "misleading, alarmist" and taken out of context. He said he had urged all the Fitzgerald people that "they'd have to do this very carefully and accurately" and even offered to help edit the finished product. "But I never heard from them again." Dr. Corbett added, in further comments to the *Free Press*, "I warned Fitzgerald's staff when they interviewed me that if they didn't do the thing credibly, they would blow it. And they blew it."

Three days later, the ads were lifted. "When I began this campaign," Fitzgerald said, "I promised the people of Michigan that if I made a mistake as a governor, I would advise the public and assume responsibility. The same goes for me as a candidate for governor." He said he had reviewed the ads before they were aired but did not notice the ambiguities because it had been clear to him that the symptoms mentioned were in animals and not people. Nevertheless, Fitzgerald concluded, "The accidental mixing of PBB into animal feed certainly is not the chief executive's fault. But when a crisis came on the scene, no one arose to meet it. It's that simple."

But now it was Fitzgerald who was on the defensive about PBB. Milliken's own ads began publicizing the withdrawn Fitzgerald ads, and featured excerpts from newspaper editorials around the state that were critical of Fitzgerald's ads.

The second—and perhaps crucial—event in October that delivered a fatal blow to Fitzgerald's hopes came with stunning surprise to the entire state.

With less than two weeks remaining before election day, a state court judge ruled flatly that low levels of PBB were not toxic to animals. After presiding over the longest trial in Michigan history, the judge, a Republican, blamed the PBB disaster on public fear created by incompetent and dishonest scientists, veterinarians, farmers and lawyers. And the judge had nothing but praise for state agencies, Michigan Chemical and Farm Bureau Services.

The suit had been filed by Roy and Marilyn Tacoma, owners of a dairy farm in Falmouth, east of Cadillac. The Tacomas never bought the heavily contaminated feeds. But in a $250,000 suit against Michigan Chemical and Farm Bureau Services, they claimed that their herd was irreparably damaged after they unknowingly gave their cows feed contaminated by low levels of PBB residue from the feed company's mixing

275

equipment. They argued that low PBB exposure was more damaging in the long run than was short-term high-level exposure. Moreover, the Tacomas said, just because their animals now have only low PBB levels does not mean they were not exposed to much higher levels earlier. The reason the Tacomas took so long to have their animals tested for PBB is because they—and many others—had been told by Farm Bureau Services that their feed never was contaminated by PBB.

The timing of the release of the opinion certainly was open to question. But the judge, William R. Peterson, explained that in releasing his ruling he hadn't thought about the election at all. He said he was worried about completing the long and complicated case—and his opinion—before something happened to him—like a heart attack—or to his notes—like a fire.

In an editorial headlined "An Ill-Timed Ruling," the Grand Rapids *Press* suggested that if Peterson indeed had harbored such concerns, he could have completed his opinion and put it, say, in a bank vault, until after the election. "With his written opinion safely locked up, the judge could easily have removed any hint of politics by delaying his decision for eleven more days," the paper said. "While we take the judge at his word that he 'didn't think about' the consequences [in releasing his opinion so close to the election], we wonder in what kind of political vacuum this elected, self-styled 'liberal' Republican judge operates. In his opinion, Judge Peterson criticized a Michigan State University pathologist: 'He wasn't living in an ivory tower, but in solitary confinement.' For the sake of public credibility, does not a judge, at the price of a small inconvenience, have the same responsibility not to live the law 'in solitary confinement'?"

Ironically, a mere week before Peterson released his opinion, CBS agreed to postpone until after the election a fictitious television show based on the PBB incident after questions were raised about its possible effect on the Milliken-Fitzgerald race. The show, entitled "Slaughter," had been scheduled for nationwide broadcast on the night before the election as a regular segment on *Lou Grant,* an hour-long Monday night series.

Donn O'Brien, CBS vice-president for program practices, said the scheduling of "Slaughter" had been purely coincidental. He said the show was postponed (until November 27) because "We felt that, in fairness to Michigan, in fairness to the election, we wouldn't air it now."

Reactions to the CBS decision were predictable. The Democrats were outraged. The Republicans were pleased. The Detroit *News* also lauded the postponement. "The network obviously did the right thing," it said in an October 22 editorial. "Perhaps now—Michigan's Democratic hierarchy permitting—the campaign for governor can serve to enlighten rather than confuse the voters on the vital issues."

Four days later, Judge Peterson's sensational ruling came out, and it did anything but help enlighten rather than confuse the voters.

It was 155 pages long, plus a 4-page preface and another 12 pages of appendices. Because the trial took place "in an atmosphere of public crisis," Peterson wrote, he had extended "great latitude to counsel in allowing discovery to continue during trial." The case was "too important" not to have allowed both sides to bring in every bit of evidence that might shed some light on the case, he said. Thus, the trial took "an inordinate amount of time to try," Peterson explained. It had begun in February of 1977. In all, sixty-three witnesses were heard. The trial transcript ran to twenty-five thousand pages. Another seventy thousand pages of exhibits were introduced. Nevertheless, Peterson conceded in his preface, "Much research into the problems dealt with herein still remains unfinished or not yet begun."

The final paragraph of Peterson's preface revealed his decision. "Finally, this opinion tells the story of a great tragedy. The evidence proved it so, but for reasons entirely different than those which the Court had supposed before the trial began. The tragedy lies in the needless destruction of animals exposed to low levels of polybrominated biphenyl and even of animals who never received any PBB. It is a terrible irony that defendant Farm Bureau unwittingly contributed to that tragedy by its initial reaction to the PBB accident in treating all cases alike, and in settling claims as if PBB were as toxic as plaintiffs have claimed. But plaintiffs' proofs have fallen shockingly short of their claims. The evidence proves, instead, that in small amounts, PBB is not toxic."

Then what did happen to cattle who ingested PBB? Peterson asked in his ruling. "To most of them," he wrote, "the answer is 'nothing that can be attributed to PBB.'"

In reaching these conclusions, Peterson relied largely on the research findings of Industrial BIO-TEST Laboratories of

Illinois and the Ohio Agricultural Research and Development Center, a branch of Ohio State University in Wooster.

Industrial BIO-TEST conducted feeding experiments involving lactating cows and calves. Only in three calves, all in the highest PBB group, was toxicosis found, the laboratory's scientists reported. Some other lesions were found, but none were related to PBB, they said. The laboratory was commissioned by Michigan Chemical.

The Ohio Agricultural Research and Development Center, known simply as OARDC, performed experiments using cows, bull calves, pregnant heifers and unbred heifers. The chief investigator was Dr. Willett, who also got funding from Michigan Chemical and Farm Bureau Services, in addition to the U.S. Food and Drug Administration. He found little, if anything, wrong with PBB in all but the animals fed extraordinary amounts of the chemical. Only the group of heifers given more than 3 million parts per billion showed definite adverse effects, such as weight loss and pregnancy complications, according to Dr. Willett. But even in this group, he said, many of the symptoms farmers blamed on PBB simply were not seen, including abnormal hoof growths, lameness, joint stiffness or discoloration of hair coat.

Judge Peterson also relied upon the conclusions of the Michigan herd survey conducted in 1975 by the Food and Drug Administration and headed by Dr. Mercer. This is the study that compared two groups of farm animals with one another—even though both had been contaminated by PBB—and then found no statistical difference of any significance between the two, thereby exonerating PBB. Peterson dismissed the higher calf mortality rate in the higher PBB group as being of no statistical significance because, he implied, the deaths of calves had been reported by farmers from memory rather than from "records."

The judge was further persuaded by the research of Dr. John Kateley, the Lansing immunologist whose work was financed largely by Farm Bureau Services and Michigan Chemical. Dr. Kateley found no damage to the immune systems of nearly seventy cows exposed to PBB over a year's time.

And finally, there were results from a Farm Bureau Services-Michigan Chemical "experimental farm" in Mason, supervised by Dr. Marvin Wastell of Farm Bureau Services. It involved about eighty cows, half of which were "controls," or unexposed cows, mostly from Wisconsin; the other half were Michigan cows with known PBB contamination. Dr. Wastell reported no difference in health, milk production or calf mortality between the two groups of cows, which were mingled and received the same treatment.

The studies by Industrial BIO-TEST, OARDC, Dr. Kateley and Dr. Wastell, besides their common sources of funding and their similar conclusions, also had other similarities.

Both the "experimental farm" animals and those in the OARDC experiments, for instance, had been fed huge amounts of feed—which tended to diminish gastro-intestinal absorption of PBB. Dr. Willett, while on the witness stand, admitted under cross-examination, that his test animals at OARDC received a diet that "definitely would not enhance toxic responses." In fact, thanks to the super ration, many of the pregnant cows in the experiments gained weight at an astounding average of 4.4 pounds a day—compared to the usual weight gain during pregnancy of 1 to 1½ pounds daily. One animal in Dr. Willett's studies put on 7.7 pounds a day during an 18-day period.

"Such PBBs as were absorbed would be sequestered in excessive amounts of fat on the animals, and would be unavailable to exert toxic effects," noted Dr. Donald P. Wallach, an enzyme specialist and senior research scientist at the Upjohn Company in Kalamazoo but who acted as a private consultant to the Tacomas.

The cows at the "experimental farm" set up by Farm Bureau Services and Michigan Chemical also were overfed, and in addition were given large doses of vitamin A. Even so, the animals in 1977 required more veterinary treatment than normal, including treatment for breeding difficulties. The lavish attention these cows received, sometimes from Michigan State University experts, Dr. Wallach said, cost $95,000 more than could be offset by milk sales. "The operation went a long way to show that Michigan's PBB afflicted farmers are right when they maintained that they can keep PBB tainted cows alive, but can't make money on them," said the scientist.

Furthermore, it turned out that the "control" animals in some of the OARDC experiments also became contaminated— as did many of the cows in Dr. Kateley's immunology study. And as for the OARDC "control" animals, not only were they contaminated, they also developed abnormal lesions. But Dr. Phillip D. Moorhead, one of the researchers, said those lesions

279

were dismissed because the control animals did not have enough PBB to make the findings "significant."

Judge Peterson, nevertheless, concluded in his opinion, "Feeding experiments seem to prove that PBB is relatively non-toxic."

It is not difficult to see why Michigan Chemical hired Industrial BIO-TEST to do PBB research. "Dr. Donald Jenkins of this organization [the lab] admitted that if the results of their studies did not please a client, they didn't get paid," Dr. Wallach said. But the outraged Dr. Wallach wasn't the only person who held Industrial BIO-TEST in low esteem.

Indeed the laboratory has been under investigation by four federal agencies for irregularities and deficiencies in its testing. It was Industrial BIO-TEST, in fact (along with two other laboratories), whose practices led the federal government in 1978 to adopt a new set of nationwide rules known as Good Laboratory Practice regulations. Two years earlier, Senator Edward M. Kennedy's subcommittee on health had exposed three notorious cases in which massive deficiencies were found in scientific data submitted to the U.S. Environmental Protection Agency and the Food and Drug Administration. One of those labs? Industrial BIO-TEST.

After looking into the practice of the three laboratories, federal investigators said they uncovered instances in which gross lesions in test animals were not properly examined or reported, and cases in which experiments were designed in such a way as to obscure whatever toxic effects a product might have. Referring to all three laboratories, Ernest Brisson, associate director for compliance in charge of FDA's new Bioresearch Monitoring Program, said: "We also encountered creative penmanship which causes test animals to appear and disappear throughout the course of the study, [events that] make us wonder who is running the show—a toxicologist or a magician."

But Judge Peterson, while conceding that "the research practices of Industrial BIO-TEST are currently under review by several federal agencies," wrote: "Nonetheless, the results of those studies are essentially consistent with the results of other research." Yet, the laboratory's performance led the federal government to terminate several contracts with it. Indeed, further testing contracts were not to be awarded to Industrial BIO-TEST by the U.S. Department of Health, Education and

Welfare or any of its component agencies (such as the FDA) without the personal approval of the assistant HEW secretary.

But what drew the wrath of Judge Peterson was not the practices of Industrial BIO-TEST, OARDC or the collaborative efforts of Michigan Chemical, Farm Bureau Services, and Michigan State University; rather it was people like Dr. Alpha Clark, the Tacomas' veterinarian, and other scientists who testified on their behalf. And Peterson spared no adjectives in his attack.

"Dr. Clark is ... emotional, partisan, unscientific and not at all objective, ... a man who, on learning about PBB leaped to a phobic conviction that it was causing every ailment seen in his clients' animals, and devoted his complete energy to the dual cause of being against sin (PBB) and aiding his clients and other claimants in obtaining financial settlements from the defendants," the judge wrote.

"...The Court felt very sorry for Dr. Clark during his testimony as he was obviously embarrassed—a man who had apparently voiced a lot of positive and extravagant statements which now, at the moment of truth, he could neither abandon nor substantiate." Peterson said Dr. Clark had been unable to provide a reliable history of the Tacomas' herd or a detailed study of the feeds that the animals had eaten. "If you didn't eat the cucumbers," he wrote, "Something else gave you gas."

The judge called another witness for the Tacomas "incompetent, biased and dishonest."

But, in the final analysis, the crucial question was what exactly happened to the dairy cows of Roy and Marilyn Tacoma.

Roy, now 40, and his father, Andrew, jointly had 35 mature cows, 31 young heifers, and their calves. Then in November 1973, they decided to go their separate ways after policy disagreements. Their herd had been housed in a barn on Andrew Tacoma's farm just down the road from Roy's place. But a new barn was finished in late 1972 at Roy's farm, so all the animals were moved there.

When they decided to go their own ways, father took with him ten cows and fifteen heifers; son kept twenty cows, sixteen heifers and all the calves, some of them still under his father's ownership.

Roy and Marilyn Tacoma grew their own corn silage, grain

and hay, but bought salt, vitamins and a special feed for young calves called Manna Mate from the Falmouth Co-Op in town.

The Falmouth Co-op has about twelve hundred members and is known historically as a pioneer in, and a model for, the agricultural cooperative movement in the American Midwest. It operates branches in Falmouth, Merritt and McBain, providing feeds, equipment and various services to farmers in the area. The independent co-op has an arrangement with Farm Bureau Services whereby it promotes Farm Bureau Service's products in exchange for services such as accounting, payroll management and bookkeeping.

Tacoma is a member of the Falmouth Co-op, which was run by his uncle, Gerritt Koster, until he retired in late 1974. The new branch manager was Russell Koster, Tacoma's cousin and son of Gerritt Koster.

There was no dispute that PBB was present in feed made by Farm Bureau Services and sold to Tacoma through the Falmouth Co-op. Right after he and his father split up their dairy operation, Roy decided to try to increase his cows' milk production and so he bought some Farm Bureau Services dairy #410 feed. Almost right away, he recalls, the animals began refusing to eat the feed, resulting in loss of milk production. Then other problems appeared: diarrhea, joint problems, lameness, runny noses and eyes, long hooves, rough hair coats and elephant-like skin. There also were breeding problems and unusual incidences of udder and uterine infections, which did not respond to treatment. Soon he stopped using the #410 feed.

Yet Tacoma actually sold more milk—for a short time. The reason turned out to be the large number of heifers that began milking after calving for the first time. He was simply milking more cows. But it didn't take Tacoma long to realize that actual milk production was dropping. By early 1974, more than a dozen cows had died. Things did not improve with the arrival of spring. Indeed the problems persisted into the fall. Five to 10 percent of the young animals were lame. Many others had overgrown hooves. Hair coats were rough; elephant-like hide developed. Some calves were stunted and deformed. And Dr. Clark could not get the animals to respond to treatment. Some of the cows were dull and depressed; but others were nervous and wild. During this period, cows that stopped producing were sent to the market.

Tacoma finally sent in some fat tissues to the Michigan Department of Agriculture for analysis. Sure enough, PBB was found, and on October 14, 1975, his farm was placed under a meat quarantine—meaning the herd's milk could be sold (since the milk did not violate the guideline levels), but the cows could not be sold until individual tests had been performed. Like many other farmers, Tacoma soon found himself in a bind by the state quarantine and the Farm Bureau Services' refusal to give him a just compensation. In mid-1976, Tacoma violated the quarantine and sold several cows for meat.

"I felt so ashamed of myself after I shipped them out," Tacoma said. "I lost sleep over it." Less than a month later, he shot 110 of the sickest animals. "I thought, 'lest I be tempted to do it again, lest I be badgered into doing it again, I just went out and shot the rest of them, so I could forget it.' In my own mind I knew that they shouldn't be going to the market." The remaining animals that he did not sell or shoot, Tacoma said, were worthless.

The Tacomas sought in court damages for the value of their entire herd, for lost profits, for extra feed and labor, for veterinary expenses, for the burial of the destroyed animals, for diminished value of their farm, for proposed cleanup costs and for lost profits in the future while they were rebuilding their dairy operation.

But Peterson denied all such claims, saying that Dr. Clark, the Tacomas' veterinarian: "Had no records, no files, no documentation to support or illustrate his claimed observations."

Even though Dr. Clark said he visited the Tacoma farm more than a hundred times in 1974, 1975 and 1976, Peterson said, the veterinarian's billing record showed only thirty-five such calls. Furthermore, the judge said, an examination of the Tacomas' income tax returns showed that they spent less for veterinary services in 1974 than in 1973, and even less in 1975. Peterson discounted the explanation given by Dr. Clark, which was that he did not bill a client for additional calls if he could not cure an animal after three visits. (Of course, Dr. Jackson likewise also did not bill Rick Halbert for the many calls and hours he devoted to help solve the animal problems at the Halbert farm.)

Peterson said his own analysis showed that the Tacomas' herd was not damaged by PBB. He said also that many of the

283

health problems as well as the decreased milk production were due to Tacoma's rush to produce calves. And even though he admitted that the farmer's 1974 calf mortality was "statistically significant," the judge said the evidence did not indicate it could be attributed to PBB.

All told, Judge Peterson wrote, the evidence "has disclosed a tragic picture ... but not the picture that the Court had anticipated at the outset. It is not merely a picture of thousands of animals being destroyed; it is a picture of animals being destroyed indiscriminately, many unnecessarily."

Peterson blamed much of the PBB tragedy on "an unhappy chain of events ... in which fear preempted the role of reason."

He wrote, "It is not surprising, in the face of the unknown and the clamor that developed in the press, that dairy farmers and veterinarians would look a second time at all the animal ailments which are ordinarily endured and forgotten, and that they and the public at large would voice a suspicion that they were caused by PBB. Rumor and exaggeration feed on themselves, nourished by fear and the self-justification of people with potential claims. Nothing could better illustrate that than this case, where professionals have forsaken objectivity and their usual standards of inquiry to accept unquestioningly, as a basis of their expressed opinions, reported facts that were not factual, and to embroider upon their own role to the extent of being untruthful.

"No case could better illustrate this point than this, in which Roy Tacoma, a man whom the Court believes to be fundamentally honest and God-fearing, is found to have told a number of inconsistent and untrue stories about what was happening to his animals. If a man of this stature could tell one person that his milk production had been cut 30 percent, and another than it had been cut in half, and that thirty-five of his forty-seven cows would not conceive, listeners would believe, and those most likely to believe and to repeat such statements would be his neighboring dairy farmers who were in the same suspicious, fearful state of mind. They told him about hyperkeratosis and he saw it is his own herd. And, if a man of his character could tell such stories, what kind of stories would others tell? And so it grew."

The judge said the initial settlement policy adopted by Michigan Chemical and Farm Bureau Services could well have

284

contributed "to the epidemic fear by encouraging the belief that any exposure to PBB, even by association, was deadly." The result was what Peterson called "indiscriminate slaughter of Michigan dairy animals without attempting to distinguish between animals that were exposed to feeds containing PBB and those that were not, or between animals exposed to insignificant levels or those which, like the Halbert, Petroshus and Crum herds, received large amounts of PBB...."

But when the companies stopped paying out settlement claims indiscriminately, the Tacomas felt cheated and discriminated against, according to Peterson.

Summing up, Peterson said, "The Court's conclusions of law are made easy by the facts. The questions of compensatory and punitive damages which the Court anticipated at the outset of the trial have not appeared."

Peterson added, "The health of their animals was not impaired, nor was their performance in milk production affected by PBB." On the other hand, he said, "the defense evidence on toxicity did show that PBB is relatively non-toxic to cattle and that animals exposed to far higher levels than were plaintiffs' animals suffered no ill effects."

Peterson also noted that the Tacomas doubled their net income from 1973 to 1974. And in 1975, he said, their net income was five times that of 1973. "Among the things that this case is not, it is not a case of an enterprise ruined by PBB," the judge wrote in a footnote.

"That's true," retorts Tacoma. "But did he check the price of milk, the rate of inflation, or check the fact that I was a young farmer trying to expand, and was working eighteen hours a day? No." In 1975, nearly half his $25,000 net income was derived from the sale of steers, Tacoma said.

"Good ol' American justice. Money and politics. Hell! We were confident as all get-out. The state quarantined us. We got PBB. We had losses. We thought the trial'd take three days!" he said.

"My cattle are still quarantined. What kind of justice is that?"

The Tacomas had rejected a settlement offer from the companies for $150,000 before the trial began. "Well," said Tacoma, "my pockets are empty, but my conscience is clean."

Judge Peterson also ordered the Tacomas to pay the court costs.

"If he didn't believe a single witness, he should have stopped the trial in December [1977, when the Tacomas rested their case]," said Schenk.

Other reactions were similarly predictable. Governor Milliken was "pleased that the judge said the state reacted properly … and agrees that rumor and exaggeration made the PBB problem far worse than it was." Senator Fitzgerald called the ruling "outrageous," and said Milliken's reaction "continues to show his inability to understand the PBB tragedy." Michigan Chemical was "elated." Farm Bureau Services hailed the verdict as "a victory for all of Michigan's great agricultural community."

The Grand Rapids *Press* reminded readers that the decision actually had a very narrow application—only as to what low levels of PBB did or did not do to Roy and Marilyn Tacoma's dairy cows. "On the broader issue—whether similarly small amounts of PBB are harmless to animals in every instance—the judge may have inadvertently led the public into thinking the decision covered an area which remains much in doubt. The fact that larger doses of PBB can be extremely toxic is beyond dispute. Judge Peterson did not, and could not, address the bottom limits of toxicity, and neither could he state absolutely that ingestion of minute quantities of PBB over long periods was harmless."

The Big Rapids *Pioneer* was more blunt. "We feel justice has not been served by his [Peterson's] action," adding, "We feel Peterson's claim … is, simply put, a crock. Granted, perhaps the Tacomas' case was not the strongest possible in proving the toxicity of PBB, and perhaps some persons have overreacted to the calamity.

"But to vindicate Farm Bureau and the state in its handling of this mess is not warranted by any stretch of the imagination. Farm Bureau has attempted continually to downplay the seriousness of the problem. The state Department of Agriculture, only after extensive prodding, took belated steps to deal with the situation…. The full story of PBB is not contained in Peterson's 155-page decision."

Peterson was roundly criticized for his timing in releasing the controversial opinion. But few questioned his motives. One who did was Gary Schenk. "The venom that was in the opinion … it's as sick and dishonest a thing as we'll ever see in Michigan legal history," he said. "People tell me I just got caught up in the politics. Nobody knew the Democrats would make such an issue of PBB."

Judge Peterson said the Tacoma case was so cut and dry that, for the first time in his career, he was able to issue an opinion without citing a single legal precedent.

"It's simple," the fifty-five-year-old judge said. "If I throw a brick at your car, it will diminish the car's value and you are owed damages. But if I throw a sponge at your car, although that may be technically wrong, you're not entitled to recover anything."

Yet, commented Rick Halbert, "whether those cows are damaged [by the sponge] is in the eyes of the beholder. Maybe they're not damaged in the eyes of the law. But that's the way our economic system works. He [Tacoma] didn't ask for PBB; his cows got it; and they should be removed."

Halbert called Peterson's verdict "courageous," adding, "the judge is trying to bring us back to our senses, and his clear implication is that we've lost them."

The judge flatly denied any political motivation in his opinion or in the timing of its release. "I don't suppose any response I make will be believed," Peterson lamented. "But my only concern throughout has been to get the decision out. I have been working twelve to fourteen hours a day for the last six weeks." Peterson said that while the trial itself ended in May, he did not receive the final briefs from the attorneys on both sides until just before Labor Day.

Going into the trial, he said, he carried a preconceived notion that "PBB was highly toxic. I'm surprised that so much effort proved so little."

The nonjury trial began in late February of 1977, shortly before the Riegle hearings were held in the state. The trial took place in the old Wexford County Courthouse, a three-story building with an imposing façade of Greek ionic columns situated on top of a hill and looking very much out of place in a residential Cadillac neighborhood.

By the time Peterson recessed the trial for eleven days over Easter, only nine witnesses had been called. And the six weeks he had allotted for the trial were gone. At the end of July, the judge recessed the trial for sixty days, asking both sides to meet with a court-appointed mediator to seek an out-of-court settlement. "It has been obvious as the trial progressed that the controversy is more complex than was originally thought and that scientific and other testimony required for completion of the case will require not merely weeks but many months," Peterson said.

But in October the trial resumed. Raymond Smith, a retired Allegan County circuit judge whom Peterson had requested to serve as mediator, reported, "We never got off dead center. Both sides were too adamant."

The previous trial record in Michigan was set in 1948 by a seven-month trial in Port Huron involving men accused of trying to kill Walter Reuther, then president of the United Auto Workers union.

Judge Peterson is a highly regarded jurist whose verdicts have been reversed only three times by higher courts in his twenty years on the bench.

He is a native of Cadillac. He was a Phi Beta Kappa graduate of Albion College and received a master's degree in economics and later a law degree from the University of Michigan. He was a law professor at the University of Missouri in Kansas City when, on a vacation, he and Mrs. Peterson returned to Cadillac and, on the spur of the moment, decided to move back to the city. He served two terms as county prosecutor and then was a probate judge before becoming judge of the Wexford County Circuit Court. He also found time to write a history of Cadillac. It was entitled *The View from Courthouse Hill.*

He later served a one-year term as president of the Michigan Judges Association.

No one was more stunned by Peterson's opinion than attorneys Schenk and Greer. But they wisely refrained from public comment over the weekend. By early the following week, however, they issued a statement in reply to the judge's verdict. None of the defense expert witnesses, they said, had examined Tacoma's animals. And the laboratory research paid for by Farm Bureau Services and Michigan Chemical had made no effort to duplicate the experiences of Tacoma's animals. "Before PBB, Tacoma had a good normal herd. After PBB they had a loss of milk production, and herd problems similar to those seen on other PBB farms in Michigan," they said.

"We believe there is a fundamental distinction between the feeding studies carried out by the defense experts designed to measure and assess the acute impact of this toxin and the chronic problem described in Michigan cattle by plaintiffs' experts years after the poisoning episode, when the acute effects would be expected to be over and done with," said Schenk and Greer.

"We believe the court adopted an unusually severe standard of proof in light of the fact that there was no question of the fault of Michigan Chemical and Farm Bureau Services in allowing the PBB to reach the Tacoma family farm in contaminated feed," they said in a joint statement. They also found it curious that Peterson had exonerated state agencies as well, since during the trial Peterson would not allow evidence to be introduced concerning the role of the state agencies, saying that the state was not on trial.

"If, in an industrial tragedy, the only proper standard of proof will be to finance experimental feeding studies in a manner beyond the means of most people who are affected by such a disaster, then, perhaps the legal system will stand as the wrong place to answer the questions which are raised," Schenk and Greer said.

Of course, they are right. The legal system is ill-equipped to decide issues involving the subtle effects of chemical contamination.

Yet, because all the other branches of government had let them down, the farmers looked to the courts as the final source of hope, and justice. The paucity of indemnification programs was appalling for PBB victims. The federal Milk Indemnity Program, for instance, applies only to victims of pesticide contamination. "Since PBB is not a pesticide, these Michigan farmers could not qualify for indemnity payment," said Richard L. Feltner, then assistant secretary of the U.S. Department of Agriculture.

Several years before the PBB poisoning began, indemnities were paid to owners of poultry slaughtered in California, but the reason for the slaughter was Newcastle's disease, a communicable disease. PBB was not. "There is no law at present permitting financial relief for losses in livestock due to the presence of chemicals or other substances that render them unwholesome," said Norman E. Ross, Jr., assistant director of the domestic council in the Ford White House in 1974. What he said in 1974 is still true today.

Indeed the only financial aid Michigan farmers got at all of any significance came not from any branch of government but from the Michigan Milk Producers Association, which made available $630,000 in interest-free loans to fifty-nine affected farmers.

Clearly, then, our laws—and the judicial system—failed the

289

PBB victims in Michigan. But similar chemical disasters inevitably will occur. And next time the victims may not be confined to the state of Michigan.

One person who was not surprised by the Peterson ruling was a bearded attorney in Washington, D.C., named Stephen M. Soble, who began pondering the question of compensation to victims of pollution even before he graduated from Harvard Law School in 1978.

"Peterson's decision was almost inevitable because the common law legal system simply is not equipped to deal with the special problems posed by toxic-substance pollution," he said.

"In a lawsuit for compensation, the victim carries the burden of proving that PBB caused damage. The burden of proving the alleged injury must be met by showing the court concrete facts. These concrete facts must be so weighty that the preponderance of the evidence supports what the victims have alleged. In a case like PBB, however, this is a standard which is almost impossible for a victim to meet," says Soble, who followed the Tacoma trial closely.

"There will always be elements of uncertainty in highly complex scientific cases. Things which our scientific tests haven't proven conclusively, even though highly probable, will be ignored." That's why, for instance, the testimony of one eminent scientist was reduced to a mere footnote in Peterson's lengthy verdict. The scientist had studied the relationship between cancer and PBB and found a strong likelihood of its carcinogenicity.

Furthermore, as the Tacoma case illuminates, the cost of litigation may effectively deter other victims from suing the culprits responsible for the contamination in the first place. Even if victims do sue, the courts are a very slow mechanism.

"To continue to rely on the ill-equipped court system to handle cases of toxic-substance pollution is to invite a repeat of the Tacoma decision in many more cases, in Michigan and across the country," says Soble. "Too often, victims of toxic-substance pollution also become victims of our legal system."

Soble, 29, is the author of an innovative proposal now being discussed in Congress that envisions a broad, industry-financed program to justly compensate victims of toxic substances pollution. Its sponsor in Congress is Michigan Representative William M. Brodhead.

Simply, the Toxic Substance Pollution Victim Compensation Act would set up a national administrative compensation system to serve victims of toxic-substance pollutions. The bill calls for a change in the traditional rules on the burden of proof and other technical legal rules in order to make the handling of evidence more fair. The bill would reduce the costs that are borne by the victims in processing their claims; it would speed up the investigation and study of injuries related to toxic-substance poisoning.

The plan would work somewhat on the principle of workers' compensation funds. Chemical producers and all handlers would be required to contribute to such a fund to reimburse future victims. The federal government would establish a schedule of fees that industry would be charged for using and handling of hazardous materials; the more dangerous the substance, the higher the charges. Revenues derived from such "use fees" would be given by the administrative board to provide compensation to victims of toxic-substance pollution.

"Once certified by the administrative board of compensation," said Representative Brodhead, "victims can file claims for compensation, including medical care, rehabilitation services, total disability, death benefits, survivors benefits, funeral expenses, attorney's fees and lost wages. ... One of the best aspects of the bill is that it encourages manufacturers to strengthen safety procedures and conduct research into the effects of dangerous products." Although the existing Toxic Substances Control Act, enacted in 1976, indeed does require some premarketing testing, it lacks the incentive contemplated in the Brodhead proposal. "A compensation system which entails a high level of self-regulation will encourage manufacturers to expend research and development efforts on issues of risk which may not be the subject of direct regulation," Soble notes.

Although the Brodhead proposal, as it is now written, would not provide compensation for property damage, it would apply to the numerous PBB personal injury suits that have been filed. And the bill includes a $500,000 appropriation to assist the state of Michigan defray the cost of medical care for those suffering from PBB poisoning. Another $750,000 is contained in the bill for the National Institute of Environmental Health Sciences to carry out further health studies in Michigan.

The plight of Michigan's PBB victims—not only Roy and Marilyn Tacoma but many, many other farm families still awaiting their day in court—provides the most eloquent argument for enactment of the Brodhead proposal.

To depend on the companies responsible for pollution to voluntarily make restitution, as Garry Zuiderveen said, is but a pipe dream.

"Nobody was prepared to help persons who lose their employment, capital and personal health to an incident of contamination," recalls Rick Halbert. "We have unemployment compensation for the worker, Social Security for the retired, workman's compensation for the worker who is injured on the job. But there was no help for victims of the PBB contamination."

# 15
# PASSAGES

In a smashing 1978 reelection victory, William Milliken became the first Republican candidate for governor since 1946 to capture Michigan's densely populated and traditionally Democratic Wayne County. Milliken's strong showing in Detroit—the home of his Democratic challenger—more than offset his losses in northern farm areas.

Oscoda County, which Milliken carried in 1970 and 1974, for instance, was won by Fitzgerald, who also captured several other surrounding and nearby counties that had voted for Milliken in the two previous elections. But most of these counties are sparsely populated, and they gave Fitzgerald an edge of only a few hundred votes, while Milliken was piling up huge pluralities in the heavily populated counties down state.

Milliken's ability to repeatedly win elections in an otherwise solidly Democratic state has gained him the admiration of national GOP leaders. And it is stirring speculation that he might seek the Republican nomination for president or vice-president in 1980 when the national party holds its nominating convention in Detroit.

In a pre-election interview with the Detroit *News*, Milliken conceded, "That [PBB], I would say, was the toughest and most elusive problem that I've coped with in the time that I've been governor. ... I think that was one of the most complex problems we've ever dealt with—there was no precedent to guide us. It is symptomatic of the age of chemicals with which we are now living. If it isn't PBB it's going to be some other problem in the future."

In other interviews, Milliken told the Grand Rapids *Press*, "I think, in looking back, had we known generally what we know today, the responses might have been different." And he conceded to the Detroit *Free Press* that his administration had not moved quickly enough in the early critical months of the disaster. He said he had not regarded PBB as a crisis until 1976. "I think the thing really developed a crisis level about that time, or at least a crisis of understanding. Nobody did understand." Milliken said he would accept his "share of responsibility" for the state government's inaction.

"No, sir," Milliken added, "I don't claim that my handling has been perfect. But I can say that I've tried in a very complicated and complex problem to deal with it responsibly."

Another winner on November 7 was William R. Peterson, who ran unopposed in his reelection bid for the twenty-eighth circuit judgship. Surprisingly, there was a strong write-in effort against Peterson. It was organized at the eleventh hour by farmers upset by the judge's ruling in the Tacoma case. Thus, a Cadillac attorney named James Herrinton unwittingly became a footnote to the state's PBB tragedy. "He just happened to be a lawyer in Cadillac that happened to be chosen, unlucky as he might have been," said Falmouth dairy farmer Bob Geering. The write-in effort spread by word of mouth.

A surprised Herrinton commented, "I'm happy practicing law and wouldn't want to be a judge." In Missaukee County, Herrinton got 23 percent of the 2,429 votes cast. In several townships, he came close to outpolling Peterson.

The 1978 election returns did provide one real note of cheer, however. Donald Albosta, the cantankerous St. Charles farmer who held the raucous PBB hearings in 1976, was elected to represent Michigan's tenth congressional district, which includes much of the north central part of Michigan. Albosta defeated incumbent Elford Cederberg, a twenty-four year House veteran whose reelection bid was supported by Gerald Ford, among other GOP stalwarts. "What we really need," Albosta said during his campaign, "is some type of federal legislation that enables farmers to get low-interest loans when such chemical catastrophes occur. Since the PBB problem has been around, I can't think of one thing that the state has done for those affected farmers, not one single thing. If anything, the state has dragged its feet."

Immediately after his resounding election victory, Governor Milliken and his staff began maneuvering to oust B. Dale Ball, the agricultural director. Ball, sixty-two, had been a state civil servant for nearly forty years and agriculture director since 1965. Milliken's desire for Ball to retire was the worst kept secret

294

in Michigan. The word was that Ball, as far as the executive office was concerned, had become a dinosaur. "Ball isn't even consulted these days—on anything. He's avoided like the plague," said one Milliken insider.

"I'd be less than honest if I said I had his full support," Ball conceded. "And it's difficult to work without someone's full support." In mid-December, Ball resigned.

The same day, Milliken announced that he would use his "clout" to select a successor to Ball. Although the director is technically named by the Agriculture Commission, three of the commission's five members were up for reappointment the same month—by the governor.

Several days later, a new agriculture director was named. He was Dean M. Pridgeon, who, as the Detroit *News* pointed out, "is no stranger to the PBB controversy ..." Pridgeon was vice-president of Michigan Farm Bureau at the height of the disaster, and had opposed efforts to impose stricter PBB guidelines. "But those things are in the past," he said. "What we need to do is look at the future. We have to try and improve relations between the governor's office, the Natural Resources Department and the Agriculture Department, and restore credibility in the whole Michigan food supply with the people of Michigan." His top priority would be to improve morale with the Agriculture Department, said Pridgeon, fifty-five. At the time of his appointment, he was chairman of the Natural Resources Commission.

Among those who had been mentioned prominently as Ball's successor was Rick Halbert, who during the heat of the election campaign joined Milliken's staff as special advisor on agriculture and toxic-substances control.

Halbert also was named by Milliken to be the staff director of an interim task force to set up Michigan's first Toxic Substance Control Commission, which was to go into business on January 1, 1979. "We need to control chemicals from the time they are manufactured, from the time they are distributed, from the time they are used, to the ultimate disposal of them and their transportation on the highway," Milliken said. "It is appropriate that Rick Halbert, Michigan's first PBB victim, should help oversee efforts to assure that society learns from the lessons of the PBB tragedy."

Halbert added, "With creation of the Toxic Substance Control Commission, Michigan has taken a step that is a model for the nation." Halbert took himself out of contention for Ball's post because he still had a lawsuit pending against Farm Bureau Services.

In early 1979, he was named as a member of the Toxic Substance Control Commission. Also named to the panel was Dr. Walter Meester, the Grand Rapids toxicologist.

The state also in 1978 created a Toxic Substance Loan Commission, authorized to make loans up to $75,000 to farmers who had suffered financial losses as a result of chemical contamination of their livestock but had not received compensation. One of the five commission members named by Milliken was Falmouth dairyman Garry Zuiderveen.

The loans are repayable over twenty years. No interest is charged during the first five years; after the fifth year, the annual interest rate is 3 percent; after the tenth year, the interest will be assessed at an annual rate of two percentage points below the average annual effective prime lending rate for commercial banks.

"It's conscience money," says Halbert. "The state realizes now that it did something wrong, even though it doesn't seem to know what it was."

The first farmer to qualify for such a loan was Clyde Clark of Sears, the older brother of Dr. Alpha Clark. Clyde Clark was among those accused by agriculture officials of trying to capitalize on PBB even though, they said, he never got PBB. Clyde Clark today has about two hundred cows buried on his farm, which he could have sold. The sponsor of legislation that created the loan commission was Francis R. Spaniola, the representative from Owosso.

The loan commission ended up being administered by the Department of Public Health. "It was said that we are the only state agency left that still had a heart," says Dr. Reizen. "The Health Department isn't ordinarily in the loan business. But when we were asked to assist the loan commission, we gave it our top priority." He added, "This program represents a high point for Michigan in an attempt to help citizens who may have suffered losses from chemical contamination through no fault of their own. It fits well with many other initiatives related to human health undertaken by the Health Department."

As a part of its long-term study, the department set up a field office in Big Rapids, an area with numerous contaminated farm families needing medical attention. The office, opened in

June of 1976 and located in a house trailer just north of town, is headed by Marvin Budd, a dedicated and sensitive bureaucrat who has earned the trust and respect of farm families.

And in late 1978, the Health Department opened two clinics to serve people with PBB-related medical problems. One is located in Sparta, just north of Grand Rapids, and the other at the Reed City Hospital.

It will be years, perhaps decades, before information gathered in the state's long-term study yields statistically significant results. More than forty-five hundred Michigan residents have been enrolled, plus another two thousand Iowa residents who will serve as a control, or comparison, study group. "If the department finds a difference between the health of the two groups of people," says Dr. Reizen, "then it must determine whether PBB caused the difference."

But even today—more than five years and a dozen health studies after the PBB blunder came to light—scientists continue to bicker over the chemical's effects, if any, on human health. But two things are clear. One is that contradictory studies will continue to proliferate for at least another generation. The other is that the conclusions of such studies will be uncannily predictable: It depends on who does them.

Studies done by, for, or in collaboration with the Michigan Department of Public Health will find little, if any, major health problems attributable to PBB—even when enlarged livers are found. On the other hand, studies have been done by independent scientists, such as Dr. Selikoff, will find significant medical problems that cannot be explained by anything but PBB.

Either conclusion, of course, may be taken at face value. But such conflicts raise serious questions. Why would state health officials downplay any untoward effects of PBB? A charitable view is that they don't want to alarm the public unnecessarily. Why do independent researchers almost unfailingly report health problems? An explanation might be their heightened concern about PBB and chemicals in general, coupled with their admitted interest in further researching such problems.

"As you know, there are many ways to analyze data," says George Van Amburg, the Health Department's chief of vital and health statistics. That is why, for instance, he saw no significance in the fact that a group of babies born in 1974—the year after the feed mix-up—weighed noticeably less than babies

297

born in years before and afterward. And so Van Amburg's analysis was never released to the public. Yet, there is another interpretation: 1974 is precisely the year such a phenomenon would show up—because babies born that year had spent the most time in the wombs of contaminated women.

Indeed, one independent scientist (Dr. James R. Allen of the University of Wisconsin) has demonstrated just such an effect among offspring of monkeys given a diet containing 300 parts per billion PBB—the same amount Michigan citizens were exposed to for more than four years, until the standard was lowered by the legislature in 1977.

The first two studies to assess PBB's human health effects, of course, were conducted by the Michigan Department of Public Health. Both found little to worry about, and one suggested "situational stress" as an explanation for many of the medical problems reported by poisoned farm families.

The third study was conducted by Dr. Irving J. Selikoff of the Environmental Sciences Laboratory of the Mt. Sinai Medical School. After studying 1,029 Michigan residents, he found that nearly one-third of them had suffered significant problems. This study had a number of offshoots. One was the finding, reported in August of 1977, of immune defects in the blood of forty-five Michigan farm residents.

Less than a year later, however, a study involving the Michigan Health Department could find no such blood abnormalities, and it suggested that the defects found by Dr. Selikoff might have arisen while the specimens were being transported from the collection site to the laboratory.

In November 1977, a study of twenty-three persons conducted for the Health Department reported nerve defects, organic brain damage and indications of liver damage. But it concluded those problems were not attributable to PBB.

Another state-sponsored study, involving forty-six persons and released in June 1978, found that 72 percent had enlarged livers. But its conclusion was that such problems could be expected in any human sampling group.

Scientists in Dr. Selikoff's November 1976 study reported that children they saw had many health problems and complaints that could not be explained by anything but PBB. But a state-sponsored children's clinic in September 1977 concluded that thirty-three contaminated children were as healthy as a group of uncontaminated youngsters.

Dr. Selikoff's studies also have found significant health problems among workers at the Michigan Chemical plant in St. Louis, Michigan. But a state-sponsored 1979 study claimed that these workers have four times fewer health problems than many farm residents—even though the workers have four times as much PBB in their bodies.

There have been two exceptions to the predictability of test results. One is a Selikoff study that found that PBB does not seem to cause sterility. The other is a study conducted as an outgrowth of the state's 1977 pediatric clinic. This study found that children with high PBB contamination did markedly worse on a battery of performance tests than children with lesser PBB.

The predictable conflict of results also holds true when it comes to PBB's effects on laboratory test animals. When the experiments are done by independent scientists, deleterious effects of PBB appear. But studies by researchers hired by Farm Bureau or Michigan Chemical turn up few, if any, problems.

Numerous other human health studies are still under way and will be reported in the days and decades ahead. Dr. Selikoff, for instance, is still analyzing several million pieces of information his research team gathered in 1978 during a study of Michigan's general population. The group's first progress report confirmed that more than 90 percent of the population have PBB in their blood.

The overriding concern, of course, is whether or not PBB will prove to be a cancer-causing agent. As yet, the answer is unknown. But animal tests to find out are under way at the National Cancer Institute. The results are expected in late 1980 or early 1981. If PBB turns out not to cause cancer, it will be the first substance to be tested in a family of synthetic chemicals called halogenated aromatic hydrocarbons that is not a carcinogen.

One group of people who have had more immediate concerns than long-term health was several hundred workers once employed by Michigan Chemical at its St. Louis factory. They all were laid off by the fall of 1978 when the company shut down the plant and left Michigan.

By then, Michigan Chemical had been absorbed by Velsicol, a subsidiary of Northwest Industries, a thriving conglomerate based in Chicago.

The company in 1976 paid a state fine of $20,000 for polluting the Pine River. The fine had been held low deliberately in return for the company's guarantee to leave Michigan, according to Stewart Freeman, an assistant attorney general. "Getting them out of Michigan was what was important." In the summer of 1978 the company made an eleventh-hour bid to stay by offering $1 million to cover the cost of cleaning up the Pine River and the Gratiot County landfill. In return, Velsicol wanted to be released from the shutdown agreement and be issued a new discharge permit.

The bid was rejected. A month later, the Department of Natural Resources found huge concentrations of PBB in a muskrat and five raccoons caught in the vicinity of the Pine River just downstream from St. Louis.

The Michigan Department of Natural Resources first heard about PBB on June 3, 1974, more than a month after agriculture officials learned about the disaster. Three days later, the department sent an inspector to tour the Michigan Chemical plant. The company's personnel told the inspector, Dennis Swanson, that only one of its twenty discharges could possibly have contained PBB and that "we have never found measurable PBBs in our discharge." But Swanson took samples of the discharge and directly from the Pine River; both contained high concentrations of PBB. Swanson, an aquatic biologist, after leaving the plant, went farther down the riverbank and captured two fish by angling. Both also turned out to have been contaminated by PBB. Eventually a ban on fishing along some thirty miles of the Pine River was imposed.

A last-minute effort by some salaried employees of the plant to purchase the factory also failed.

Michigan Chemical in late 1976 was merged into the Velsicol Chemical Corporation, then an obscure subsidiary of Northwest Industries, which was headed by Ben W. Heineman, Sr., one of the nation's most respected businessmen. Heineman's son, Ben, Jr., is now a top aide to Joseph A. Califano, Jr., who was attorney for Michigan Chemical prior to becoming Jimmy Carter's Secretary of Health, Education and Welfare. The elder Heineman himself has been frequently mentioned as a possible cabinet appointee in several Democratic administrations.

In 1956, Heineman took over a struggling Chicago and North Western Railroad and made it the basis for a widely diversified holding company whose products include Cutty Sark Scotch whisky and Fruit of the Loom underwear. Today,

300

Northwest Industries' annual sales are about $2 billion. Heineman's 1965 acquisition of both Velsicol and Michigan Chemical were the company's first nonrailroad ventures.

But starting in the 1970s, the chemical companies have caused nothing but headaches for Heineman. In December 1977, both Velsicol and Farm Bureau Services were indicted by a federal grand jury in Grand Rapids on four counts of criminally adulterating animal feed, a misdemeanor. Each company ended up paying serveral thousand dollars' fine.

That same month, six former and present employees of Velsicol were indicted by another federal grand jury, in Chicago, on charges that they concealed from the U.S. Environmental Protection Agency results of tests showing that two of Velsicol's best-selling pesticides, chlordane and heptachlor, could cause cancer. The indictment was dismissed by a federal district judge in Chicago on April 20, 1979.

Velsicol's plant in Bayport, Texas, near Houston, also has attracted unwanted attention stemming from a federal investigation into neurological disorders suffered by its employees during the production of leptophos, another pesticide, between 1971 and 1976. Later the U.S. Occupational Safety and Health Administration recommended fines amounting to $40,000 against Velsicol for alleged workplace violations. A December 1976 report by the staff of a U.S. Senate committee criticized Velsicol for permitting the manufacture of leptophos to continue at Bayport even after it had been warned that its employees were falling ill.

Velsicol also was a major producer of Tris, a flame retardant that was banned for use in children's sleepwear in 1977 after studies suggested it could cause cancer.

At the end of April, 1979, a federal grand jury in Detroit indicted Velsicol and two of its employees for conspiracy to defraud a federal investigation of the PBB accident. And the two-count indictment charged that Velsicol covered up its role in the mixup for more than two and a half years.

The indictment was returned in the nick of time, too. In a matter of days, the five-year statute of limitations would have expired, meaning the company could not then have been charged. A separate investigation of Farm Bureau Services' role continued into spring.

"I'm a little surprised by the indictment," said Judge Peterson, whose controversial ruling against farmer Tacoma

301

also said Velsicol, Farm Bureau Services, and state agencies had acted responsibly in the aftermath of the disaster. Indeed, when Tacoma's attorneys during the Cadillac trial had presented much the same information that later was heard by the Detroit grand jury, Peterson had called their charges "flagrantly irresponsible."

Hearing of the indictment, Doc Clark commented, "I'm glad the grand jury used that information, because Peterson sure didn't."

Named in the indictment were Charles L. Touzeau, plant manager, and William Thorne, operations manager. They were charged with falsely claiming that the livestock feed and PBB had been produced and then stored in different buildings a quarter-mile apart. The indictment said no such second building existed.

One count of the indictment charged that Velsicol and Touzeau and Thorne "falsified, concealed, and covered up by trick, scheme, and device, material facts relating to the potential and actual contamination and adulteration of food and drug products...."

Count two charged that they "willfully and unlawfully did combine, conspire and agree together and with one another, and with diverse other persons whose names to the grand jury are unknown, to defraud" the federal government.

Each count carries a maximum prison term of five years, plus a $10,000 fine.

Nearly six months after Velsicol closed its St. Louis factory, John Broder, a Detroit *News* reporter, visited St. Louis and spoke with many former Michigan Chemical employees.

"Three-quarters of the workers who lost their jobs when the plant was shut down are still out of work," complained one of them, Ron Orwig. "The governor's made all sorts of promises but I don't know of one job the state has gotten us."

Milliken in the fall of 1978 created a task force of officials from the labor and commerce departments to study ways to create jobs in Gratiot County, historically one of the most depressed areas in Michigan—with an average unemployment rate of 16 percent for the last five years. The governor's task force produced two reports, but no jobs.

Among those who lost a paycheck was Tom Ostrander, thirty-one, who had not worked since March of 1977 but was kept on the Velsicol payroll. Ostrander was so sick that the company had sent him to the Mayo Clinic in Rochester, Minnesota. The diagnosis was that Ostrander probably was suffering from PBB poisoning, for he had 3,600 parts per billion in his body.

Velsicol issued a report to the state's workmens' compensation bureau, blaming Ostrander's disability on PBB. But the company later withdrew the report and then began paying Ostrander his full salary although no longer requiring him to report for work. Today Ostrander is barred from collecting unemployment pay because he is unable to work; but he is also ineligible for workmens' compensation benefits because the Michigan Department of Labor continues to refuse to accept "PBB syndrome" as a "compensable work-related injury."

Earlier this year, state Representative Dana Wilson, who headed a special House committee looking into ways to help former Velsicol workers, proposed that loans be made to them similar to those now available to the farmers. Wilson's other proposals include mandatory licensing and inspection of chemical companies doing business in Michigan, and requirements that such firms tell their employees about the hazards involved, which Velsicol did not do with PBB.

Workers at the St. Louis plant had been allowed to eat lunch in the dust-filled room where PBB was made and allowed to work for years without respirators or other protective measures—even after workers demanded them. "The state should require these companies to come out of the Dark Ages and let their employees know if they are exposed to health risks," Wilson said.

Former workers at the plant have filed a $250 million lawsuit against Velsicol, charging the company with failure to inform them of the dangers of PBB. They also have filed a second suit for the same amount, against the state Health Department.

Meanwhile, the state of Michigan has a $120 million lawsuit pending against Farm Bureau Services and Michigan Chemical to recover costs incurred by the state as a result of the disaster.

There are still scores of other farmers who have lawsuits pending against Farm Bureau Services and Michigan Chemical, seeking to recover damages caused by PBB. Among them is Patricia Miller of Reed City. "We're not backing down. When you know you're right, you don't quit. You just keep on going."

303

After Peterson's ruling came out, she and other members of the PBB Action Committee created a legal fund to raise money for Roy and Marilyn Tacoma to help pay for their court costs and for future expenses in their own lawsuits. "We're asking for support. And I believe eventually we will be vindicated of the charges that we are alarmists and liars," she said. The first contribution came from Bud Freeman, the freelance writer in Los Angeles who had written the script of "Slaughter." The check was for $1,000.

The lawsuits may drag on for years. "The system has to respond faster," says Halbert. "And I don't know how it can be done within the legal framework. I don't think it can." What may take even longer than the litigation is the process of healing the wounds in the farm community as a result of the PBB controversy. Take, for instance, the church attended by Roy and Marilyn Tacoma. "There is a deep division here," says the Reverend Stephen Sietsema of the Aetna Christian Reformed Church in Falmouth.

The Reverend Sietsema says he thinks he serves more PBB victims than any other church in Michigan, and attributes the split in his congregation to the fact that some members, like the Tacomas, felt unfairly treated while others were satisfied with their treatment.

The two groups quickly began viewing each other with hostility and deep suspicion. "The first sign was when people started talking about each other in not-too-pleasant tones," recalls the Reverend Sietsema. "The anxiety dredged up bitterness of years gone by.... The people I'm acquainted with are really hurt. This thing is hurting in an emotional, spiritual way. It's going to affect them for the rest of their lives."

In Gregory, dairyman Tom Butler finally succeeded in obtaining additional life insurance, but at twice the expected premium because of his "added risk"—PBB contamination.

As for the many farms heavily contaminated by PBB, a team of researchers reported in mid-February of 1979 that they may never be free of the chemical. Among those involved in seeking ways to rid such farms of PBB is Dr. George Fries, the federal government scientist who first identified PBB as the mysterious ingredient in Rick Halbert's feed.

Also doing PBB research now is Dr. Isadore Bernstein, chairman of the governor's 1976 PBB scientific advisory panel. At the University of Michigan, he is experimenting with animals in search of a way to rid the human body of PBB.

At the Ohio Agricultural Research and Development Center, Dr. Lynn Willett is continuing his PBB studies with cows. Part of his research grant had come from the U.S. Food and Drug Administration, thanks to the agency's Dr. Dwight Mercer, whose backing of Dr. Willett led the FDA to award him the grant without considering other bids. Dr. Mercer later went back to Ohio State University to complete a doctorate's degree. While there, he served as the toxicologist in Dr. Willett's experiments.

In Ann Arbor, Dr. Thomas Corbett, who was so instrumental in raising the public awareness about the hazards of PBB in 1974, has become embittered by his experiences. He has left the University of Michigan and the Veterans' Administration Hospital to go into private practice in Toledo, Ohio. "I'm making more money than ever before. After fighting for four years, you become cynical," he says. "I made a lot of enemies; many didn't like my going to the press. But the disenchantment is mutual."

"Maybe we needed a prophet like that," Dr. Reizen says of Dr. Corbett. "But that kind of person is terribly hard on us bureaucrats. The lesson the state has learned is to be more responsive."

There is one further interesting footnote involving Dr. Corbett. His isoflurane studies could not be duplicated by researchers in California. The reason later became clear: the mice in his isoflurane experiments had become contaminated by PBB—via mice feed. So what caused the mice to develop tumors perhaps was not isoflurane but PBB.

In March of 1978, Edie Clark, the Democratic legislative aide who had done so much for PBB-affected farmers, left Michigan. She married Kenneth D. Rosenman, a tall young doctor who was a member of Dr. Selikoff's research team at the Environmental Sciences Laboratory. They moved to Springfield, Massachusetts, where Dr. Rosenman began his residency training. Edie, meantime, began studying at the University of Massachusetts to earn a master's degree in public health.

One other key figure in the PBB tragedy left Michigan in 1978. He was Lou Trombley, the husky, angry farmer from Hersey. In late August, he and his wife, Carol, and four of their six children loaded up what was left of their lives into two borrowed trucks and left the state where both Lou and Carol had been born and reared.

"I'm very bitter," Trombley, forty, said. "I planned to live on this farm for the rest of my life. Now I've lost everything. I have less now than when I started twenty-five years ago. I worked all my life to get this place."

Trombley had lost his 375-acre farm to the Farmers Home Administration after he was no longer able to meet his mortgage payments. He had tried for a year to sell his farm, appraised at $620,000. But the stigma of PBB drove away potential buyers. "Nobody would touch it because it was a contaminated farm," Trombley said. "Once the word PBB was mentioned, they didn't want anything to do with it."

Before they left, the Trombleys auctioned off their dairy herd of 150 cows, farm equipment and even furniture and personal belongings, raising $80,000 to pay off some of their debts. But that still left them more than $200,000 in debt.

"Nothing's ever been done for us in the state except covering up this PBB mess. There's nothing for us here anymore," Trombley said.

They moved to Salem, Missouri, where Trombley has not been able to borrow the necessary funds to go back into farming. For the time being, he is working as a carpenter. "They said we didn't have enough farming experience," said Carol Trombley.

The Trombleys still have a suit pending against Farm Bureau Services and Michigan Chemical. "They're going to pay for every damned dime I've lost in the past five years," said Trombley. "If not in my lifetime, then in my kids' or my grandkids' lives. Somebody's got to sue them bastards for everything they've done to us. It was a good life before PBB."

Shortly before the Trombleys moved to Missouri, a letter arrived from Robert Mitchell, the new state director of the U.S. Farmers Home Administration. The letter turned out to be one of the most prized items the Trombleys took with them to Missouri.

It read:

Dear Lou:
Just a personal note to express my best wishes to you and your family, as you move to a new area.

I'm sure the last few years have been the most trying years of your life as a result of the contamination of your cattle and family with PBB. It will be difficult for people

306

outside of Michigan to understand the hardships, complexities and confusion still surrounding the worst chemical contamination of the food chain in Michigan history.

The farmers were left alone by this disaster. Neither the state nor the federal government really offered the kind of assistance needed by farmers to withstand the tremendous economic loss.

Certainly you are entitled to be disappointed by the way things developed in your struggle to survive. But you can hold your head high knowing you have fought a good fight against insurmountable odds. This is true not only in your efforts to overcome PBB on your farm but in your efforts with the PBB Action Committee.

The record of success that you had established before PBB contamination was indeed noteworthy. In fact, the local Farmers Home Administration county supervisor was planning on recommending you as the Farmers Home Administration Farmer-of-the-Year. PBB hit and, for a long time after, most people could not understand what was happening. So the recommendation was never submitted. But I can tell you that the people in this agency were impressed with your farm operation and production. Also the staff was pleased with your cooperation and attitude in working with this agency. There was one major controversy between the Farmers Home Administration staff and yourself before I became state director. Of course, that involved the question of what to do with the contaminated cattle. I cannot and will not defend this agency's position back then of encouraging farmers to sell their contaminated cattle for human consumption. You took a courageous and unpopular stand by deciding to destroy the cattle, and I commend you for making that tough decision.

I know you will go on to start over and that you will enjoy the success that would have been yours in Michigan if it had not been for PBB. Please keep in contact and let me know how things are going for you.

Mitchell's letter now hangs, framed, on the wall of the Trombley's rented home in Missouri. "People here can't believe that we've been married as long as we have and have so little," Carol Trombley said after living in Salem for six months.

Shortly after the Trombleys got to Missouri, another letter arrived. It was written by state representative Francis R. Spaniola.

It said:

Dear Lou,

I was sincerely saddened to learn that you had found it necessary to leave the state of Michigan. It certainly is a sad commentary on the officials in this state who, by their negligence, have forced you to find a haven in Missouri.

Lou, I hope and pray that the day will come soon when those who have caused you so much misery will be held publicly accountable. You know much better than I how important it is to rid this state of uncaring and/or dishonest public officials. I promise I will do all I can to call them to account.

You are a true profile in courage. You spoke out when it was not popular to do so. You were dishonestly branded as a television glory seeker by officials of this state. But most important of all, you would not sell sick animals to poison me or my children. Economically, you destroyed your business to protect me and others in this state.

When I read of your decision to leave Michigan I felt that in many ways I had failed you. Surely my bills were good but much too late. I wish that I could have accomplished more for you and your friends. I want you to know, for whatever it may be worth, that I know you to be a good farmer and an honest man and a person of extreme courage. I am proud to have known you....

# 16
# POISONED NATION

The popular perception is that only Michigan's environment and its 9 million citizens have been contaminated by PBB. But that is not so.

Through a variety of means, millions of other Americans have been exposed to the chemical.

It is well known that anyone in Michigan who ate anything but a strict vegetarian diet became contaminated by PBB—particularly from mid-1973 on, and lasting well into 1975. During just this two-year span, at least 30 million out-of-state tourists spent time in Michigan.

Furthermore, PBB now has been detected in the environment—including the food supply—of thirteen states besides Michigan, plus fish from at least one major waterway.

One way people in other states got PBB, of course, was through consuming products that originated in Michigan; these include not only milk and meat but many processed foods such as canned chicken soup, butter, eggs, cheese, cream and even infant formula. Feeds contaminated in Michigan also were sent to many other states, where they were consumed by farm animals, who, in turn, passed PBB on to people.

Additional routes of human exposure include soap and even influenza vaccine, including possibly during the ill-fated 1976 swine flu program.

But despite these data demonstrating an environmental disaster of monumental proportions—one that has spread far beyond Michigan—no concerted effort has been made to ascertain the true dimensions of the PBB contamination.

The few early attempts to gauge the spread of PBB beyond Michigan came too late, and were conducted at a time when laboratory analytical capabilities were still poor. Thus PBB presence in other states easily could have escaped detection, as in Michigan.

309

But even so, PBB turned up in September and October of 1974 in beef in Iowa, duck in Wisconsin, turkey in Indiana, chicken in Alabama, Mississippi, New York and Texas. The samples contained PBB at levels between 10 and 110 parts per billion. They had been collected as a part of the U.S. Department of Agriculture's animal and plant health inspection service's national residue sampling program that covers thirty-four states.

Also in late 1974 and early 1975, the U.S. Food and Drug Administration surveyed some food products and animals feeds on a nationwide basis. Eleven samples turned up positive; they were from Indiana, Pennsylvania and Ohio.

In follow-up studies in 1975 and 1976, 9 out of 597 samples of food products in other states still had PBB.

But it wasn't only meats and milk that were contaminated. Countless processed foods also were tainted and ended up being consumed. And a thorough check on these products was never conducted.

Many dairy plants in Michigan, after the PBB incident became known, refused to buy any milk whatsoever from the contaminated farms—even when the milk met the PBB standards. Hence, many of these farms had no choice but to sell their milk to manufacturers of processed foods, such as butter, cheese, powdered and nondry fat milk and condensed skim milk. And these products went all over the country in the months before the PBB accident was discovered.

Three lots of cheese, for instance, were shipped from Michigan Farm Cheese Dairy, Inc., in Fountain, Michigan, to the Farm Food Company of Chicago on May 20, 1974. They contained up to 1,500 parts per billion PBB, but had been sold before they could be seized. Additional lots were sampled at the Fountain plant, but contained only trace levels of PBB and the cheeses were allowed for sale.

A number of lots of evaporated milk made by the Carnation Company in Sheridan, Michigan, were shipped to Indiana and Ohio on April 3, 1974. Three shipments were recalled after the accident was discovered, and they contained up to 2,530 parts per billion PBB.

Two lots of butter manufactured by the Kalamazoo Creamery were shipped to Atlanta in late May of 1974 and later were found to contain 350 and 890 parts per billion PBB. But no action was taken since the federal guideline then was 1,000 parts per billion.

310

Subsequent testing turned up PBB in butter, milk, eggs and feed in Indiana and in milk in Pennsylvania. The actual quantities of PBB-contaminated foods that were distributed all across the nation before the accident was discovered are simply inestimable.

PBB even turned up in Enfamil, an infant formula made by Mead Johnson and Company. But the levels of contamination were deemed safe—between .04 and .9 part per billion—and thus sold.

As late as February of 1978, a farm in Michigan was found to have been sending highly contaminated products to a food processor—in Indiana.

"They all said it didn't spread into Indiana, which I knew wasn't so because for the first eight months—I'm three miles from the Indiana border—I would say 80 percent of the cows that are sold for butcher go to Shipshewana or Topeka, which are in Indiana," said Dr. Susan Jacoby, the Constantine veterinarian. "For eight months we didn't even know we had PBB. All those cows went to Indiana. I'm sure on the eastern side of Michigan, they go to Ohio. ... I know that a lot of chickens that had got PBB exposure went into Campbell soup. People had contact with soup manufacturers and sent the eggs all over the United States." (Research has shown that, through cooking, chicken meat loses between 37 to 45 percent of PBB; but one-third of the loss ends up in the broth.)

Adds Donald J. Albosta, the ex-Michigan state representative, "Contaminated meat has gone outside Michigan. In fact, one herd of cattle that was quarantined left the state and went to Wisconsin, to Green Bay, and was processed there. I called the Wisconsin Department of Agriculture ... and found they knew nothing about that."

And farther to the west, a dairy farmer in southwestern Minnesota in the summer of 1978 discovered PBB in his cattle feed and in a side of beef. The feed contained 240 parts per billion PBB. The farmer had suffered headaches, nausea, fatigue, and minor wounds that healed very slowly.

Feeds in Illinois and Indiana have also turned up with PBB.

One possibility of how PBB-contaminated feeds might have reached other states is through feed brokers. These are middlemen who unknowingly purchased contaminated feeds in Michigan and then transported them to other states for sale. Another is the widespread use of Aureomycin Crumbles, an

311

antibiotic feed that was sold all over the country. Several shipments of the feed were sent to Pennsylvania, Ohio and Indiana, and had up to 280 parts per billion PBB.

Countless Michigan farm animals over the years ended up in rendering plants, where they emerged as ingredients for animal feed, pet food and tallow. Tallow is a nearly colorless, tasteless solid fat extracted from animals and used to make candles, soaps, margarine and lubricants.

Even the cattle Dr. George Fries used in his PBB experiments in Beltsville, Maryland, ended up in the human food supply. "It was a slipup," Dr. Fries admitted. "I was a little slipshod on that."

But for the general U.S. population, the major route of PBB exposure may have been through influenza vaccine, starting in late 1974.

Parke, Davis and Company, one of the country's largest drug manufacturers and based in Detroit, received tens of millions of eggs from a highly contaminated poultry farm in St. Clair County, beginning in early 1974. The first batch of vaccine produced from these eggs became available during the 1974-75 flu season.

And because the poultry farm went through a cleanup process of dubious efficacy (and because Parke, Davis continued buying millions of eggs from this farm), it is not unreasonable to think that PBB also got into some of the 30 million doses of swine flu vaccines Parke, Davis produced in 1976.

Parke, Davis, as it does with all the vaccines it produces, tested batches of influenza vaccine for unwanted residues, such as proteins. But it did not test for PBB—even after it realized one of its major egg suppliers had been a heavily contaminated farm and that the chickens that produced these eggs had to be destroyed. (Research later showed that up to 58 percent of a laying hen's PBB is passed on into the eggs.)

Although there is a much quicker turnover rate of chickens on a poultry farm than cows on a dairy farm, special circumstances involving the St. Clair poultry operation strongly suggest that its new chickens—and eggs—continued to be contaminated by PBB for a long time.

This farm, one of the largest in Michigan, purchased twenty to thirty tons of Farm Bureau Services feed ingredients, such as proteins, vitamins and trace minerals—all of which, of course, were contaminated by PBB residues at the Climax plant. The poultry owner had his own elevator and feed mixing equipment, and mixed his own chicken feed. Thus the equipment became contaminated, and passed off PBB residues to all subsequent feeds, even after he stopped buying Farm Bureau Services products in late 1974.

The farm was quarantined in late May, 1974, when one laying hen showed 3,900 parts per billion PBB.

The poultryman said he gave his buildings "a good washing job," which consisted of "just high-pressure water—rinsing everything down." He did no steam cleaning. All these precautions, and more, had failed to clean the Farm Bureau Services plant; and the poultry farmer also had his own mixing equipment. This farm also sold countless spent hens to fowl processors, who in turn did business with chicken soup manufacturers.

The St. Clair poultry farmer went as far as to Colorado to obtain replacement flocks. And even though he stopped buying Farm Bureau Services' products, his new chickens also became contaminated, tests revealed. "None of the flocks were clean," he said.

In an average year, he sells Parke, Davis close to 4 million eggs. But he sold the drug company far more than that in 1976 because Parke, Davis, which usually makes about 10 million doses of influenza vaccine annually, that year more than tripled its vaccine production to meet the swine flu immunization program.

The St. Clair poultryman said Parke, Davis in 1974 knew the eggs it used for vaccine production during the first half of the year had come from contaminated hens. "They really sweated it out, and we kept it quiet."

But C. R. Shelton, a Parke, Davis spokesman, said, "We really don't think there was any PBB in the eggs we used." And he said the company's five vaccine purification processes, in any case, would have eliminated any PBB from the final product.

Yet, a scientist intimately involved in the process conceded, "I guess they [the eggs] could have [been contaminated]." While also adding that the purification steps likely would have eliminated PBB, he admitted that the company was never "looking specifically for PBB" in the vaccines.

On June 17, 1977, the Environmental Protection Agency announced that it had found PBB in human hair, fish, plants, soil and water in the vicinity of two PBB manufacturing plants in northern New Jersey and a factory that used PBB in Staten Island, New York.

The two PBB makers are the White Chemical Company in Bayonne and the Hexcel Corporation in Sayreville, which produced a total of about 1 million pounds of the chemical for export to Europe. The New York plant that used PBB in its wire coatings was the Standard T Company.

One human hair sample contained 1,000 parts per billion PBB; another had 3,500 parts per billion. In the hair oil, the PBB presence was even more alarming: up to 315,000 parts per billion.

A swamp containing runoff water from the Hexcel plant showed 135 parts per billion. Reeds in the swamp had up to 37,000 parts per billion. A turtle captured nearby contained 30 parts per billion.

Fish taken from water near White Chemical contained up to 160 parts per billion, and 220 parts per billion from near Standard T. The soil near the two manufacturers had up to 4,600 parts per billion.

Less than two months after the New York-New Jersey contaminations were discovered, news came that PBB had been found in catfish taken from the Ohio River near Parkersburg, West Virginia. "There are catfish restaurants all up and down the Ohio River," said Congressman Thomas A. Luken of Ohio.

"The reason that we decided to look in that area is because of the presence of one of the users of PBBs" explained Dr. I. Eugene Wallen, deputy director of the Environmental Protection Agency's office of toxic substances. The contaminated catfish had been taken from the river in the vicinity of the Borg-Warner Corporation's plant, where PBB was used in the production of thousands of television cabinets.

It was unclear just how or when the fish had become poisoned, since the Borg-Warner plant had stopped using PBB in 1974 and the fish were gathered in 1977. Subsequent tests found that most fish from the waterway were not contaminated, although some still contained traces.

The Borg-Warner plant in West Virginia was only one of more than 130 domestic users of PBB.

"We didn't check earlier because we didn't know PBB was a problem outside Michigan," said Dr. Wallen. "Now we have evidence it may well be a national problem. Yes, PBB now is a

314

concern nationwide. And these findings certainly move us in the direction of totally banning PBB."

Public hearings on this question were held in late 1977 in Lansing and in early 1978 in Edison, New Jersey, by the Environmental Protection Agency. But PBB was not banned. "We decided not to regulate PBB because no one in the United States is making it anymore. And there are no imports of PBB," said John DeKany, deputy assistant administrator for chemical control in the EPA's office of toxic substances.

"We're more concerned about PBB substitutes," he said. "There already are forty-five derivatives of PBB—at least. And there's no data on any of them whatsoever. PBB is just one of about eight hundred chemical fire retardants."

After his PBB hearings in 1977, Senator Riegle introduced legislation to create a "chemical emergency response team." The bill authorized formation of a federal interagency strike force comprised of scientists and medical personnel who, at a moment's notice, can be mobilized to identify, control and eliminate chemical contamination once it has occurred.

"It would be a team that could go out without delay into any environment where an accident has happened," the senator said. "Given the assault of toxic chemicals on our very fragile environment and now on the human system, it would pay us to have the capability at the federal level to come into any situation with all the equipment to be able to get a handle on this as quickly as we can, so that we can make some rational public policy decisions."

Halbert agreed. "The lesson I draw is we really need some very high-level professional, technical capability in a task force effort, so that the machinery and the know-how and the expertise that we would need with these very complicated chemical issues is in place," he said.

Support for the Riegle proposal came from many federal agencies and their top officials. One was Carol Tucker Foreman, assistant secretary for food and consumer services of the U.S. Agriculture Department. "It is clear that all of the [federal] agencies whose programs may be affected by these accidents have to improve their actions in order to deal with them. And I think it would be naïve for us to assume that we are not going to continue to have these kinds of problems, these kinds of accidents," she said.

Dr. David P. Rall, director of the National Institute of

315

Environmental Health Sciences, also supported the Riegle proposal. But he cautioned, "One of the problems [with PBB] was the ambiguity of the signals from the state of Michigan. I am sympathetic to the concept of a response team. But it requires a clear signal from the local government, saying we need help."

Senator Riegle's bill became law but has not received funding from the Carter administration. "The OMB [Office of Management and Budget] killed it from the fiscal year 1980 budget," said a Riegle aide.

If such a chemical response strike force had existed in 1974, Riegle says, "I think we could have contained the problem and prevented a lot of hardships and suffering that has resulted since."

The entire Michigan episode involved only about two thousand pounds of PBB, of which some 12 million pounds were produced, notes Dr. Selikoff. "It has been used in hundreds of other places around the country, and there hasn't even been time yet for most of it to leak into the environment. Similar to other experiences, PBB that is presumably locked into other products, such as plastics, may in time leak back into the environment," says Dr. Selikoff.

"Indeed," adds one of his Mt. Sinai colleagues, Dr. Kingsley Kay, the toxicologist, "it may ultimately be found that the pattern of environmental transport of PCB applies also to aspects of human exposure to PBB in the broad public health context."

Later a report by the Environmental Protection Agency cautioned, "While PBBs are effective fire retardants in thermoplastics, they can pose a health hazard because flameless combustion of the consumer product (e.g., in a garbage dump or an office fire) causes volatilization of intact PBBs."

"The unintentional release of a chemical contaminant into the food supply is not a new or unique problem," says Halbert. "Since 1969, this country has experienced two dozen separate major incidents which resulted in the contamination of the food supply. They were probably only the tip of the iceberg of contamination, since any new or exotic material will go unnoticed in even the most thorough of laboratory examinations."

Speaking again of the Michigan tragedy, Halbert concludes: "...tens of millions of dollars in property damage has been done. The entire population of the state has been exposed to PBB. And thousands of farm residents have had their health and well-being compromised. This is a legacy we have left for future generations—a stain that no amount of scrubbing will remove.

"The lesson that Sandy and I have learned is how vulnerable we all are. When something strikes, we used to think—assume—that there'd be a way, some mechanism to help the individual, be it the federal government, the local government, the church. Whoever. But no. There isn't. If something strikes you as an individual, as a single person, there is nothing. That's what we've learned: the absolute vulnerability of an individual. If something odd happens, he can be wiped out without knowing what hit him."

# INDEX

320

Smith, Elton, 206, 254
Smith, Raymond, 287
Soble, Stephen M., 290–291
Society for Toxicology, 37
Sodium Chloride, 34
Spaniola, Francis R., 162, 171–172, 248; legislation, 249–252, 264, 296, 307–308
Sparta, Michigan, 297
Speth, Gus, 113–114, 118
Spies, Frank, 101
Spike, Dr. Thomas E., 210
Springer, Clyde, 137
Standard T Company, 314
Stanwood, Michigan, 166
Stariha, Kathy, 160, 199, 202, 217
State assistance, 128; food stamps, welfare, 130
Stevens, E. Dan, 221–222
Stockman, Dr., 102
Strabo, 111
Strauss Meat and Packing House, 137
Sturgis, Michigan, 99, 210
Swanson, Dennis, 300
Swine cholera, 128–129
Swine herds or farms, 59, 78
Szeluga, Charles, 42–44

Tacoma, Andrew, 281
Tacoma, Marilyn, 275, 279, 281–282, 285–286, 289, 292, 304
Tacoma, Roy, 45, 99, 181, 275, 279, 281–289, 292, 301–302, 304
Tallow, 135, 312
Tanner, Dr. Howard, 131, 189, 257, 259
Tephly, Dr. Thomas, 199, 207
Terrian, Dr. James, 170–173, 195
Texas, xiv, 310; Bayport, Houston, 301
Thomas, Ron, 109–110, 250
Thorne, William W., 44, 302
Three Rivers, Michigan, 138
Tilson, Dr. H. A., 267
Time magazine, 94
Touzeau, Charles L. 302
Toxic Substance Pollution Victim Compensation Act, 291–292
Toxic Substances Control Act, xii, 261, 291
Traverse City, 66–67, 130, 152, 192; Health Department, 67
Trenton, Michigan, 176
Tri-County Veterinary Clinic, 95

Tris, 301
Trombley, Carol, 177, 305–306
Trombley, Lou, 163–165, 175–177, 184, 230, 305–306
Tuberculosis, 226
Turney, William, 259
Tustin, Michigan, 146

United Auto Workers union, 193, 248, 272, 288
University of Detroit, 37
University of Iowa, 199
University of Massachusetts, 305
University of Michigan, 61, 63, 76, 197, 218, 221, 241–242, 267, 288, 304–305
University of Missouri, 288
University of Parma, 111
University of Western Ontario, 77
University of Wisconsin, 139, 266, 298
Upjohn Company, 34, 198, 279
Upton, Dr. Arthur C., 116
Urea, 9, 11, 105
U.S. Center for Disease Control, xvi, 83–84, 115, 201, 215, 217, 223, 232, 266
U.S. Council on Environmental Quality, 113, 118
U.S. Department of Agriculture, 8, 19, 29–30, 32, 55–56, 59, 120, 128, 140, 178, 181, 253, 267, 272, 289, 310, 315
U.S. Department of Health Education and Welfare, 226, 232, 235, 263, 280–281, 300
U.S. Department of Justice, 270
U.S. Environmental Protection Agency, 59, 228, 258, 280, 301, 313–316
U.S. Farmers Home Administration, 183, 306–307
U.S. Food and Drug Administration, 22–25, 29–30, 39, 46, 55, 57, 59, 61, 64, 66, 70, 72, 80, 84, 88, 100–101, 103–104, 106, 108, 116–117, 136, 143–144, 174, 177, 179–181, 200–201, 207, 215, 217, 237–238, 253, 263–264, 268, 272, 278, 280–281, 305, 310; health survey, 85–87, 214, 264; inspection of Farm Bureau Services, 104–105; inspection of Michigan Chemical, 39–40; low-level herd survey, 142–143, 153, 278; toler-

328